MW00835204

Artificial Intelligence in Radiation Oncology

ARTIFICIAL INTELLIGENCE IN RADIATION ONCOLOGY

Editors

Seong K Mun
Virginia Tech, USA

Sonja Dieterich
University of California, Davis, USA

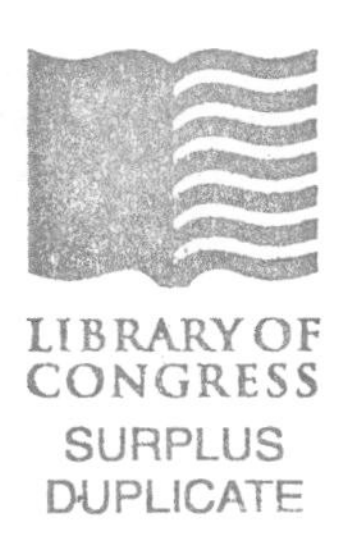

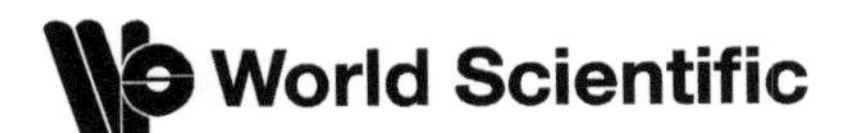
NEW JERSEY • LONDON • SINGAPORE • BEIJING • SHANGHAI • HONG KONG • TAIPEI • CHENNAI • TOKYO

Published by

World Scientific Publishing Co. Pte. Ltd.
5 Toh Tuck Link, Singapore 596224
USA office: 27 Warren Street, Suite 401-402, Hackensack, NJ 07601
UK office: 57 Shelton Street, Covent Garden, London WC2H 9HE

Library of Congress Control Number: 2022942258

British Library Cataloguing-in-Publication Data
A catalogue record for this book is available from the British Library.

ARTIFICIAL INTELLIGENCE IN RADIATION ONCOLOGY

ISBN 978-981-126-353-8 (hardcover)
ISBN 978-981-126-354-5 (ebook for institutions)
ISBN 978-981-126-355-2 (ebook for individuals)

For any available supplementary material, please visit
https://www.worldscientific.com/worldscibooks/10.1142/13060#t=suppl

Desk Editor: Joseph Ang

Typeset by Stallion Press
Email: enquiries@stallionpress.com

Preface

Radiation oncology is a technology-intensive field of medicine undergoing rapid changes. It offers a rich research and development platform to move the system toward precision and personalized therapy. Artificial intelligence (AI) or deep learning is a powerful technology with many subfields in the era of big data to address a variety of issues in medicine. AI tools can be used to improve decision-making, productivity, precision, safety, and professional satisfaction in various clinical settings.

There are many good teaching materials available for teaching the basics of Artificial Intelligence. There is also an exponentially increasing body of peer-reviewed literature on AI applications in Radiation Oncology. What was missing was a text bridging the gap between basic didactics and frontline research: a book which would bridge this gap and set the foundation for applying sophisticated Artificial Intelligence tools in Radiation Oncology.

We, together with the contributors, collectively wanted to develop a book that defines the future and identifies the problems suitable for AI applications as well as AI tools and experiences from other fields such as radiology imaging and a new research environment enabling AI research.

In designing the book, we have tried to balance the depth of science and technology of AI with the breadth of applications within radiation oncology. The book also includes assessment, evaluation, and ethics. The excellence of a book depends on the quality of its contributors.

World-class experts in AI, radiation oncology, and related fields have collaborated to develop this book. Each chapter was peer-reviewed by other authors for the book, and that process greatly enhanced the relevance of the material through cross-discipline pollination.

The book chapters are grouped into six sections: Defining the Future, Strategy, AI Tools, AI Applications, Assessment, and Outcomes.

This book is the result of the efforts of dedicated professionals with highly sophisticated expertise working together to share their knowledge with the greater radiation oncology community. We thank them all. We have been very fortunate to have such a team of more than 30 world-class experts in physics, science, engineering, patient care, ethics, assessment from academia and industry. We all learned from each other, resulting in a book of high value for the radiation oncology community.

Sonja and I feel immensely honored to have such a satisfying experience as stewards of the contributed expertise in radiation oncology for the book.

Seong K. Mun and Sonja Dieterich

List of Contributors

Michael J. Baine
Department of Radiation Oncology, University of Nebraska Medical Center, Omaha NE, USA

William Bennett
Department of Biomedical Informatics, University of Arkansas for Medical Sciences, Little Rock AR, USA

Ashish Chawla
Inova Schar Cancer Institute, Falls Church VA, USA

Leigh Conroy
Department of Radiation Oncology, University of Toronto, Princess Margaret Cancer Centre, 700 University Ave, Toronto, ON M5G 1X7, Canada

Quan Chen
Radiation Oncology, City of Hope Comprehensive Cancer Center, 1500 E Duarte Rd, Duarte, CA 91010, USA

Joseph O. Deasy
Department of Medical Physics, Memorial Sloan Kettering Cancer Center, New York NY, USA

Parin Dalal
Advanced, AI, Varian Inc, USA

Sonja Dieterich
Radiation Oncology, UC Davis, Sacramento CA, USA

Jiajin Fan
Inova Schar Cancer Institute, Falls Church VA, USA

Xue Feng
Carina Medical LLC, 145 Graham Ave, A168, Lexington, KY 40506, USA

Alexander Hyun
Department of Arts and Humanities, Minerva University, San Francisco CA, USA

Julian C. Hong
Bakar Computational Health Sciences Institute, University of California, San Francisco, San Francisco CA, USA

Department of Radiation Oncology, University of California, San Francisco, San Francisco CA, USA

UCSF-UC Berkeley Joint Program in Computational Precision Health, Berkeley CA, USA

University of California San Francisco Department of Radiation Oncology, San Francisco CA, USA

Megan Hyun
Department of Radiation Oncology, University of Nebraska Medical Center, Omaha NE, USA

Gretchen Purcell Jackson
Associate Professor of Surgery, Pediatrics, and Biomedical Informatics, Vanderbilt University Medical Center, Nashville TN, USA

Intuitive Surgical, Sunnyvale CA, USA

Ed Kline
RadPhysics Services LLC, Albuquerque NM, USA

Sangkyu Lee
Department of Medical Physics, Memorial Sloan Kettering Cancer Center, New York NY, USA

Shih-Chung Lo
Arlington Innovation Center: Health Research, Virginia Tech: Washington DC Region, Arlington VA, USA

Seong K. Mun
Arlington Innovation Center: Health Research, Virginia Tech: Washington DC Region, Arlington VA, USA

Lisa Ni
University of California San Francisco Department of Radiation Oncology, San Francisco CA, USA

Jung Hun Oh
Department of Medical Physics, Memorial Sloan Kettering Cancer Center, New York NY, USA

Christina Phuong
University of California San Francisco Department of Radiation Oncology, San Francisco CA, USA

Dalong Pang
Department of Radiation Medicine, Georgetown University Medical Center, Washington, DC 20007, USA

Fred Prior
Department of Biomedical Informatics, University of Arkansas for Medical Sciences, Little Rock AR, USA

Thomas G. Purdie
Departments of Radiation Oncology and Medical Biophysics, University of Toronto, Princess Margaret Cancer Centre, 700 University Ave, Toronto, ON M5G 1X7, Canada

Agam Sharda
Flash Solutions, Varian, USA

Srijan Sengupta
North Carolina State University, Raleigh NC, USA

Maria Thor
Department of Medical Physics, Memorial Sloan Kettering Cancer Center, New York NY, USA

Gabriel S. Vidal
Department of Radiation Oncology, University of Oklahoma, Oklahoma City OK, USA

Department of Medicine, University of Oklahoma, Oklahoma City OK, USA

Roy Vergis
Associate Partner and Clinical Leader, IBM Healthcare Consulting, London, UK

Expert in Digital Health, World Health Organization, Geneva

Honorary Consultant in Clinical Oncology, Mount Vernon Cancer Centre, London, UK

Andrew Wilson
Oncology Informatics Solutions, Elekta, Inc., Sunnyvale CA, USA

Christopher Wardell
Department of Biomedical Informatics, University of Arkansas for Medical Sciences, Little Rock AR, USA

Kenneth Wong
Arlington Innovation Center: Health Research,
Virginia Tech: Washington DC Region, Arlington VA, USA

Corey Zankowski
Primum Health, New York, USA

Dandan Zheng
University of Rochester Medical Center, Rochester NY, USA

Dongyang Zhang
Oncology Informatics Solutions, Elekta, Inc., Sunnyvale CA, USA

Xiaofeng Zhu
Inova Schar Cancer Institute, Falls Church VA, USA

Contents

Part 1

Define the Future

Chapter 1

Clinical Radiation Oncology in 2040: Vision for Future Radiation Oncology from the Clinical Perspective

Gabriel S. Vidal*,† and Julian C. Hong‡,§,¶

**Department of Radiation Oncology, University of Oklahoma, Oklahoma City OK, USA*
†Department of Medicine, University of Oklahoma, Oklahoma City OK, USA
‡Department of Radiation Oncology, University of California, San Francisco, San Francisco CA, USA
§Bakar Computational Health Sciences Institute, University of California, San Francisco, San Francisco CA, USA
¶UCSF-UC Berkeley Joint Program in Computational Precision Health, Berkeley CA, USA

Abstract

Oncology has seen tremendous advancements over the past 10 to 30 years through the development of a variety of technologies to improve personalization and precision in cancer care. Artificial intelligence (AI) and, more specifically, machine learning (ML) have the potential to push this transformation further. The chapters that follow will take a deep dive into describing areas where AI will advance care. This chapter will synthesize these to formulate a blue-sky vision for radiation oncology practice in 2040 and the accompanying role of AI, and more broadly, novel computational and statistical technologies. A critical eye and rigorous data (including randomized controlled trials in many cases) will be imperative as these technologies are evaluated and implemented in the clinic (James *et al.*, 2022), and barriers to implementation remain a challenge (Beede *et al.*, 2020; Kang *et al.*, 2020; Morse *et al.*, 2020). Nevertheless, early randomized controlled data have demonstrated that once these challenges are faced, cancer care delivery can be made safer, more efficient, more affordable, more inclusive, and more equitable with AI (Hong *et al.*, 2020b; McIntosh *et al.*, 2021). These technologies are poised to play a larger and more central role in the radiation oncology clinic workflow.

As in other fields of medicine, oncology practices are faced with a staggering amount of healthcare data for each patient. AI has the potential of harnessing this clinical data and providing methods to both understand and deliver better precision care for cancer at the individual level. It also offers promise in improving the delivery of cancer care and providing more systematic and accessible care across the spectrum of practices. Overall, these advances will improve many of the tasks involved in cancer care to enable physicians to focus on the most important aspect of oncology: the patient.

In this chapter, we will lay out an ambitious vision for the radiotherapy of 2040, driven by the continued advances in computational technologies. To best characterize this, we will follow the journey of a patient through the most typical elements in the oncology (specifically radiation oncology) pathway: screening and diagnosis, staging and risk stratification, clinical decision-making, radiotherapy planning, treatment delivery, and clinical management.

1. The Diagnosis

A number of cancers are identified through the use of screening via laboratory tests, imaging studies, or procedures. Common screen-detected cancers with national guidelines include breast, colorectal, lung, cervical, and prostate cancers (Duffy *et al.*, 2020; Mottet *et al.*, 2021; Team, 2011; Zauber *et al.*, 2021). Cancer screening is currently delivered with some adjustment for risk (age, heritability, exposures, etc.), as well as prior testing (prior colonoscopy or imaging findings, human papilloma virus detection on pap smears). AI promises to improve the accuracy and personalization of this process, and potentially advance the lead time with which cancers may be anticipated.

Breast cancer screening, for example, is one of the areas which has attracted the most AI-based attention. Importantly, all advances in AI technology will demand that we learn from lessons of computer-aided diagnosis for screening mammography, which, despite years of use and reimbursement in routine clinical practice, was ultimately demonstrated to have limited — and potentially negative — utility in the diagnosis of breast cancers (Lehman *et al.*, 2015). Novel AI has laid out a particularly ambitious agenda in breast cancer screening, as a recent mammography-based risk model assessed internationally was shown to accurately predict future breast cancer (Yala *et al.*, 2021). Such approaches, if validated, will enable potential early interventional strategies and better streamline the screening process.

Colorectal cancer screening has potentially seen the most rigorous clinical evaluation of the use of AI, with multiple randomized trials demonstrating the benefit of computer vision technologies to improve the detection and quality of exams (Gong *et al.*, 2020; Su *et al.*, 2020; Wang *et al.*, 2020; Wu *et al.*, 2019). Similarly, in lung cancer, pre-clinical work with computational image analysis approaches have demonstrated promise in improving the current use of radiologist-assessed pulmonary nodule size and morphology for risk stratification based on the Fleischner Society guidelines (MacMahon *et al.*, 2017). Numerous studies have been carried out with the goal of characterizing benign and malignant pulmonary nodules (Heuvelmans & Oudkerk, 2019; van Griethuysen *et al.*, 2017).

2. In 2040, AI will Facilitate Anticipatory Predictions to Improve Early Detection

The diagnosis of cancer relies on tissue confirmation, an important step in defining the biology of a cancer and subsequently both its commensurate prognosis and best treatment strategy. Traditionally, tissue has been interpreted via gross histologic examination by expert pathologists, but molecular and genomic biomarkers have allowed clinicians to formulate a more tailored treatment approach for breast and prostate cancers (Feng *et al.*, 2021; Mamounas *et al.*, 2020; Rakovitch *et al.*, 2021; Solin *et al.*, 2013). In particular, the use of genomic tools have already been clearly validated in randomized studies and impacted clinical care in breast cancer (Kalinsky *et al.*, 2021; Sparano *et al.*, 2018). We anticipate that prostate cancer, where genomic tests are already playing a role among early adopters, and other cancers will be close behind. A number of other AI-driven approaches to analyzing biological samples are emerging and will likely play an important role. These include digital pathology and circulating tumor DNA.

The process of pathology review is importantly impacted by inter-rater variability (Allsbrook *et al.*, 2001a, 2001b), which is persistent, though reduced, among specialized experts despite standardized grading guidelines (Ginter *et al.*, 2021). AI-based digital pathology approaches are capable of reducing the interobserver variability often noted in histopathological evaluation (Luchini *et al.*, 2022). However, the important promise of AI is in its potential to go beyond interpretation and provide additional risk stratification, which may offer opportunities to better stratify treatment (Takamatsu *et al.*, 2022; Yu *et al.*, 2016).

3. In 2040, AI-based Approaches will Improve Consistency and Accessibility of High Quality Pathology Interpretation, and Provide Prognostic and Predictive Functionality with Greater Randomized Supporting Data

Once a cancer diagnosis is established, the extent and risk of a disease are usually assessed in the staging process. Traditional cancer staging incorporates several variables to provide risk stratification and prognosis, with a focus on anatomic characteristics. Treatment options vary greatly depending on staging. Early signs of the contributions of computational approaches to define staging have already become apparent in clinical practice. The ICON-S study created a more meaningful staging classification for oropharynx cancers based on recursive partition analysis (RPA) using an international cohort (O'Sullivan *et al.*, 2016). The results of this study have since been used to define the oropharynx cancer staging system.

4. In 2040, Advanced Statistical Approaches will Drive or Provide Critical Characteristics in Staging

In addition to the risk stratification of staging, prognostication is one of the variables considered during the initial visit, critically important to balance the risks and benefits of potentially toxic therapies. This impacts both eligibility for systemic therapies and best approaches in balancing toxicity of therapy and treatment goals. AI algorithms and statistical models in general have long been targeted toward prognosis (Avati *et al.*, 2017; Charlson *et al.*, 2022; Dosani *et al.*, 2018; Mojica-Márquez *et al.*, 2020; Peterson *et al.*, 2012). These models have a journey ahead over the coming decades to improve their accuracy, robustness, and generalizability as they can be brittle depending on clinical context (Wu *et al.*, 2021). Nevertheless, they are likely to find an avenue where they can contribute, in light of typically optimistic clinician-estimated prognoses (Sborov *et al.*, 2019). As it is important that these tools do not become self-fulfilling and adjust with improvements in therapy, one reasonable avenue is to improve palliative care referrals and serious illness conversations (Manz *et al.*, 2020).

5. In 2040, AI will Provide Improved Decision Support to Improve Appropriate Personalized Treatment, and Drive Targeted Areas in Patient-Centered Goals of Care

Finally, AI also has the important promise to also practically impact the clinical data review process at the point of care. Clinicians currently are required to synthesize these large swaths of data through manual review and make orders and documentation in the electronic health record (EHR). A number of studies have begun to focus on the metadata describing physician interaction with the EHR, referred to as the audit log. This audit log carries significant potential to identify physician pain points, potentially offering solutions to ease the burden on physicians and subsequent burnout, reduce areas for errors, and improve care delivery (Huilgol *et al.*, 2022).

6. In 2040, Algorithmic Tools Built into EHR Systems will Ease the Process of Record Review, Ordering, and Documentation

6.1. *Radiotherapy planning*

Once a patient is on the path toward radiotherapy, they will undergo the simulation and treatment planning process. Target and normal tissue segmentation remain a labor-intensive task in the radiation oncology workflow. This process of delineation, particularly for clinical target volumes, can be subject to significant variability (Michalski *et al.*, 2010).

Autosegmentation has been in the pipeline for commercial products for some time, with advances based on deep learning. These processes may be further advanced through the aggregation of "crowd sourced" data (Mak *et al.*, 2019). We ultimately anticipate that these products will be ready for broad use in the near future, particularly as treatment volumes are subject to clinician review before treatment delivery. However, we expect that the AI-assisted radiotherapy of the future will not only apply autosegmentation approaches for known targets, but also improve target delineation by informing areas of risk for recurrence.

Similarly, dose constraints to vital organs remain an important component for radiation planning. Building on the experience of Quantitative Analysis of Normal Tissue Effects in The Clinic (QUANTEC), ML offers avenues, particularly in standardized settings, to improve the identification of clinically meaningful dosimetric goals (Polizzi *et al.*, 2021). Statistical approaches similarly enable potential identification of appropriate dose constraints for normal tissues (Thor *et al.*, 2021).

Knowledge-based treatment planning (KBP) and other similar auto-planning approaches have the potential of reducing overall treatment planning times while delivering plans that are non-inferior to the current standard. We predict that automated planning will become standard across many disease sites. Current prospective studies have already demonstrated that KBP is non-inferior to human-driven plans across multiple disease sites (Cornell *et al.*, 2020), and that ML-based planning can generate clinically acceptable treatment plans (McIntosh *et al.*, 2021). We anticipate, as time progresses, this trend will continue and that AI will advance both the ability to achieve optimal radiotherapy plans (Bitterman *et al.*, 2022) and advance the efficiency of the planning process (Li *et al.*, 2021). These advances will also expand the accessibility of high-quality planning to practices with fewer resources and improve access to radiotherapy.

It is worth highlighting a significant advancement in the treatment delivery in the form of online adaptive radiotherapy, ushered in by the MRI-guided linear accelerator (LINAC) systems with online adaptive radiotherapy, by which physicians can generate a new radiotherapy plan prior to each treatment fraction delivery based on anatomical changes. The need for resegmentation and replanning is a natural fit for the benefits of rapid, AI-assisted segmentation and planning.

7. In the Year 2040, AI-Assisted Segmentation and Treatment Planning will be Commonplace and Improve the Quality and Accessibility of Radiotherapy Plans, with Particular Impacts on Access to Care and Active Replanning

7.1. *Clinical management*

Patient care remains at the forefront of radiation oncology, and in particular oncology practice demands the management of patient symptoms and quality of life, whether related to disease, treatment, or other comorbid conditions. AI has the potential of improving clinical management by helping to focus care to improve standardization and equity and reduce the cognitive burden on physicians.

The System for High Intensity EvaLuation During Radiation Therapy (SHIELD-RT) was a randomized controlled study implementing ML-guided management during radiotherapy at Duke University (Hong *et al.*, 2018; Hong *et al.*, 2020b). In that study, ML accurately triaged patients undergoing treatment and identified those who had a higher risk of requiring acute care. High-risk patients were randomized to mandatory supplemental evaluations during treatment, reducing both rates of acute care and their associated costs in half.

Clinical management during radiotherapy treatment will also be impacted by the influx of patient-generated health data (PGHD). PGHD in particular includes data such as patient-reported outcomes (PROs), frequently captured in an electronic format, and consumer devices that track patient activity and vital signs (Purswani *et al.*, 2019). The clinical impact of PROs has already been demonstrated, with improved survival for patients with metastatic cancers receiving chemotherapy. These are being increasingly reported via digital format, and the next two decades will see particular efforts toward improving access and reducing disparate use of patient portals (Sinha *et al.*, 2021), which play an integral role in capturing PROs in most healthcare centers. These efforts will be critical to realizing the potential of these systems.

Data from consumer devices such as wearables are much more limited. One of the larger experiences at Montefiore Einstein Cancer Center implementing activity monitoring demonstrated the prognostic value of step counts during chemoradiotherapy (Ohri *et al.*, 2017, 2019). This is the subject of the broader upcoming cooperative group NRGF-001 (NCT04878952), which aims to improve supportive care and decrease the rate of adverse clinical events by monitoring daily step counts during the course of concurrent chemoradiotherapy for patients with locally advanced non-small cell lung cancer.

Project Persist is a current prospective, single-institution trial at the Stephenson Cancer Center at the University of Oklahoma. This study currently uses a novel smartphone app to track emotional, physical, and behavioral symptoms as well as cancer treatment side effects. Patients are enrolled before radiation treatment starts, and eligible patients must be scheduled to receive a minimum of four consecutive weeks of radiation treatments. Patients are randomized on a 1:1 basis to receive anxiety/depression treatment components within the app. Patients are provided with a smartphone if they do not own one.

Finally, a number of medical specialties have advanced surveillance efforts to identify drug-related adverse events based on natural language processing (NLP) applied to clinical documentation. These approaches have been externally validated to identify National Cancer Institute (NCI) Common Terminology Criteria for Adverse Events (CTCAE) encoded toxicities in radiotherapy notes (Hong *et al.*, 2020a). Prior manually reviewed correspondence from patients via patient portals have suggested that specific topics are correlated with the early discontinuation of hormone therapy for breast cancer (Yin *et al.*, 2018). One could easily envision a future where NLP may offer automated mechanisms for surveillance of both physician- and patient-generated text to direct symptom management during cancer therapy.

8. In 2040, AI will Enable the Use of Multiple Sources of Data to Help Physicians Better Manage Patient Quality of Life

We are enthusiastic about the potential AI has to transform radiation therapy by the year 2040. While much work and evaluation are needed before these approaches are ready for prime time, the foundational steps are coming into focus today. AI will likely impact a number of elements in the care of patients with cancer, and it will be important for the community to evaluate this progress and its benefit in clinical practice. We have laid out an ambitious agenda over the next couple of decades and are optimistic that AI will free clinicians and care teams from certain tasks to focus their attention on delivering patient-centric care.

References

Allsbrook, W. C., Jr, Mangold, K. A., Johnson, M. H., Lane, R. B., Lane, C. G., & Epstein, J. I. (2001). Interobserver reproducibility of Gleason grading of prostatic carcinoma: general pathologist. *Human Pathology*, *32*(1), 81–88. https://doi.org/10.1053/hupa.2001.21135

Allsbrook, W. C., Mangold, K. A., Johnson, M. H., Lane, R. B., Lane, C. G., Amin, M. B., Bostwick, D. G., Humphrey, P. A., Jones, E. C., Reuter, V. E., Sakr, W., Sesterhenn, I. A., Troncoso, P., Wheeler, T. M., & Epstein, J. I. (2001b). Interobserver reproducibility of Gleason grading of prostatic carcinoma: Urologic pathologists. *Human Pathology*, *32*(1), 74–80. https://doi.org/https://doi.org/10.1053/hupa.2001.21134.

Avati, A., Jung, K., Harman, S., Downing, L., Ng, A., & Shah, N. H. (2017, 13–16 Nov. 2017). Improving palliative care with deep learning. 2017 IEEE International Conference on Bioinformatics and Biomedicine (BIBM).

Beede, E., Baylor, E., Hersch, F., Iurchenko, A., Wilcox, L., Ruamviboonsuk, P., & Vardoulakis, L. M. (2020). A human-centered evaluation of a deep learning system deployed in clinics for the detection of diabetic retinopathy. In *Proceedings of the 2020 CHI Conference on Human Factors in Computing Systems* (pp. 1–12). Association for Computing Machinery. https://doi.org/10.1145/3313831.3376718

Bitterman, D. S., Selesnick, P., Bredfeldt, J., Williams, C. L., Guthier, C., Huynh, E., Kozono, D. E., Lewis, J. H., Cormack, R. A., Carpenter, C. M., Mak, R. H., & Atkins, K. M. (2022). Dosimetric planning tradeoffs to reduce heart dose using machine learning-guided decision support software in patients with lung cancer. *International Journal of Radiation Oncology*Biology*Physics, 112*(4), 996–1003. https://doi.org/https://doi.org/10.1016/j.ijrobp.2021.11.009

Charlson, M. E., Carrozzino, D., Guidi, J., & Patierno, C. (2022). Charlson Comorbidity Index: A Critical Review of Clinimetric Properties. *Psychotherapy and Psychosomatics, 91*(1), 8–35. https://doi.org/10.1159/000521288

Cornell, M., Kaderka, R., Hild, S. J., Ray, X. J., Murphy, J. D., Atwood, T. F., & Moore, K. L. (2020). Noninferiority Study of Automated Knowledge-Based Planning Versus Human-Driven Optimization Across Multiple Disease Sites. *International Journal of Radiation Oncology, Biology, Physics, 106*(2), 430–439. https://doi.org/10.1016/j.ijrobp.2019.10.036

Dosani, M., Tyldesley, S., Bakos, B., Hamm, J., Kong, T., Lucas, S., Wong, J., Liu, M., & Hamilton, S. (2018). The TEACHH model to predict life expectancy in patients presenting for palliative spine radiotherapy: external validation and comparison with alternate models. *Supportive care in cancer: official journal of the Multinational Association of Supportive Care in Cancer, 26*(7), 2217–2227. https://doi.org/10.1007/s00520-018-4064-x

Duffy, S. W., Tabár, L., Yen, A. M., Dean, P. B., Smith, R. A., Jonsson, H., Törnberg, S., Chen, S. L., Chiu, S. Y., Fann, J. C., Ku, M. M., Wu, W. Y., Hsu, C. Y., Chen, Y. C., Svane, G., Azavedo, E., Grundström, H., Sundén, P., Leifland, K., Frodis, E., … Chen, T. H. (2020). Mammography screening reduces rates of advanced and fatal breast cancers: Results in 549,091 women. Cancer, 126(13), 2971–2979. https://doi.org/10.1002/cncr.32859

Feng, F. Y., Huang, H. C., Spratt, D. E., Zhao, S. G., Sandler, H. M., Simko, J. P., Davicioni, E., Nguyen, P. L., Pollack, A., Efstathiou, J. A., Dicker, A. P., Todorovic, T., Margrave, J., Liu, Y. S., Dabbas, B., Thompson, D., Das, R., Dignam, J. J., Sweeney, C., Attard, G., … Tran, P. T. (2021). Validation of a 22-Gene Genomic Classifier in Patients With Recurrent Prostate Cancer: An Ancillary Study of the NRG/RTOG 9601 Randomized Clinical Trial. JAMA oncology, 7(4), 544–552. https://doi.org/10.1001/jamaoncol.2020.7671

Ginter, P. S., Idress, R., D'Alfonso, T. M., Fineberg, S., Jaffer, S., Sattar, A. K., Chagpar, A., Wilson, P., & Harigopal, M. (2021). Histologic grading of breast carcinoma: A multi-institution study of interobserver variation using virtual microscopy. *Modern Pathology*, *34*(4), 701–709. https://doi.org/10.1038/s41379-020-00698-2.

Gong, D., Wu, L., Zhang, J., Mu, G., Shen, L., Liu, J., Wang, Z., Zhou, W., An, P., Huang, X., Jiang, X., Li, Y., Wan, X., Hu, S., Chen, Y., Hu, X., Xu, Y., Zhu, X., Li, S., Yao, L., ... Yu, H. (2020). Detection of colorectal adenomas with a real-time computer-aided system (ENDOANGEL): a randomised controlled study. *The lancet. Gastroenterology & hepatology*, *5*(4), 352–361. https://doi.org/10.1016/S2468-1253(19)30413-3

Heuvelmans, M. A., & Oudkerk, M. (2019). Deep learning to stratify lung nodules on annual follow-up CT. The Lancet. *Digital health*, *1*(7), e324–e325. https://doi.org/10.1016/S2589-7500(19)30156-6

Hong, J. C., Niedzwiecki, D., Palta, M., & Tenenbaum, J. D. (2018). Predicting Emergency Visits and Hospital Admissions During Radiation and Chemoradiation: An Internally Validated Pretreatment Machine Learning Algorithm. JCO clinical cancer informatics, 2, 1–11. https://doi.org/10.1200/CCI.18.00037

Hong, J. C., Fairchild, A. T., Tanksley, J. P., Palta, M., & Tenenbaum, J. D. (2020). Natural language processing for abstraction of cancer treatment toxicities: accuracy versus human experts. *JAMIA open*, *3*(4), 513–517. https://doi.org/10.1093/jamiaopen/ooaa064

Hong, J. C., Eclov, N., Dalal, N. H., Thomas, S. M., Stephens, S. J., Malicki, M., Shields, S., Cobb, A., Mowery, Y. M., Niedzwiecki, D., Tenenbaum, J. D., & Palta, M. (2020). System for High-Intensity Evaluation During Radiation Therapy (SHIELD-RT): A Prospective Randomized Study of Machine Learning-Directed Clinical Evaluations During Radiation and Chemoradiation. *Journal of clinical oncology: official journal of the American Society of Clinical Oncology*, *38*(31), 3652–3661. https://doi.org/10.1200/JCO.20.01688

Huilgol, Y. S., Adler-Milstein, J., Ivey, S. L., & Hong, J. C. (2022). Opportunities to use electronic health record audit logs to improve cancer care. Cancer medicine, 10.1002/cam4.4690. Advance online publication. https://doi.org/10.1002/cam4.4690

James, C. A., Wachter, R. M., & Woolliscroft, J. O. (2022). Preparing Clinicians for a Clinical World Influenced by Artificial Intelligence. *JAMA*, *327*(14), 1333–1334. https://doi.org/10.1001/jama.2022.3580

Kalinsky, K., Barlow, W. E., Gralow, J. R., Meric-Bernstam, F., Albain, K. S., Hayes, D. F., Lin, N. U., Perez, E. A., Goldstein, L. J., Chia, S. K. L., Dhesy-Thind, S., Rastogi, P., Alba, E., Delaloge, S., Martin, M., Kelly, C. M., Ruiz-Borrego, M., Gil-Gil, M., Arce-Salinas, C. H., . . . Hortobagyi, G. N. (2021). 21-gene assay to inform chemotherapy benefit in node-positive breast cancer. *New England Journal of Medicine*, *385*(25), 2336–2347. https://doi.org/10.1056/NEJMoa2108873

Kang, J., Morin, O., & Hong, J. C. (2020). Closing the gap between machine learning and clinical cancer care — first steps into a larger world. *JAMA Oncology*, *6*(11), 1731–1732. https://doi.org/10.1001/jamaoncol.2020.4314

Lehman, C. D., Wellman, R. D., Buist, D. S. M., Kerlikowske, K., Tosteson, A. N. A., Miglioretti, D. L., & for the Breast Cancer Surveillance, C. (2015). Diagnostic accuracy of digital screening mammography with and without computer-aided detection. *JAMA Internal Medicine*, *175*(11), 1828–1837. https://doi.org/10.1001/jamainternmed.2015.5231

Li, X., Wang, C., Sheng, Y., Zhang, J., Wang, W., Yin, F. F., Wu, Q., Wu, Q. J., & Ge, Y. (2021). An artificial intelligence-driven agent for real-time head-and-neck IMRT plan generation using conditional generative adversarial network (cGAN). Medical physics, 48(6), 2714–2723. https://doi.org/10.1002/mp.14770

Luchini, C., Pantanowitz, L., Adsay, V., Asa, S. L., Antonini, P., Girolami, I., Veronese, N., Nottegar, A., Cingarlini, S., Landoni, L., Brosens, L. A., Verschuur, A. V., Mattiolo, P., Pea, A., Mafficini, A., Milella, M., Niazi, M. K., Gurcan, M. N., Eccher, A., Cree, I. A., … Scarpa, A. (2022). Ki-67 assessment of pancreatic neuroendocrine neoplasms: Systematic review and meta-analysis of manual vs. digital pathology scoring. *Modern pathology: an official journal of the United States and Canadian Academy of Pathology, Inc*, *35*(6), 712–720. https://doi.org/10.1038/s41379-022-01055-1

MacMahon, H., Naidich, D. P., Goo, J. M., Lee, K. S., Leung, A., Mayo, J. R., Mehta, A. C., Ohno, Y., Powell, C. A., Prokop, M., Rubin, G. D., Schaefer-Prokop, C. M., Travis, W. D., Van Schil, P. E., & Bankier, A. A. (2017). *Guidelines for Management of Incidental Pulmonary Nodules Detected on CT Images: From the Fleischner Society 2017. Radiology*, *284*(1), 228–243. https://doi.org/10.1148/radiol.2017161659

Mak, R. H., Endres, M. G., Paik, J. H., Sergeev, R. A., Aerts, H., Williams, C. L., Lakhani, K. R., & Guinan, E. C. (2019). Use of crowd innovation to develop an artificial intelligence–based solution for radiation therapy targeting. *JAMA Oncology*, *5*(5), 654–661. https://doi.org/10.1001/jamaoncol.2019.0159

Mamounas, E. P., Mitchell, M. P., & Woodward, W. A. (2020). Molecular predictive and prognostic markers in locoregional management. *Journal of Clinical Oncology*, *38*(20), 2310–2320. https://doi.org/10.1200/JCO.19.02905

Manz, C. R., Parikh, R. B., Small, D. S., Evans, C. N., Chivers, C., Regli, S. H., Hanson, C. W., Bekelman, J. E., Rareshide, C. A. L., O'Connor, N., Schuchter, L. M., Shulman, L. N., & Patel, M. S. (2020). Effect of integrating machine learning mortality estimates with behavioral nudges to clinicians on serious illness conversations among patients with cancer: A stepped-wedge cluster randomized clinical trial. *JAMA Oncology*, *6*(12), e204759–e204759. https://doi.org/10.1001/jamaoncol.2020.4759

McIntosh, C. A.-O., Conroy, L., Tjong, M. C., Craig, T., Bayley, A., Catton, C., Gospodarowicz, M., Helou, J., Isfahanian, N. A.-O., Kong, V., Lam, T., Raman, S., Warde, P., Chung, P., Berlin, A. A.-O., & Purdie, T. A.-O. (2021). Clinical integration of machine learning for curative-intent radiation treatment of patients with prostate cancer.

Michalski, J. M., Lawton, C., El Naqa, I., Ritter, M., O'Meara, E., Seider, M. J., Lee, W. R., Rosenthal, S. A., Pisansky, T., Catton, C., Valicenti, R. K., Zietman, A. L., Bosch, W. R., Sandler, H., Buyyounouski, M. K., & Ménard, C. (2010). Development of RTOG consensus guidelines for the definition of the clinical target volume for post-operative conformal radiation therapy for prostate cancer. *International journal of radiation oncology, biology, physics*, *76*(2), 361–368. https://doi.org/10.1016/j.ijrobp.2009.02.006

Mojica-Márquez, A. E., Rodríguez-López, J. L., Patel, A. K., Ling, D. C., Rajagopalan, M. S., & Beriwal, S. (2020). External validation of life expectancy prognostic models in patients evaluated for palliative radiotherapy at the end-of-life. *Cancer medicine*, *9*(16), 5781–5787. https://doi.org/10.1002/cam4.3257

Morse, K. E., Bagley, S. C., & Shah, N. H. (2020). Estimate the hidden deployment cost of predictive models to improve patient care. *Nature Medicine*, *26*(1), 18–19. https://doi.org/10.1038/s41591-019-0651-8.

Mottet, N., van den Bergh, R. C. N., Briers, E., Van den Broeck, T., Cumberbatch, M. G., De Santis, M., Fanti, S., Fossati, N., Gandaglia, G., Gillessen, S., Grivas, N., Grummet, J., Henry, A. M., van der Kwast, T. H., Lam, T. B., Lardas, M., Liew, M., Mason, M. D., Moris, L., ... Cornford, P. (2021). EAU-EANM-ESTRO-ESUR-SIOG Guidelines on prostate cancer-2020 update. Part 1: Screening, diagnosis, and local treatment with curative intent.

O'Sullivan, B., Huang, S. H., Su, J., Garden, A. S., Sturgis, E. M., Dahlstrom, K., Lee, N., Riaz, N., Pei, X., Koyfman, S. A., Adelstein, D., Burkey, B. B., Friborg, J., Kristensen, C. A., Gothelf, A. B., Hoebers, F., Kremer, B., Speel, E. J., Bowles, D. W., Raben, D., … Xu, W. (2016). Development and validation of a staging system for HPV-related oropharyngeal cancer by the International Collaboration on Oropharyngeal cancer Network for Staging (ICON-S): a multicentre cohort study. *The Lancet. Oncology*, *17*(4), 440–451. https://doi.org/10.1016/S1470-2045(15)00560-4

Ohri, N., Kabarriti, R., Bodner, W. R., Mehta, K. J., Shankar, V., Halmos, B., Haigentz, M., Jr., Rapkin, B., Guha, C., Kalnicki, S., & Garg, M. (2017). Continuous activity monitoring during concurrent chemoradiotherapy.

Ohri, N., Halmos, B., Bodner, W. R., Cheng, H., Guha, C., Kalnicki, S., & Garg, M. (2019). Daily step counts: A new prognostic factor in locally advanced non-small cell lung cancer?.

Peterson, J. C., Paget, S. A., Lachs, M. S., Reid, M. C., & Charlson, M. E. (2012). The risk of comorbidity. *Annals of the rheumatic diseases*, *71*(5), 635–637. https://doi.org/10.1136/annrheumdis-2011-200473

Polizzi, M., Watkins, R. W., & Watkins, W. T. (2021). Data-driven dose-volume histogram prediction.

Purswani, J. M., Dicker, A. P., Champ, C. E., Cantor, M., & Ohri, N. (2019). Big Data from small devices: The future of smartphones in oncology.

Rakovitch, E. A.-O., Sutradhar, R., Nofech-Mozes, S., Gu, S., Fong, C., Hanna, W., & Paszat, L. (2021). 21-Gene assay and breast cancer mortality in ductal carcinoma in situ.

Sborov, K., Giaretta, S., Koong, A., Aggarwal, S., Aslakson, R., Gensheimer, M. F., Chang, D. T., & Pollom, E. L. (2019). Impact of accuracy of survival predictions on quality of end-of-life care among patients with metastatic cancer who receive radiation therapy. *Journal of Oncology Practice*, *15*(3), e262–e270. https://doi.org/10.1200/JOP.18.00516

Sinha, S., Garriga, M., Naik, N., McSteen, B. W., Odisho, A. Y., Lin, A., & Hong, J. C. (2021). Disparities in Electronic Health Record Patient Portal Enrollment Among Oncology Patients. *JAMA oncology*, *7*(6), 935–937. https://doi.org/10.1001/jamaoncol.2021.0540

Solin, L. J., Gray, R., Baehner, F. L., Butler, S. M., Hughes, L. L., Yoshizawa, C., Cherbavaz, D. B., Shak, S., Page, D. L., Sledge, G. W., Jr., Davidson, N. E., Ingle, J. N., Perez, E. A., Wood, W. C., Sparano, J. A., & Badve, S. (2013). A multigene expression assay to predict local recurrence risk for ductal carcinoma in situ of the breast. *Journal of the National Cancer Institute*, *105*(10), 701–710. https://doi.org/10.1093/jnci/djt067

Sparano, J. A., Gray, R. J., Makower, D. F., Pritchard, K. I., Albain, K. S., Hayes, D. F., Geyer, C. E., Dees, E. C., Goetz, M. P., Olson, J. A., Lively, T., Badve, S. S., Saphner, T. J., Wagner, L. I., Whelan, T. J., Ellis, M. J., Paik, S., Wood, W. C., Ravdin, P. M., ... Sledge, G. W. (2018). Adjuvant chemotherapy guided by a 21-gene expression assay in breast cancer. *New England Journal of Medicine*, *379*(2), 111–121. https://doi.org/10.1056/NEJMoa1804710

Su, J.-R., Li, Z., Shao, X.-J., Ji, C.-R., Ji, R., Zhou, R.-C., Li, G.-C., Liu, G.-Q., He, Y.-S., Zuo, X.-L., & Li, Y.-Q. (2020). Impact of a real-time automatic quality control system on colorectal polyp and adenoma detection: a prospective randomized controlled study (with videos). *Gastrointestinal Endoscopy*, *91*(2), 415–424.e414. https://doi.org/https://doi.org/10.1016/j.gie.2019.08.026

Takamatsu, M., Yamamoto, N., Kawachi, H., Nakano, K., Saito, S., Fukunaga, Y., & Takeuchi, K. (2022). Prediction of lymph node metastasis in early colorectal cancer based on histologic images by artificial intelligence. *Scientific Reports*, *12*(1), 2963. https://doi.org/10.1038/s41598-022-07038-1

Team, T. N. L. S. T. R. (2011). Reduced lung-cancer mortality with low-dose computed tomographic screening. *New England Journal of Medicine*, *365*(5), 395-409. https://doi.org/10.1056/NEJMoa1102873

Thor, M., Iyer, A., Jiang, J., Apte, A., Veeraraghavan, H., Allgood, N. B., Kouri, J. A., Zhou, Y., LoCastro, E., Elguindi, S., Hong, L., Hunt, M., Cerviño, L., Aristophanous, M., Zarepisheh, M., & Deasy, J. O. (2021). Deep learning auto-segmentation and automated treatment planning for trismus risk reduction in head and neck cancer radiotherapy. *Physics and Imaging in Radiation Oncology*, *19*, 96–101. https://doi.org/10.1016/j.phro.2021.07.009

van Griethuysen, J. J. M., Fedorov, A., Parmar, C., Hosny, A., Aucoin, N., Narayan, V., Beets-Tan, R. G. H., Fillion-Robin, J. C., Pieper, S., & Aerts, H. (2017). Computational radiomics system to decode the radiographic phenotype. *Cancer Res*, *77*(21), e104–e107. https://doi.org/10.1158/0008-5472.Can-17-0339

Wang, P., Liu, X., Berzin, T. M., Glissen Brown, J. R., Liu, P., Zhou, C., Lei, L., Li, L., Guo, Z., Lei, S., Xiong, F., Wang, H., Song, Y., Pan, Y., & Zhou, G. (2020). Effect of a deep-learning computer-aided detection system on adenoma detection during colonoscopy (CADe-DB trial): a double-blind randomised study. *The Lancet Gastroenterology & Hepatology*, *5*(4), 343–351. https://doi.org/https://doi.org/10.1016/S2468-1253(19)30411-X

Wu, L., Zhang, J., Zhou, W., An, P., Shen, L., Liu, J., Jiang, X., Huang, X., Mu, G., Wan, X., Lv, X., Gao, J., Cui, N., Hu, S., Chen, Y., Hu, X., Li, J., Chen, D., Gong, D., ... Yu, H. G. (2019). Randomised controlled trial of WISENSE, a real-time quality improving system for monitoring blind spots during esophagogastroduodenoscopy. *Gut*, *68*(12), 2161. https://doi.org/10.1136/gutjnl-2018-317366

Wu, S. Y., Yee, E., Vasudevan, H. N., Fogh, S. E., Boreta, L., Braunstein, S. E., & Hong, J. C. (2021). Risk stratification for imminent risk of death at the time of palliative radiotherapy consultation. *JAMA Network Open*, *4*(7), e2115641–e2115641. https://doi.org/10.1001/jamanetworkopen.2021.15641

Yala, A., Mikhael, P. G., Strand, F., Lin, G., Satuluru, S., Kim, T., Banerjee, I., Gichoya, J., Trivedi, H., Lehman, C. D., Hughes, K., Sheedy, D. J., Matthis, L. M., Karunakaran, B., Hegarty, K. E., Sabino, S., Silva, T. B., Evangelista, M. C., Caron, R. F., ... Barzilay, R. (2021). Multi-institutional validation of a mammography-based breast cancer risk model. *Journal of Clinical Oncology*, JCO.21.01337. https://doi.org/10.1200/JCO.21.01337

Yin, Z., Harrell, M., Warner, J. L., Chen, Q., Fabbri, D., & Malin, B. A. (2018). The therapy is making me sick: How online portal communications between breast cancer patients and physicians indicate medication discontinuation. *Journal of the American Medical Informatics Association: JAMIA*, *25*(11), 1444–1451. https://doi.org/10.1093/jamia/ocy118

Yu, K.-H., Zhang, C., Berry, G. J., Altman, R. B., Ré, C., Rubin, D. L., & Snyder, M. (2016). Predicting non-small cell lung cancer prognosis by fully automated microscopic pathology image features. *Nature Communications*, *7*(1), 12474. https://doi.org/10.1038/ncomms12474

Zauber, A. G., Winawer, S. J., O'Brien, M. J., Lansdorp-Vogelaar, I., van Ballegooijen, M., Hankey, B. F., Shi, W., Bond, J. H., Schapiro, M., Panish, J. F., Stewart, E. T., & Waye, J. D. (2012). Colonoscopic polypectomy and long-term prevention of colorectal-cancer deaths. *The New England journal of medicine*, *366*(8), 687–696. https://doi.org/10.1056/NEJMoa1100370

Chapter 2

A Vision for Radiation Oncology in 2030

Sonja Dieterich*, Parin Dalal†, Agam Sharda‡ and Corey Zankowski§

Radiation Oncology, UC Davis, Sacramento CA, USA
†*Advanced, AI, Varian Inc, USA*
‡*Flash Solutions, Varian, USA*
§*Primum Health, New York, USA*

Abstract

By 2030, clinicians will routinely interact and collaborate with Artificial Intelligence (AI) software that leverage closed-loop continuous learning systems to extend the reach of radiotherapy. Cancer incidence and demand for treatment continues to outpace the growth of radiation therapy, which is one major driver for the adoption of AI. Another is the continued pressure to reduce the total cost of healthcare as the developed world embraces value-based care. AI is expected to further the dramatic automation of workflows within the radiation oncology department, making it possible to plan and deliver higher-quality care more quickly at lower costs.

Today, despite recent advances in techniques and technologies, radiation therapy remains a fundamentally manual process, reliant on individual expertise, and characterized by subjectivity. In some parts of the world where training and infrastructure are limited, radiation therapy is virtually non-existent. Early use of machine learning tools has demonstrably reduced variability, improved quality, and increased efficiency. We predict that AI will eliminate many barriers to the adoption of radiotherapy and enable a rapid expansion in global access to high-quality radiation oncology, resulting in millions of additional cancer patients' lives saved.

1. Introduction

1.1. *The growing cancer burden*

Cancer continues to be one of the biggest global health challenges. In 2012, a staggering 14.1 million new cases of cancer were reported worldwide, a number that could rise to 24.6 million by 2030 (Bray *et al.*, 2012). Cancer causes one of every six deaths globally. In 2018, at least 9.6 million people died from the disease, according to the World Health Organization (WHO).

Cancer is, by and large, the disease of the aged with 66 years being the median age of cancer patients at diagnosis while 80–84 years being the modal age group for incidence (Institute, N.C.). In the list of risk factors, advancing age stands alone as being the most important. The past two centuries, and specifically the past five decades, have created the foundation for an increasing cancer burden that the coming five decades will experience. Since 1950 we have witnessed the widening of the global population pyramid that, when combined with reduced population growth rates, suggests a 'filling up' of the pyramid — a substantial increase in the number of older people (see the figure in the next page for reference). Based on current population trends, the compounded annual growth rate for people over 65 years of age is expected to be almost triple that of people under 65 years of age over the coming 20 years.

This data predicts that global cancer incidence will continue to rise. Developing economies will rightly focus infrastructure and resources on controlling and preventing communicable diseases, which would result in people living longer. An aging population increases the need for cost

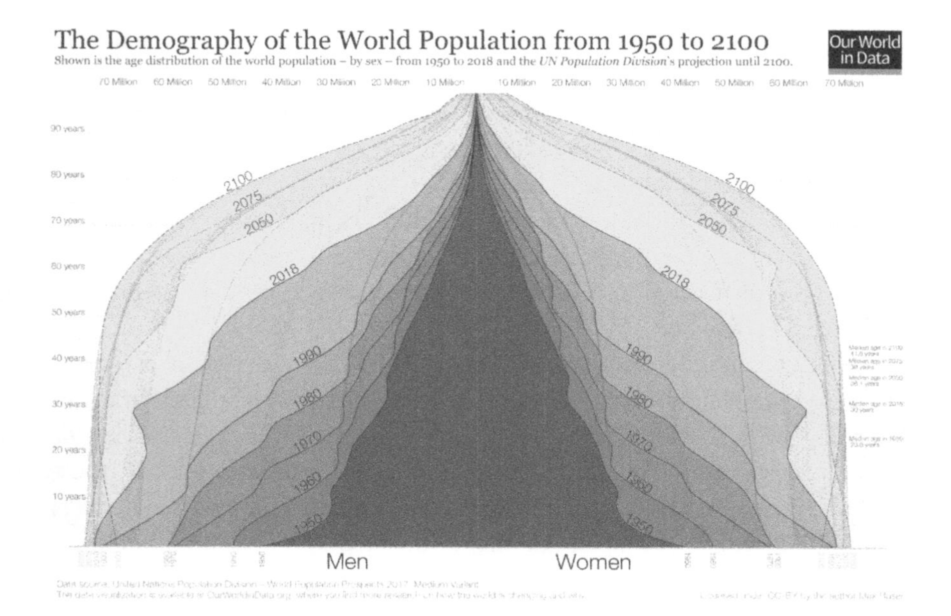

effective and socio-economically beneficial ways of managing the expected increasing cancer burden.

The Lancet Oncology Commission found radiotherapy to be indispensable for half or more cancer patients; essential for the effective treatment of most common cancers in low- and middle-income countries; and used to cure more than half of all localized cancer cases in high-income countries (Atun *et al.,* 2015). Yet, worldwide access to radiotherapy is very low, especially in low- and middle-income countries. Scaling up radiotherapy capacity could save 26.9 million life years, if done by 2035, according to the Lancet Oncology Commission, and give countries a net economic benefit of USD $278.1 billion. However, increasing access to care requires more than simply installing equipment. Physicians and well-educated staff are needed to operate radiation therapy equipment safely and effectively.

To increase access to cost-effective cancer care, radiation therapy stakeholders are trying to accomplish several goals simultaneously: simplify treatment planning and delivery, raise the quality of care, increase the efficiency of treatments, and lower the total cost of care. While no magic solution can address all these goals, the application of Artificial Intelligence (AI) technology to radiation therapy may offer new hope for the global cancer care community, given the exponential acceleration of this promising technology.

Innovation in radiation therapy technology has progressed broadly along two vectors: higher precision in dose delivery (improved outcomes), and the simplification and standardization of processes and technology (increased access and utilization).

It is encouraging that most such studies were undertaken before an explosion in technologies such as Artificial Intelligence and Machine Learning, which have created significant systemic efficiencies in several other industries. What might the large-scale introduction of these technologies offer radiation oncology and, indeed, the field of cancer therapy at large? This chapter and the following book seek to explore these possibilities.

1.2. *The growing data challenge*

As researchers, clinicians, and industry continuously develop new cancer diagnostic and treatment solutions, it creates an information challenge for clinicians. Additionally, medical information doubles nearly every 73 days (Sharon & Lucivero, 2019). Under these circumstances, one must ask how can oncologists incorporate the avalanche of data generated by these new solutions? How can they determine the optimal care strategy for the patient? New solutions are rendered irrelevant when care teams drown in data, wasting precious time trying to decide how to manage the patient. AI is already proving to be a valuable tool in tackling the data challenge and allowing cancer care teams to make faster and better-informed decisions.

2. A Vision for the Future

For AI to help address the global cancer challenge, it will likely pass through three phases of evolution: automation, augmentation, and amplification of human capabilities. Each phase involves the combination of people, data, and technology working together.

2.1. *Automation*

Automation is the simplest phase in the adoption of AI, which emphasizes completing tasks faster. The net result is to save time for the oncologist to do other work. An important benefit of automation is lower process variation by eliminating the potential for human error. In the automation phase, algorithms automate repetitive and error-prone manual activities, such as outlining healthy organs like the liver or heart in a medical image.

Many AI automations can be introduced safely in the Quality Assurance of human-driven processes. As evidence of its performance compared to clinicians is collected, the AI automation tools may be introduced into the primary workflow as productivity tools — helping to accelerate the care process.

2.2. *Augmentation*

The next step up is the augmentation of human skills. This phase allows people to solve higher-order problems. AI might expand what a person can do, for example, scan large volumes of data to identify best practices for every patient. Augmentation may manifest as AI that explores multiple treatment plans, each following a different technique to find the best treatment strategy.

In emerging markets, skill augmentation might boost the abilities of caregivers to deliver high-quality care. This could enable relatively low-skilled technicians to deliver advanced patient treatments, such as IMRT that is enabled by automatic image segmentation. Similarly, in developed markets, AI-fueled augmentation might boost the expertise of average physicians or heighten the skills of less expensive staff.

2.3. *Amplification*

In this, AI confers "superhuman" abilities onto caregivers, for example, the identification of signs that indicate which patients will — or will not — respond to certain treatments. These signs would be too subtle for even an expert oncologist to spot without the aid of a smart algorithm. But, once identified, these signs might be easily screened for. Being able to identify them could make the difference between life and death for individual patients, regardless of the market in which they reside.

AI might ultimately be built into radiotherapy equipment, adjusting treatments on the fly. (Lightning-fast smart algorithms might reshape the radiation beam to concentrate radiation on the target and away from healthy tissues. They might even change dose settings.)

The power of AI to automate, augment, and amplify routine processes will enable the care team to focus on complex knowledge work needed for optimal care. AI will automatically contour both healthy and malignant tissues in images obtained throughout the care continuum — the context of each image session will be known, and each new image of a patient will be automatically registered to previous patient images to form a longitudinal model of the patient, the Digital Patient Twin. The Digital Patient Twin can quantify and visualize changes in patient anatomy, physiology, and metabolism over time. AI will adjust radiation therapy plans automatically to account for changes in the patient between or during treatments, quantifying the treatment dose on the Digital Patient Twin. Recording the dose in this way will render therapy more precise and outcomes more accurate, leading to higher quality of life through treatments that are more convenient and comfortable.

In emerging markets, nurses and technicians might use AI to augment their skills so they can cover for scarce oncologists. In developed markets, these same algorithms will be used to reduce the cost of care by accelerating the care process. As AI elevates the capabilities of physicians and their staff, while making the treatment process more efficient, it will enable the three hallmarks of value-based medicine — improved quality and better patient outcomes at reduced cost.

The use of AI, therefore, could standardize radiation therapy as sites administer care of equal quality, regardless of their locations. In sum, AI has the potential to expand access to quality radiation therapy, increase quality while decreasing variability, and reduce costs.

3. The Radiation Oncology AI Toolkit

3.1. *Training and learning paradigms*

Supervised learning assumes an *i.i.d.* (independent, identically distributed) set of input data, x_i, paired with a label y_i. As with any statistical learning, a training paradigm appropriate to the task needs to be selected or engineered to produce a stable equilibrium of trained parameters, to predict y from x, or more generally predict the probability distribution $p(y_i \mid x_i)$. This criterion is often evaluated against a held-out set of x_i and y_i to gauge the generalizability of the model and to ensure a means to stop overtraining.

Unsupervised learning finds the essential features or latent space of a group of unlabeled samples, x_i. This learning can then be leveraged for supervised tasks later. Oftentimes, a very high-dimensional input space can be reduced to a lower-dimensional feature space that preserves reconstruction as well as some desirable properties appropriate to future tasks. For example, Auto-encoder (AE), and various styles of Variational Auto-encoders (VAEs), such as the popular Vector Quantized Variational Auto-encoder (VQ-VAE), can train a latent space that may be exploited for many purposes, e.g., transfer learning (explained in what follows) compression, disentangling of style features from object features, or even outlier detection.

In *semi-supervised learning* a small subset of the data is labeled, or their labels are trusted, and a larger corpus of data is unlabeled, or other labels are not trustworthy. Semi-supervised learning seeks to train features on the unlabeled data to transfer-learn and fine-tune with the labeled data to avail itself of the probability prior of the input data, x_i.

In *active learning* an agent decides when to ask a human being to label a specific sample in order to learn efficiently. Active learning always presents a trade-off between the cost of a human query and the generalized accuracy of a model. Active learning has been found to collapse the number of labeled samples needed for non-medical segmentation; however, human variability and multiple ground truths within images and image labels has prevented similar uptake in radiation therapy. Active learning can also refer to specific exploration–exploitation, trade-offs in working with knowledge already gained and attempting to gain new knowledge through possible failure.

Self-supervised learning essentially plays a series of "games" to supervise a machine learning model when it is presented with only unlabeled data. In the case of image processing without labeled data, one may attempt to reconstruct random holes created from images or look to provide full resolution out of a low-resolution subsampling. These games allow machine models to quickly learn the salient features of a data set, particularly when the number of parameters of the model is very high, as in Transformers. A very popular form of self-supervised learning constitutes the creation of an embedding: for example, word2vec (and more recently data2vec) converted words into tensor objects representing the relationships between them and compressed the dimensionality of their input.

Self-distillation is a modern method of self-supervised learning where models may be trained without contrasting pairs. In these models, a teacher and a student or "twins" train each other taking great care not to "collapse" the training between them. These techniques form modern state of the art, harnessing the power of many unlabeled examples before training on supervised sets.

Generative Modeling seeks to predict the joint probability of the input space and labels $p(x_i, y_i)$ so that new samples may be generated synthetically from the same distribution. Optionally, these samples can be hardened through an adversary that attempts to distinguish generated samples from real samples. Generative models can provide a means for regularizing networks so as to achieve higher generalizability. Adversarial models can probe for robustness of different predictive networks.

Medical data often cut across a variety of patient cases and treatments that can introduce many confounders to monolithic statistical training. These data are referred to as "long-tail" data, meaning there are diminishingly few of the same contexts even though there are many total samples. In these cases, one often uses *Multi-Task learning* so that certain parameters are shared in training to represent learnings independent of confounders; yet certain task-specific parameters will continue to contextualize predictions. Meta-learning refers to the ability to quickly learn a new context given training on previous contexts.

Deep reinforcement learning is over 50 years old but has found great recent success with the advent of deep networks. In essence, reinforcement learning allows one to produce a statistically biased optimizer as an output from training on different scenarios where the sample set is determined by the prediction. Samples are not *i.i.d.* so they require a great deal of care to ensure stability between the predicting model and the correlated training samples of that model.

In *dimensionality reduction*, a high-dimensional input space is transformed into a low-dimensional manifold that allows one to relate different samples. Such relations allow humans or other machine learning to explore possible trials or assert possible relationships.

3.2. *Toolkit selection*

The role of an AI scientist in using the above tools to classify the nature of the automation, augmentation, or amplification at hand into one or more canonical AI tasks (examples): Classifying (e.g. Diagnosing malignant versus benign tumors), Interpolating, Embedding (using machine-learned imaging features in Knowledge-Based planning), Forecasting (estimating the future positions of organs under patient-specific breathing patterns and sensors), Controlling (changing the machine sequence of instructions based on movement of the patient), Simulating (modifying therapy based on physical simulations of particle transport or biological outcomes), Recommending (placing the users' preferred machine at the top of the list), Interacting (providing contour autocompletion when drawing PTV borders), and Designing (modifying the style of the treatment plan, rather than optimizing an objective).

This may result in a hybrid or novel AI task type. As with any statistical learning a training appropriate to the task needs to be engineered to produce a stable equilibrium of trained parameters across known data tests, training, and validation sets.

The **Inductive Bias** of a neural network describes how its initial architecture captures the statistics of the problem. For example, popular Convolutional-style Neural Networks exploit the statistical, spatial relationships of real-world 3D objects in the filters of learned convolutional functions, while Transformer-style Neural Networks exploit the attention affinity of specific elements of high-dimensional inputs. In general, the engineering of networks must reflect the known inductive biases of the radiation therapy workflow, such as particle transport, anatomical features, usual interventional modalities, usual sparing modalities, and typical trade-off strategies.

When one problem is automated through a sufficient domain of data, **Transfer Learning** allows for a fast jump start on a new problem with far less data. In the context of radiation therapy, it confers a fast means of understanding the anatomy of a new patient in the context of previous patients, or learning to automate a new interventional process given previous interventions, or quickly learning a new preference or recommendation given previous recommendations. **Transfer Learning** is ubiquitous in Machine Learning as it derives from its underpinning in statistical learning theory. Interventional planning execution in engineering terms may be thought of as control theory: sensing or diagnosing, reasoning, actuating, and then sensing, etc. in a closed loop. Control theory does a poor job of leveraging previous control decisions to inform new ones. **Reinforcement Learning (RL)** brings this ability to train control algorithms that statistically learn or train on previous control loops to optimize the speed and training time of new ones.

Inevitably, certain controls cannot be expressed in a real-time training gym for RL algorithms due to a lack of modeling and a lack of prospective RCT data. **Causal Inference** is a field that estimates the probability of a causal relationship between a series of events or a time-series of data and can suggest the minimal experiments that would be needed to support those claims further. It is achieved through Perl Causality, Granger Causality, or Directed Information, or Synthetic Control analysis. Such analysis can refine inclusion and exclusion criteria in new prospective trials and has recently formed the basis of RWE for the FDA when lacking large-scale RCT trials.

4. The Trajectory of AI Tools into 2030

Currently, the AI tools of choice in radiotherapy surround means of contour automation, knowledge-based planning, motion management, and specific transfer learning. These will greatly evolve and change by 2030.

When we envision the use of AI in radiotherapy, we need to distinguish between solutions that could be implemented realistically in the next 3–5 years versus those that need significantly more research and development to be deployed safely outside major research institutions. In the immediate future, AI tools extending existing methods to increase automation for routine tasks are the most likely candidates for successful, robust implementation.

The care process starting when the patient is seen for their first radiotherapy consultation and ending on the last day of treatment is highly complex, having multiple, interactive feedback loops. While the general steps of a typical workflow, as described in the AAPM TG-100 report, are applied similarly in different departments, there are significant variations between radiotherapy clinics worldwide. In the clinical implementation of automation and AI, the AI tools must distinguish between desirable variations that benefit an individual patient and undesirable variations that lower quality and safety. The following paragraphs describe current sources of detrimental variations in care and how AI could improve the clinical process.

Accurate patient staging is the foundation of an evidence-based treatment plan. As more is discovered about cancer genetics, this new information influences staging. Staging systems evolve with science. To practice evidence-based medicine, Radiation Oncologists must memorize hundreds of treatment recommendations based on patients' pathology, cancer staging, age, co-morbidities, and other factors (Hansen & Roach, 2010). As new clinical trial results are published, many studies have shown the challenge and multi-year delays to move the best new evidence into routine clinical practice (Grol & Grimshaw, 2003; Ploeg *et al.*, 2007; Szulanski, 1996). For example, more than 30% of women with N2/N3 breast cancer in the US still do not receive the recommended post-mastectomy radiation, increasing the local recurrence rate by 20–27% and reducing overall survival by 8–9% (Chu *et al.*). Clinicians in developing countries face additional barriers in implementing new evidence, because they often do not have the resources to access peer-reviewed literature or attend conferences to update their clinical expertise.

EMR-based collaborative intelligence (CI) decision support software using natural language processing (NLP) will be able to assist with accurate staging and solve the problem of delayed and insufficient implementation of evidence-based treatment. CI software based on natural language processing combined with web scraping is in development (Saiz *et al.*, 2021) to assist physicians with literature review and developing treatment plans. Based on the patients' relevant EMR data, CI decision support software will pull the applicable society recommendations and clinical trials results and present the resulting treatment recommendations in a user-friendly graphical user interface (GUI).

Contouring is one of the best examples of an area at the forefront of benefiting patients. Contouring is a time-intensive and repetitive task, which is where automation excels. There is also a vast body of literature exploring the substantial inter-observer variation even between expert physicians in both organ-at-risk (OAR) and target contours. Early studies have shown that AI-based contouring tools can significantly reduce the variability of OAR contours. AI-based segmentation is a well-developed subspecialty within AI and is relatively mature compared to other AI applications. The track record and lessons learned from using AI-based segmentation and structure labeling in Diagnostic Radiology transfer directly to Radiation Oncology applications.

In addition to reducing contour variability and saving clinician time, AI-based segmentation can significantly impact three major areas over the next decade. First, AI segmentation tools can facilitate standardized nomenclature along the recommendations published by AAPM TG-263 and adopted by clinical trial groups. This in turn facilitates research based on big data science by reducing data pre-processing needs.

Second, AI-based algorithms can support the faster adoption of contouring atlases and guidelines published by clinical trial groups. Currently, it takes a conscientious effort by physicians and dosimetrists to seek out these guidelines and implement them in their practices. An AI tool could integrate updated contouring recommendations into future software releases, proactively bringing these standards to physicians when and where they need them. Thirdly, and most significantly, AI-based segmentation algorithms could be a training tool. Similar to contouring clinics available in high-resource regions of the world, AI software could coach residents and clinicians moving from 2D to volumetric-based radiation therapy using customized feedback and adapting the coaching to the local environment:

- The specific equipment a clinic owns. A large radiotherapy center that routinely provides adaptive radiotherapy, SBRT, MR-guided simulation and treatment, and complex interstitial brachytherapy services will have different workflows than a clinic with older equipment.

- The amount of staffing for the various specialties. A small satellite facility that hires consulting physicists a few days a week may assign dosimetrists and therapists tasks that a larger department would assign to physicists. In some countries such as Japan, the profession of medical physics is new, others have a well-established professional role.
- Local regulations and reimbursement methods will drive some of the practice variations. For example, reimbursement for third-party device-based measurement and routine in-vivo dosimetry for IMRT QA affects the number of resources allocated to safety and quality.

Real-time optimization: Currently the creation of a treatment plan can be a time-intensive process, particularly with complex cases, such as head and neck. The essential iterations that take place between an optimizer that does not speak the language of the clinician, and the clinician that must learn the vagaries of an optimizer, lead to poorer outcomes. Clinical plans are often those that fit within a time box and are deemed acceptable. In the future, machine learning will provide nearly instantaneous optimizations. They will rely on scalable distributed GPU computing in the cloud and algorithms that exploit prior strategic reasoning born of Reinforcement Learning rather than simple standard deviations of optimization lines in knowledge-based planning and absolute prioritization of weight in lexicographic ordering.

Causal Inference-based planning: Today's standard in treatment planning has components of style and anecdotal experience. This is largely due to the huge scalability gap between data-based outcome analysis and rigorous clinical, prospective trials. In the future all such longitudinal data will be available electronically and will be able to detect how anatomical, sub-anatomical, and biological outcomes can be optimized directly without the style and individual trainings of a radiation oncologist or medical physicist. All of the confounders that would otherwise mask the signal from the noise will be eliminated using causal inference.

Scheduling is critical for timely access to medical services and efficient use of staff and equipment resources. Queuing theory, routinely applied to operations management, traffic control, and staffing models to improve customer service, has yet to find its way into routine use in healthcare facilities. Radiation Oncology, with treatment courses running over 4–6 weeks, is a prime model for testing the use of advanced scheduling software algorithms in clinical practice.

Radiation Oncology scheduling has two distinct areas where automation could benefit the clinic: the staff-intensive scheduling for initial consultation and simulation, which requires coordination of insurance authorization, other providers such as Oncology, and more. The treatment course scheduling requires optimization of the linac schedule based on treatment length, patient preference, and staffing availability.

For the first aspect, initial scheduling, AI-supported scheduling could reduce the cognitive workload and task tracking for front office staff. Unsupervised learning algorithms could take on tasks such as initiating insurance authorization requests and coordinating schedules with other departments such as Oncology, nutritionists, and social support services. For routine scheduling, ML software will track actual linac time needed for classes of treatments such as breast or H&N, including parameters such as patient age and mobility. Optimizing machine schedules based on large datasets of time required for similar procedures, optimizing patient distribution among machines, adjusting schedules based on patient preferences, and quickly adjusting schedules for machine downtime will increase resource use while reducing wait times and increasing patient satisfaction.

To realize the above-described implementation of AI into clinics, we also need to describe what conditions must be in place for successful AI implementation. There are lessons learned from Diagnostic Radiology, the IBM Watson project, and on a smaller scale the current rate of adoption for commercially available AI solutions in our field.

First, implementation of AI requires IT resources and support. Currently, many hospital IT systems are structured such that the data flow between the clinic and outside entities is severely restricted. The reasons for these restrictions are maintaining Cybersecurity and adhering to HIPAA laws. Within these constraints, implementation of AI will require building strategies for access to cloud-based computing, HIPAA-compliant data sharing for software relying on big data, and developing a framework for open-source software development. In addition to the IT infrastructure, personnel resources are required to implement, commission, and maintain AI tools. Like the installing and continued maintenance of hardware solutions, software and processes also need continued maintenance and improvement.

Second, vendors should aim to build AI tools which can be widely adopted in daily clinical practice given the constraints most clinics face. To achieve this goal by 2030, vendors need to learn where current barriers and pitfalls are, and how product design can create robustness against failure. The major challenge for the vendor is their intrinsic removal from clinical processes. Unless product managers and software designers are embedded in a variety of clinics, it will be difficult to grasp where their products are not integrating well with humans. Technology offers a possible solution here as well: automated workflow monitoring software could learn to flag where deviations from the ideal process are larger than desired, which in turn could initiate focused clinical immersion of a vendor/clinician team to diagnose the issue. Another challenge vendors face is that AI tool development and implementation is currently driven by high-resource institutions. Multi-institutional consortiums that work with vendors for clinical implementations rarely include small or under-resourced centers. To achieve widespread adoption of AI by 2030 to reduce health disparities, vendors and low-resource clinics need to find a way to communicate their respective needs and solutions.

5. Summary

In summary, we can expect the pace of AI tool adoption in clinical practice to accelerate in the coming decade. As we improve our knowledge of how to build robust algorithms that can be commissioned for local needs and are robust in the face of data creep, the safe use of these algorithms will reach resource-constrained clinics. As we step through automation, augmentation, and amplification to support clinicians, AI tools in Radiation Oncology will increase access to cancer care and lower the cost for currently under-served patient populations.

References

Atun, R. *et al.* (2015). Expanding global access to radiotherapy. *The Lancet Oncology, 16*(10), 1153–1186.

Bray, F. *et al.* (2012). Global cancer transitions according to the Human Development Index (2008–2030): A population-based study. *The Lancet Oncology, 13*(8), 790–801.

Chu, Q. D. *et al.* (2015). Postmastectomy radiation for N2/N3 breast cancer: Factors associated with low compliance rate. *Journal of the American College of Surgeons, 220*(4), 659–669.

Grol, R. and Grimshaw, J. J. T. I. (2003). From best evidence to best practice: Effective implementation of change in patients' care. *The Lancet Oncology, 362*(9391), 1225–1230.

Hansen, E. K. and Roach, M. (2010). *Handbook of Evidence-based Radiation Oncology*. Vol. 4. Cham: Springer.

National Cancer Institute (Webpage). Available from: https://www.cancer.gov/about-cancer/causes-prevention/risk/age.

Ploeg, J. *et al.* (2007). Factors influencing best-practice guideline implementation: Lessons learned from administrators, nursing staff, and project leaders. *Worldview of Evidence-Based Nursing, 4*(4), 210–219.

Saiz, F. S. *et al.* (2021). Artificial intelligence clinical evidence engine for automatic identification, prioritization, and extraction of relevant clinical oncology research. *JCO Clinical Cancer Informatics*, 5, 102–111.

Sharon, T. and Lucivero, F. (2019). *Introduction to the Special Theme: The Expansion of the Health Data Ecosystem — Rethinking Data Ethics and Governance*. London, England: SAGE Publications Sage UK, p. 2053951719852969.

Szulanski, G. J. S. M. J. (1996). Exploring internal stickiness: Impediments to the transfer of best practice within the firm. *Strategic Management Journal, 17*(S2), 27–43.

Part 2

Strategy

Chapter 3

Lessons from Artificial Intelligence Applications in Radiology for Radiation Oncology

Seong K. Mun, Shih-Chung Lo and Kenneth Wong

Arlington Innovation Center: Health Research, Virginia Tech: Washington DC Region, Arlington VA, USA

Abstract

Artificial intelligence (AI) promises to bring dramatic changes in all industries as new industries are created and existing industries undergo digital transformation to meet future demands. The evolution of AI has experienced high expectations at times, followed by multiple disappointments over the past 50 years. Meanwhile, the development rate of AI science and technology is accelerating. Practitioners of AI and the user community understand the pitfalls of some unbounded expectations. AI is a set of powerful tools to solve many problems in a data-rich chaotic healthcare system. Radiology has been the first healthcare community to invest in developing imaging AI tools aggressively. However, after more than 25 years of research and development that resulted in many FDA-approved products, the radiology community's adoption of these AI tools remains in its infancy. This chapter reviews the lessons of AI in radiology and offers some strategic suggestions to the radiation oncology community on development and deployment so that AI as a whole can become meaningfully intelligent. We are used to thinking in terms of technology push, but AI strategy should be demand-driven and match the AI tools to solve significant problems sustainably. The successful digital transformation must focus on value creation through productivity improvement for the entire service chain.

1. Evolution of the Artificial Intelligence Ecosystem

1.1. *Expectations and disappointments of AI*

The idea of learning machines began with the concept of the McCulloch–Pitts mathematical model of a biological neuron (McCullouch & Pitts, 1943). It remained mainly within the academic community until the recent big data era. To recap, Artificial Intelligence (AI) is a broad term describing a software system designed to identify patterns and make decisions without human interventions. Machine Learning (ML) is a subset of AI that includes more advanced models and techniques where the programs can learn from examples. Deep Learning (DL) is an evolution of ML-based on multi-layered artificial neural networks.

There have been two significant concepts in the evolution of AI:

(1) AI as a symbolic representation and formal logic expressed as expert systems and the development of a family of high-level computer programming languages such as LISP, which became a common program language for AI in the 1960s and
(2) Conceptualization and mathematical frameworks mimicking neurons in the brain, which have evolved to the technique of artificial neural networks.

During the 1960s and 1970s, some successful applications of AI in the form of expert systems generated excitement in the industry. But the community realized that early successes that worked in well-structured narrow problems failed to generalize to the broader category of applications or deliver operationally valuable systems. This period is commonly known as the AI winter.

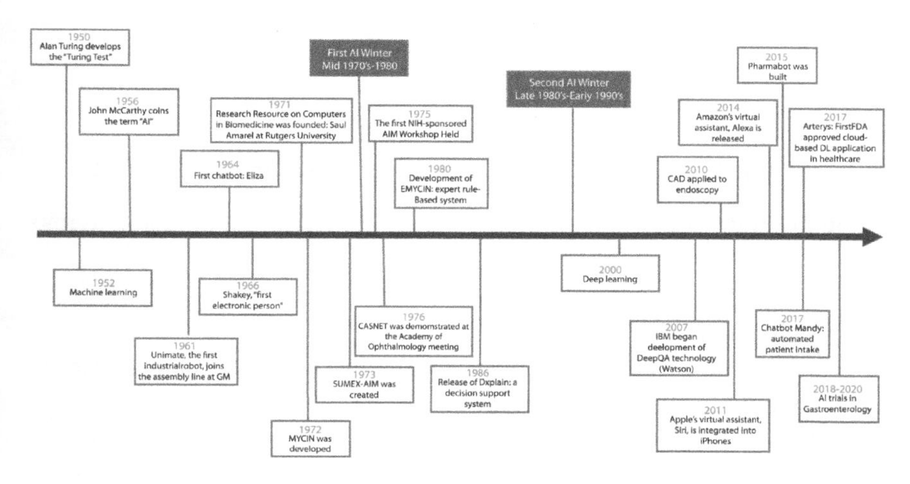

Fig. 1. Timeline of the development and the use of AI in medicine.

During the AI winter, the various disciplines of computer science, probability, mathematics, and AI came together to overcome the initial failures of AI. In particular, techniques from probability and signal processing and optimization were incorporated into AI architecture, resulting in the field known as machine learning (ML). Popular ML techniques include random forests, boosting, support vector machines, and artificial neural networks. Around 2010, AI began its spectacular global resurgence largely fueled by internet industries such as Google and Amazon, with AI becoming a core investment area by governments, industries, and academia. Figure 1 shows the timeline of development and the use of AI since 1950, including two AI winters (Kaul *et al.*, 2020).

Artificial convolutional neural networks (CNN) have recently dominated machine learning by solving computational problems in training neural networks and the availability of data necessary for training. The resulting systems are called deep learning (DL) systems and showed significant performance improvements over prior generations of algorithms. This has generated the next cycle of hype. While we grow out of the AI Winter, we must maintain a balanced perspective. We should not overstate utility. It is prudent to maintain cautious optimism based on a disciplined strategy for development and deployment, as AI will have ups and downs in many industries, including healthcare (West & Allen, 2018).

1.2. *Technical ecosystem helping research and development in AI*

There are four main reasons why AI research and development activities have exploded.

(1) Availability of Massive Datasets:
Machine Learning algorithms require large quantities of training data to produce high-performance AI models. For example, some facial recognition AI systems can now routinely outperform humans. Still, to do so, they require tens of thousands or millions of labeled images of faces for training data. More data are becoming available from many industries to develop training and testing data sets that match the real-world operational situations.

(2) Increased Computing Power:
Machine Learning AI systems require a massive computing power to process, store, and manage the data. A new computer architecture, Graphics Processing Units (GPUs), was developed around 2010 for massively parallel processing necessary for AI modeling. The GPU system can increase this AI training process by a factor of 20, obviating the need for supercomputers.

The development of cloud computing is also beneficial for AI since organizations can rapidly access massive computing resources on-demand and limit purchases of computing power to only what they need when they need it.

(3) Improved Machine Learning Algorithms:
The first Machine Learning algorithms are decades old, and some decades-old algorithms remain useful. However, researchers have developed many new algorithms that have accelerated advances in AI capabilities in recent years. These new algorithms have made Machine Learning models more flexible, more robust, and more capable of solving different types of problems.

(4) Open Source Code Libraries:
Machine Learning was a specialized niche within computer science for a long time.

Developing Machine Learning systems required many specific expertise and custom software development that only a few organizations could afford. Now, however, there are many open-source code libraries and developer tools that allow organizations to use and build upon the work of external communities. So today, no team or organization has to start from scratch. Furthermore, non-experts and beginners can create useful AI tools if they have access to high-quality data. Depending on specific applications of AI, especially in medical imaging, some of these open-source codes will require further development for optimum performance. A critical aspect of an open-source system is allowing users ease of collaboration, which is vital in AI development and testing.

2. Different Types of Machine Learning Tools

As the ML field advances, there is a growing number of many different types. However, the following are more common approaches to Machine Learning algorithms:

- Supervised Learning System
- Unsupervised Learning System
- Reinforcement Learning System
    (1) Supervised learning uses example data that human "supervisors" have labeled. Supervised learning has incredible performance, but getting sufficient labeled data can be difficult, time-consuming, and expensive.
    (2) Unsupervised Learning uses data but doesn't require labels for the data. As a result, it has lower performance than Supervised Learning for many applications, but it can also tackle problems where Supervised Learning isn't viable.
    (3) Reinforcement Learning has autonomous AI agents that gather their data and improve based on their trial and error interaction with the environment. An AI agent learns how to do a task by relentless trial and error in reinforcement learning. The agent

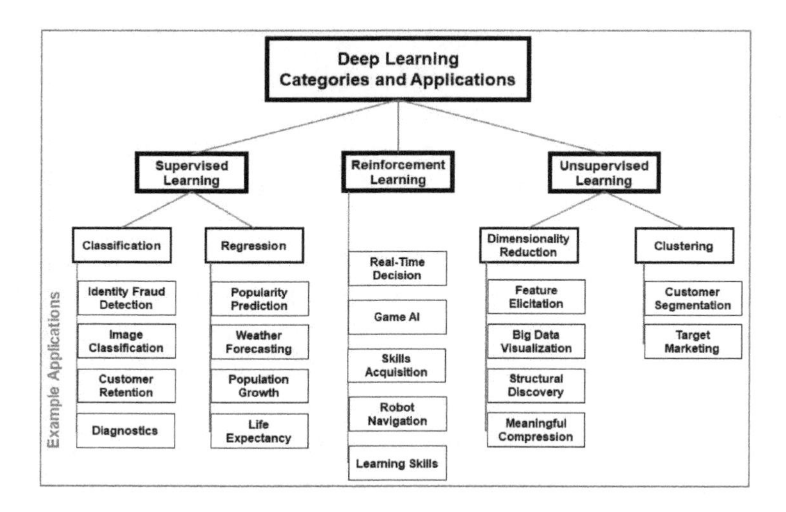

Fig. 2. Three types of Machine Learning categories and their applications.

figures out the best solution via millions of attempts. Once it is successful, it earns a reward. Reinforcement learning has been popular in video games where the system beats humans. It is a subject of intense basic research, but it is yet to be adopted for real-world problems.

Figure 2 shows three major types of machine learning categories and possible applications.

3. Digital Transformation of Radiology and Computer-Aided Diagnosis (CAD)

Radiology was one of the first healthcare specialties to adopt digital technology, an essential foundation for any application of AI. Since the 1970s, radiology has adopted many new digital imaging modalities such as Computed Tomography (CT), Magnetic Resonance Imaging (MRI), Positron Emission Tomography (PET), Single Photon Emission Computed Tomography (SPECT), Digital Ultrasound, Digital Mammography, and many others. These digital images were initially printed on films for interpretation, sharing, and archiving. Computed Radiography (CR) replaced the film-based conventional x-ray images (aka Roentgenography). As digital technologies for data capture, storage, image display, and transmission improved, radiology operations converted to a filmless digital environment in the late 1990s. Today, x-ray films are gone, and the Picture Archiving and Communication System (PACS) manages all digital radiological images (Mun *et al.*, 1993). These digital images opened the era of image processing for various specialty applications beyond diagnostic radiology (Mun *et al.*, 2007). Radiation oncology is a specialty area where advances in digital imaging, mainly cross-sectional imaging such as CT and MRI, have transformed the entire therapy process.

3.1. *Computer-aided diagnosis*

As more digital radiology images became available, the radiology community began to explore the concept of an artificial convolution neural network for image pattern recognition (Lo *et al.*, 1995). Some began to develop computer-aided diagnosis (CAD) as a possibility to assist radiologists (Doi, 2007). At the same time, the computer science community was developing computer vision technology. Computer vision, a domain of computer science, attempted to replicate the human visual process. Softwares were developed to segment, identify, and track objects in still and moving images. The computer vision and interpretation of radiology images by radiologists seemed to offer a considerable overlap of technical tools and applications of those tools dealing with images.

The concept of CAD research in radiology imaging has evolved into two distinct clinical applications; computer-aided diagnosis (CADx) and computer-aided detection (CADe) (Geiger *et al.*, 2008). CADx means the computer provides a diagnosis for physician review as needed. On the other hand, CADe means the computer highlights the area of concern (i.e., cancer) for further diagnostic evaluation without providing a diagnosis. For example, the CADe screens lung cancer or breast cancer for the asymptomatic but higher-risk population. The patients will undergo additional precision diagnostic studies if cancer is suspected from the screening study. The CADe as a detection algorithm to identify abnormality is based mainly on segmentation, pattern recognition, normal structure identification, and feature analysis. CADx as a classification algorithm to categorize disease severity or prognosis would focus on image pattern recognition, feature differences, as well as patient information. In many situations, particular low-resolution image of a single modality or even high-resolution image does not possess sufficient information to develop a clinically viable CADx algorithm.

Additionally, the radiological computer aided triage and notification (CADt) software is intended to aid in prioritization and triage of radiological medical images. It notifies a designated list of clinicians of the availability of time sensitive radiological medical images for review based on computer aided image analysis. Marking, highlighting, or directing users' attention to a specific location in the original image may not be provided by a CADt. It should be noted that FDA recently classified CADt as class II software.

A family of CAD tools that propelled the dramatic increase in interest and imaging AI investments is computer-assisted screening mammography. The government's interests in women's health in the 1990s created a massive demand for breast cancer screening and the need to read a large number of screening mammograms. As a result, the US government allowed a higher reimbursement rate for AI for computer-assisted screening mammography than conventional mammography to improve clinical service capacity and the quality of screening services. This financial incentive associated with CADe increased clinical adoption of CADe tools throughout the US. The success of AI in screening mammography excited the AI research community and spurred the research and development of many new AI products for radiology. In the public press, some speculated that robots would soon replace radiologists.

However, a major study involving 271 radiologists and 323,973 women between Jan 2003 and Dec 2009 compared reading mammograms with and without CADe. The study concluded that CADe does not improve diagnostic accuracy in mammography. It increased false positives (Lehman *et al.*, 2015). A more recent study by Schaffter and colleagues conducted a crowd-sourced trial on the use of deep learning in digital mammography involving 300,000 mammograms from the US and Sweden. The project had 126 teams from 44 countries to see if AI could meet or beat the radiologists' performances. They concluded that AI tools again did not perform better than radiologists without AI tools (Schaffter *et al.*, 2020).

One successful AI application in radiology is lung cancer screening. With the use of CADe for low-dose CT images for lung cancer screening, the sensitivity can be improved, and at the same time, the radiologist's reading speed can be improved by 30% (Lo *et al.*, 2018). In lung cancer screening CT, AI tools can reduce the blood vessel interference with potential lung nodules and improve the interpretation speed. This significant productivity improvement is a considerable incentive for clinical use.

After more than a decade of intense research and development in AI in radiology and the availability of more than 100 FDA-approved imaging AI products, the clinical adoption of these tools has been slow (Tadavarthi *et al.*, 2020). AI, in general, has not made any significant impacts on radiology despite having a massive digital infrastructure. As a result, some in the radiology community see the current situation as AI "winter," similar to that the greater machine vision community has experienced over the past 50 years, as shown in Fig. 1.

It is improbable that additional reimbursements will be allowed for the use of AI tools in radiology; thus, the productivity improvements, as in the case of lung cancer screening and cost savings, may become drivers for the clinical adoption of AI tools. There are many opportunities for AI to optimize and automate the workflow to improve overall productivity.

3.2. *Technical lesson learned from radiology AI*

The AI application in radiology has been the exclusive use of the supervised learning model mentioned in the early part of the chapter. However, several aspects of this process will need additional improvements.

3.2.1. *Limitations of CNNs*

The neural network as a part of the DL concept is based on the architecture of the multilayer perceptron. The convolution neural network (CNN) consists of a series of convolution layers equivalent to compositional convolution layers with a set of large kernels. A CNN acts as a feature learning model based on spatial features with multiple channels. They were initially developed for the recognition of alphanumerical handwriting. General image pattern recognition relies on essential graphic pattern features (e.g., edges), orientations, and size. However, medical image pattern recognition depends more on gray intensity distribution and size but not orientation (Lo *et al.*, 2018). The common difficulties in the traditional CNN approach for medical imaging can be grouped into three categories;

(i) inability to separate normal from ill-defined abnormal structures in the past;
(ii) inability to differentiate disease patterns, particularly in subtle cases from a broad spectrum of normal structures; and
(iii) inability to establish an integrated system between compositional and divide-and-conquer models.

Additional research and developments in the CNN community will be required to optimize CNN for medical imaging applications, especially CADx. The strength of CNN is to learn features automatically with millions of convolutions involving short and long regional pixels' correlation (tensor) as long as a sufficient number of samples is provided rather than limited number of defined formula. Radiomics is really a conventional approach as we have used in the field CAD.

3.2.2. *Data quality and pre-processing*

In any data science project, one can spend a significant effort to "clean" the data, and medicine is no exception. The data must be of sufficient quality and acquired with uniform parameters to validate conclusions. The image quality in patient care settings can vary depending on the time and day of imaging, image protocol, imaging system set up, patient conditions, and clinical practice standards in different departments. While human vision can adapt to reading through the images of varying qualities, AI tools generally cannot. One important task to produce a systematic image AI performance is image pre-processing, including image quality optimization, noise reduction, clutter removal, and enhancement of essential features for differentiation. In addition, there is an increasing number of AI tools to standardize image quality.

Thus, a radiology AI tool for screening or diagnosis of the disease consists of several components:

(i) pre-processing such as image normalization;
(ii) image segmentation or region of interest (ROI) extraction; and
(iii) potential disease pattern identification and classification.

Image segmentation is of particular interest when contrasting radiology and radiation oncology because the role of segmentation and identification in radiation oncology is far more prominent. For many radiology exams, segmentation is either not needed or is limited to measuring the size and shape of a tumor and may have little bearing on the final diagnosis. By contrast, segmentation in radiation oncology will usually involve several contiguous or overlapping organs and the treatment target, and these volumes are critically crucial for assessing the quality of the treatment plan.

3.2.3. *Data volume and data mix*

There are two data issues: access to a sufficient volume of data and enough data diversity representing a realistic case mix of the clinical, operational environment (Yamashita, 2018).

The imaging data requirement in radiology is relatively modest compared with non-medical applications, less than 10,000 cases per disease category. For example, in the case of the recent AI tool development for lung cancer screening with CT images, approximately 2,000 cases consisting of 300,000 CT images were sufficient for training. Around 300 cases of 45,000 images with about 20% subtle cases tested by more than ten radiologists were sufficient for an FDA-specified clinical trial (Lo *et al.*, 2018a). For different disease types and imaging modalities, these numbers would be different. If the clinical problem has many subtle features, the required data volume could be much higher.

Biases in AI can be thought of as a specific type of generalizability problem, although one which is more insidious because if the bias in an AI system matches the bias of human practitioners, it is effectively invisible because no one will notice. Moreover, because of the frequent need to draw upon human experts when labeling or interpreting image data, human biases can become enshrined into an AI system at a foundational level, making them very difficult to root out. The bias problem is further compounded by structural inequalities which affect access to healthcare.

3.2.4. *Expert labeling and curation*

In radiological imaging, the supervised learning approach is the most popular tool, and it requires labeled data for training and validation (Lo *et al.*, 2018a). Expert radiologists must do the labeling of images manually. This process is very labor-intensive and very costly. In addition, the truth panel for images is established by having 2 out of 3 radiologists agree on the diagnoses and clinical determinations. Non-experts cannot do this truth labeling.

3.3. *Lessons from poor clinical adoption of AI tools in radiology*

The radiology imaging community has been very active in developing computer-aided diagnosis (CAD) tools since the early 1990s, long before the imagination of artificial intelligence (AI) fueled many unbounded expectations in medicine and other industries. Today there are more than 100 FDA-approved AI imaging products in the US, but clinical adoption of these products has been very slow.

A number of hindering factors for AI implementation (Strohm, 2020) of traditional CAD were identified as follows:

- Inconsistent technical performance of AI algorithms (false positives and false negatives);
- Lack of planning and monitoring AI implementation;
- Lack of empirical evidence on the effect of AI application on the radiology workflow;
- Uncertain funding due to lack of evidence of benefits;
- Widely varying acceptance and trust;
- Legal and regulatory issues.

Traditional CAD efforts in radiology have narrowly focused on interpreting diagnoses by radiologists. However, diagnostic imaging services are

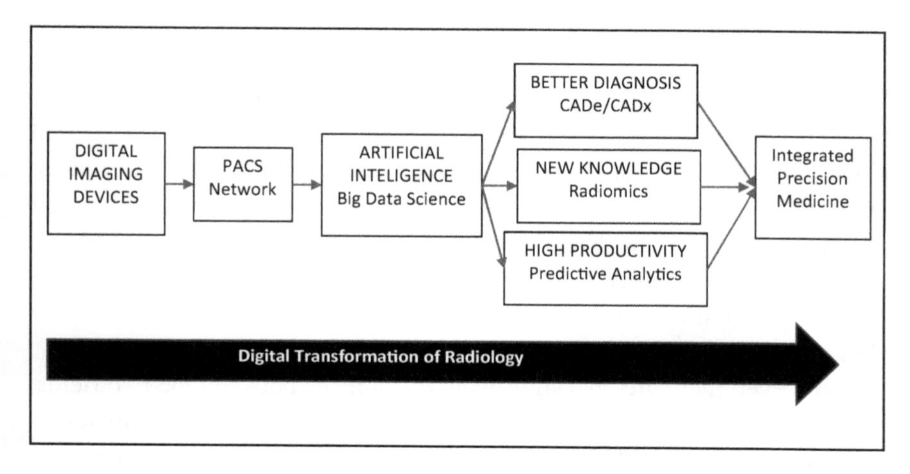

Fig. 3. Three potential pathways for AI adoption in Radiology services.

far more than just aiding interpretation of diagnoses by radiologists. One has to address issues in the entire workflow.

As mentioned earlier, AI is a set of powerful tools with multiple capabilities beyond pattern recognition. Current research in imaging AI has three parallel tracks, as shown in Fig. 3:

1. Next Generation CAD:
   Improving the technical performance of traditional CAD
2. Radiomics:
   Creating new knowledge through quantitative imaging, also known as radiomics
3. Productivity:
   Workflow optimization to improve overall productivity with predictive analytics

Though the CAD and radiomics are mentioned separately for historical reasons, the work in radiomics will improve the performance of CAD in the future. Therefore, the rest of the chapter will discuss radiomics for new knowledge creation and productivity, and workflow optimization will be addressed as two essential target areas for AI application for radiology and radiation oncology.

4. Comparing Radiology and Radiation Oncology

When considering applications of AI, it is helpful to draw some comparisons and contrasts between Radiation Oncology and Radiology. At first glance, the applications of AI in radiology and radiation oncology appear very similar. Both fields make extensive use of medical images as their primary source of data. Therefore, large image archives with rapid access to the data are essential. Expert labeling and curation are challenging to obtain because they require the work of highly trained individuals who are already very busy.

However, there are also significant differences between the two fields. Table 1 compares and contrasts the two fields along several parameters.

One significant difference relevant to the workflow for the department is the number of major devices during the patient care process. Generally, in radiology, we deal with a single imaging device per study. In radiation oncology, many major components have to work in concert. The following

Table 1: Comparison chart showing key differences between radiology and radiation oncology. These differences should inform and guide the development of AI algorithms in their respective fields.

Radiology	Radiation Oncology
Emphasis on detection and diagnosis	Emphasis on treatment and cure
Must recognize a very wide range of potential disease states	Relatively narrow range of disease states
Screening of asymptomatic patients is an important goal	Does not deal with asymptomatic patients
Patient encounters are typically short and require only one session	Patients may be treated over several days or weeks
Diagnostic imaging follows specific protocols with relatively low variation from patient to patient.	Treatment plans are highly individualized to a specific patient and may change during the course of treatment.
Simpler workflow with fewer personnel	Complex workflow involving many personnel
Image generation and interpretation are not typically dependent on computational optimization.	Lengthy history of using computational methods for treatment optimization

are the major components: treatment simulator, treatment planning system, verification system, treatment system, and information management system. During the course of treatment, some systems are used multiple times for the same patient. These enterprise related issues will be further discussed in the later section.

5. Quantitative Imaging; For New Insights

One area of shared research interest between radiology and radiation oncology is quantitative imaging, also known as radiomics (Kuhl & Truhn, 2020).

Quantitative imaging extracts features from radiological images that may or may not be visualized by radiologists. It intends to quantify the abnormality, the degree of severity, or the status of a disease relative to normal based on phenotype characteristics or tensor features in an automated high-throughput manner. A semi-automatic operation is necessary, particularly in the segmentation of region of interest. It has been hypothesized that such analysis may help prognosticate, predict treatment outcomes, and assess images of potential disease tissues including the malignancy or benignity of lesions.

The value of AI in radiomics is two-fold.

First, AI can be used for automated image analysis at scale, enabling rapid evaluation of hypothetical radiomic features. Whereas comparison studies involving human radiologists should take into account a wide range of ergonomic and perception factors (such as the required number of readers or the need to provide time between different readings of the same image), a comparison of radiomics algorithms is only limited by computational speed and power. Similarly, new features can easily be tested against existing data sets.

Second, unsupervised learning methods can be used to search for new radiomic features that might be very different from what would be noticed by a human observer. In essence, AI can take on the role of discovery and extract new and valuable patterns within existing data.

Radiomics offers the appeal of objective analysis and the ability to detect features or qualities in the image that would either be too subtle for a human observer or too difficult/time-consuming to compute without assistance. But only a few approaches in this regard have some breakthroughs so far. The current issue of the quantitative imaging approach is that it is still unable to fully recognize patterns/features identified by expert observers, particularly when the image contains substantial clutters or structure or non-structure noises.

Out of many technical issues, to make radiomics effective and scalable, there is an urgent need to standardize factors in processes involved in the quantitative analysis. The Image Biomarker Standardization Initiative (IBSI) (IBSI, 2022) is a new organization to address many challenges in the following areas:

- standard nomenclature and common radiomic features,
- radiomics image processing schemes,
- provide data sets for validation and calibration, and
- set of reporting guidelines.

This group defined 174 radiomics features commonly used to quantify the morphologic characteristics, and numerous others needed to determine the quantitative information clearly. In addition, the group is trying to standardize the image processing steps of data conversion, post-acquisition processing, segmentation, interpolation, masking, etc. It is expected that such standardization will eventually make radiomics clinically useful and scalable for imaging application for radiology, and radiation oncology.

Radiomics can offer non-invasive diagnoses by exploring more refined imaging properties such as tumor heterogeneity and biological characteristics of a tumor (Vaugier *et al.*, 2020).

6. Productivity Improvement and Workflow Optimization

Much of the AI effort in radiology has focused on diagnostic decision support. However, potential applications of AI in radiology beyond image

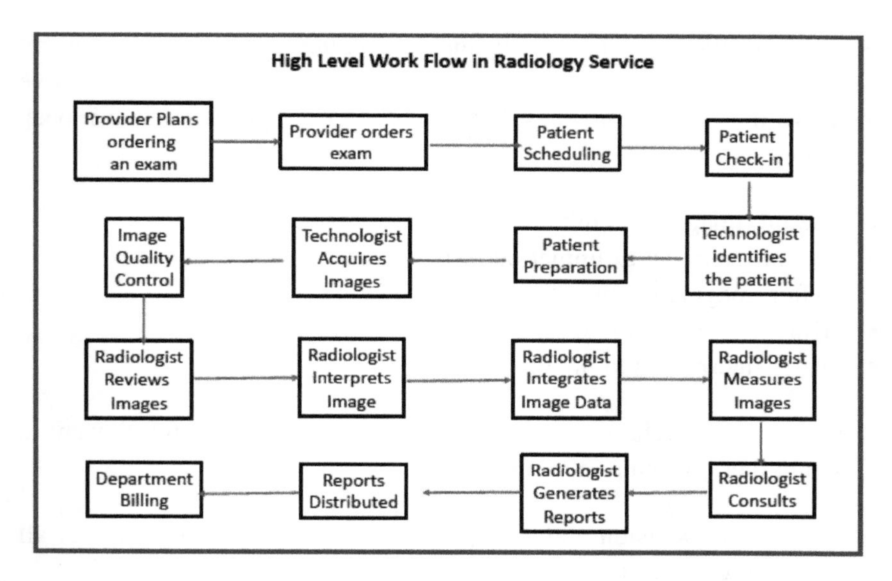

Fig. 4. A typical series of activities in a Radiology service workflow.

analysis and classification can become increasingly more important from the perspective of entire radiology and radiation oncology operations involving radiologists, therapists, technologists, managers, referring physicians, and patients. Figure 4 shows a typical radiology workflow conducting activities from ordering images to billing.

Radiology service is changing from the traditional concept of "reading images" to creating, organizing, and conveying relevant information with greater accuracy, faster speed, and lower cost. The department-wide issues and end-to-end productivity should be a problem-rich environment for AI innovations.

Most of the AI work in radiology has been primarily focused on radiologists' efforts in establishing diagnoses, which is only a small portion of the entire workflow of the department. There are many segmented components where information flows from one sub-system to the next and the next. Productivity improvement is rarely a popular area of academic research. The research literature on the issues dealing with operational efficiency and productivity in imaging services is limited compared with research topics on diagnosis and cure of diseases. However, from the AI perspective, there are increasing interests (Choy *et al.*, 2018) in using AI to improve the workflow (Letourneau *et al.*, 2020). The following five areas with multiple subareas for potential AI applications have been identified:

- Before imaging examination or procedures;
- During imaging examination or procedures;
- After imaging examination or procedures;
- During interpretation;
- After interpretation, including billing.

A recent article (Huynh, 2020) proposed the use of AI for the entire radiation therapy chain in six parts:

- Treatment Decision with decision support tools for integration of all relevant clinical information;
- Simulation to optimize dose efficiency with improved image quality;
- Treatment planning with automated segmentation and optimal dose prediction;
- Plan approval and QA that can detect errors and time saving for approval and QA;
- Radiotherapy delivery with enhanced image guidance, motion management, clinical efficacy, and patient outcomes;
- Follow up care with a more accurate prediction of response and adverse effect management.

The changes in reimbursement models and emphasis on the quality of care will be a strong driver to optimization of workflow and improvement of productivity, which will be a rich area of AI application in radiation oncology in the near future. There are several shortcomings and discrepancies in Medicare's current fee-for-service payment model for radiation oncology service. They include different payment systems, known as site-of-service payment differential, based on the therapy delivery settings, free-standing therapy centers versus hospital outpatient departments. At the same time, the current fee-for-service payment system encourages volume of service over the values of service, which may discourage the adoption of some evidence-based practices such as hypofractionation based on modern technology. The Center for Medical Service began to develop an alternative payment model to address these shortcomings (Meeks *et al.*, 2021). The proposed episode-based payment system is prospective, site-neutral, and modality agnostic, resulting in high-value radiation therapy care. Some fear that this new model could result in a reduction in reimbursement.

As the debate for a new payment model intensifies, the productivity of the radiation oncology service will emerge, becoming an essential issue in managing the practice of radiation oncology. A recent survey reported the survey results on staffing, productivity, revenue, and expenses as well as a salary survey of 27 oncology-specific positions (Bourbeau *et al.*, 2020). This report offers an initial framework of looking at the productivity of radiation oncology at the systems level. Changes in payment model coupled with advances in science and technology for radiation oncology will form a rich data source for successful AI applications. Needless to say, successful AI application will require a sufficient volume of high-quality data from multiple data points in the chain of radiation oncology.

7. Integration of AI Tools into Workflow and New Intelligence Management System (IMS)

Workflow improvements will involve many systems and components throughout the radiology department. They could include hospital information system, electronic health records, imaging devices, radiology information system, radiology workstations, billing and collection system, staffing system, radiology reporting system, and, indeed, PACS, to name a few.

Eventually, there can be many specific AI tools for specific disease types. Integration of these AI tools matched with disease cases and radiologists would require massive integration work involving multiple vendors. It might be prudent to start with PACS, which manages the bulk of workflow and work distribution to reading stations.

Systems integration of many innovative AI solutions in radiation oncology is expected to be much more challenging than in radiology. As mentioned earlier, the radiation therapy process involves many more subsystems, and some are used multiple times for the same patients during the course of therapy. In radiology, PACS has been used as system-wide workflow optimization tool. However, today's PACS is a centralized architecture of past generations. In order to integrate AI tools to many different parts of the workflow chain, we will need a distributed intelligence management system (IMS) with similar functionalities to edge computing or internet of things (IOT). This evolution of digital transformation in radiology will require collaboration between academia for better tools and industry for a new IT platform for intelligence management. Radiation oncology, where the workflow is more complex compared with radiology, will also need a new IT platform to manage intelligence for the entire service chain.

8. Ten Principles for Good Machine Learning Practice

The imaging community has accumulated a significant amount of AI research and development knowledge (Larson, 2021). The US Food and Drug Administration (FDA), Health Canada, and the United Kingdom's Medicine and Healthcare Products Regulatory Agency (MHRA) have jointly identified ten guiding principles that can inform the development of Good Machine Learning Practice (GMLP) (FDA, 2021). These guiding principles aim to help develop safe, effective, and high-quality products that use artificial intelligence and machine learning (AI/ML) technologies. The principles have not been operationalized as regulations yet. However, they represent the accumulated lessons on evaluation of AI/ML products over 20 years. They also offer a roadmap for developing and testing AI/ML products in the future. The 10-point principles are:

1. Multi-Disciplinary Expertise Is Leveraged Throughout the Total Product Life Cycle.
2. Good Software Engineering and Security Practices Are Implemented.
3. Clinical Study Participants and Data Sets Are Representative of the Intended Patient Population.
4. Training Data Sets Are Independent of Test Sets.

5. Selected Reference Data sets Are Based Upon Best Available Methods.
6. Model Design Is Tailored to the Available Data and Reflects the Intended Use of the Device.
7. Focus Is Placed on the Performance of the Human–AI Team.
8. Testing Demonstrates Device Performance During Clinically Relevant Conditions.
9. Users Are Provided Clear, Essential Information.
10. Deployed Models Are Monitored for Performance and Re-training Risks Are Managed.

These principles will evolve into a powerful and effective roadmap in developing clinically acceptable AI products for radiology and radiation oncology.

9. Conclusion

The radiology and radiation oncology workload is increasing, and technology is getting more sophisticated. Precision medicine demands higher accuracy and better outcome. Both services will be expected to do more with less. At the same time, there is a constant pressure of limiting reimbursement. Therefore, using AI tools, productivity improvement will become a core function of digital transformation.

The major lessons from radiology can be summarized as follows:

- Think productivity. The AI offers powerful predictive analytics to improve the productivity of the entire clinical operation.
- Think quantitative imaging. The use of radiomics offers new insights into cancer that can contribute to precision medicine.
- Plan for new digital imaging platforms for integrated AI tools.

Acknowledgments

The authors thank Coleman Rosen, MS, and Shijir Bayarsaikhan, MS, for their valuable suggestions in developing this chapter. Appreciation is also due to Fred Prior, PhD, for internal critical review of the manuscript.

References

Bourbeau, B., Harter, D., & Towle, E. (2020). Results from the ASCO 2019 survey of oncology practice operations. *JCO Oncology Practice, 16*(5), 253–262. https://doi.org/10.1200/OP.20.00009.

Choy, G., Khalilzadeh, O., Michalski, M., Do, S., Samir, A. E., Pianykh, O. S., Geis, J. R., Pandharipande, P. V., Brink, J. A., & Dreyer, K. J. (2018). Current applications and future impact of machine learning in radiology. *Radiology, 288*(2), 318–328. https://doi.org/10.1148/radiol.2018171820.

Doi, K. (2007). Computer-aided diagnosis in medical imaging: Historical review, current status and future potential. *Computerized Medical Imaging and Graphics: The Official Journal of the Computerized Medical Imaging Society, 31*(4-5), 198–211. https://doi.org/10.1016/j.compmedimag.2007.02.002.

Food and Drug Administration (FDA) USA, Center for Devices and Radiological Health. (2021). Good machine learning practice for medical device development. Retrieved February 1, 2022, from https://www.fda.gov/medical-devices/software-medical-device-samd/good-machine-learning-practice-medical-device-development guiding-principles

Geiger, M. L., Chan, H. P., & Boone, J. (2008). Anniversary paper: History and status of CAD and quantitative image analysis: the role of Medical Physics and AAPM. *Medical Physics, 35*(12), 5799–5820. https://doi.org/10.1118/1.3013555.

Huynh, E., Hosny, A., Guthier, C., Bitterman, D. S., Petit, S. F., Haas-Kogan, D. A., Kann, B., Aerts, H., & Mak, R. H. (2020). Artificial intelligence in radiation oncology. *Nature Reviews. Clinical Oncology, 17*(12), 771–781. https://doi.org/10.1038/s41571-020-0417-8.

IBSI. (2022). https://theibsi.github.io.

Kaul, V., Enslin, S., & Gross, S. (2020). The history of artificial intelligence in medicine. *Gastrointestinal Endoscopy, 92*(4). https://doi.org/10.1016/j.gie.2020.06.040.

Kuhl, C. K. & Truhn, D. (2020). The long route to standardized radiomics: Unraveling the knot from the end. *Radiology, 295*(2), 339–341. https://doi.org/10.1148/radiol.2020200059.

Larson, D. B., Harvey, H., Rubin, D. L., Irani, N., Tse, J. R., & Langlotz, C. P. (2021). Regulatory Frameworks for Development and Evaluation of Artificial Intelligence-Based Diagnostic Imaging Algorithms: Summary and Recommendations. *Journal of the American College of Radiology, 18*(3A), 413 -424. https://doi.org/10.1016/j.jacr.2020.09.060

Lehman, C. D., Wellman, R. D., Buist, D. S., Kerlikowske, K., Tosteson, A. N., Miglioretti, D. L., *et al.* (2015). Diagnostic accuracy of digital screening mammography with and without computer-aided detection. *JAMA Internal Medicine, 175*(11), 1828–1837. https://doi.org/10.1001/jamainternmed.2015.5231.

Lo, S. B., Chan, H.-P., Lin, J.-S., Li, H., Freedman, M. T., & Mun, S. K. (1995). Artificial convolution neural network for medical image pattern recognition. *Neural Networks, 8*(7–8), 1201–1214. https://doi.org/10.1016/0893-6080(95)00061-5.

Lo, S. B., Freedman, M. T., Gillis, L. B., White, C. S., & Mun, S. K. (2018a). JOURNAL CLUB: Computer-aided detection of lung nodules on CT with a computerized pulmonary vessel suppressed function. *American Journal of Roentgenology,* 210(3), 480–488. https://doi.org/10.2214/AJR.17.18718.

Lo, S. B., Freedman, M. T., & Mun, S. K. (2018b). Transformationally identical and invariant convolutional neural networks by combining symmetric operations or input vectors. *arXiv preprint arXiv:1807.11156.*

Letourneau-Guillon, L., Camirand, D., Guilbert, F., & Forghani, R. (2020). Artificial Intelligence applications for workflow, process optimization and predictive analytics. *Neuroimaging Clinics of North America, 30*(4), e1–e15. https://doi.org/10.1016/j.nic.2020.08.008.

McCullouch, W. & Pitts, W. (1943). A logical calculus of the indeas immanent in nervous activity. *Bulletin of Matherical Biophysics*, *5*(1943), P. 115–139.

Meeks, S. L., Mathews, R., Mojica, J., Shah, A. P., Kelly, P., & Dvorak, T. (2021). Impact of radiation oncology alternative payment model on community cancer centers. *JCO Oncology Practice*, *17*(12), e1949–e1957. https://doi.org/10.1200/OP.21.00298.

Mun, S. K., Prior, F., Caramella, D., & Ratib, O. (2007). Guest editorial introduction to the special section on image management in the healthcare enterprise. *IEEE Transactions on Information Technology in Biomedicine, 11*(1), 1–6.

Mun, S. K., Freedman, M., & Kapur, R. (1993). Image management and communications for radiology. *IEEE Engineering in Medicine and Biology Magazine, 12*(1), 70–80.

Schaffter, T., Buist, D. S. M., Lee, C. I., Nikulin, Y., Ribli, D., Guan, Y., *et al.* (2020). Evaluation of combined artificial intelligence and radiologist assessment to interpret screening mammograms. *JAMA Netw Open, 3*(3), e200265. https://doi.org/10.1001/jamanetworkopen.2020.0265.

Strohm, L., Hehakaya, C., Ranschaert, E.R. et al. (2020). Implementation of artificial intelligence (AI) applications in radiology: hindering and facilitating factors. *European Radiology 30*, 5525–5532 (2020). https://doi.org/10.1007/s00330-020-06946-y

Tadavarthi, Y., Vey, B., Krupinski, E., Prater, A., Gichoya, J., Safdar, N., *et al.* (2020). The state of radiology AI: Considerations for purchase decisions and current market offerings. *Radiology: Artificial Intelligence, 2*(6), e200004.

Vaugier, L., Ferrer, L., Mengue, L., & Jouglar, E. (2020). Radiomics for radiation oncologists: Are we ready to go? *BJR Open*, *2*(1), 20190046. https://doi.org/10.1259/bjro.20190046.

West, D. and Allen J. How artificial intelligence is transforming the world, Brooking Report, April 24, 2018. https://www.brookings.edu/research/how-artificial-intelligence-is-transforming-the-world//.

Yamashita, R., Nishio, M., Do, R.K.G. et al. (2018). Convolutional neural networks: an overview and application in radiology. *Insights Imaging 9*, 611–629. https://doi.org/10.1007/s13244-018-0639-9.

Chapter 4

Open Access Data to Enable AI Applications in Radiation Therapy

Fred Prior and William Bennett

Department of Biomedical Informatics, University of Arkansas for Medical Sciences, Little Rock AR, USA

Abstract

Training, testing, and validation of AI algorithms applied to enhance radiation therapy require large quantities of high-quality, well-curated, and labeled data. For algorithms to generalize they must train on a representative sample of the human population including both the varying presentations of the target disease and healthy controls. What constitutes labeled data depends on the research question being addressed. Thus, AI applications differ in their definition of and requirements for labeled data. This adds complexity to curation, data management, and query or semantic search requirements imposed on data repositories that attempt to make such data widely available.

Open-access data repositories that support the FAIR and TRUST principles provide the types of high-quality data required for AI applications and are essential for the rapid advancement of the field. Open access is hampered by international privacy regulation differences, e.g., HIPAA vs. GDPR and intellectual property and regulatory requirements that force data sequestration. Approaches based on distributed machine learning where the data is not shared are being developed as an alternative. Consistent data quality assurance and curation must still be employed.

The bulk of Radiation Therapy data are collected and communicated according to the DICOM standard, which also provides profiles for proper de-identification of this data for research use and open reuse. Acquisition, quality assurance, de-identification, and curation tools based on DICOM are key to the success of open data repositories as well as distributed machine learning approaches which combine data from multiple repositories since in all cases reusable, well-documented data are required.

1. Introduction

Radiation oncology is an integral component of cancer care with nearly 70% of all cancer patients being treated with radiation therapy as part of the management of their disease. Modern radiation therapy is planned using multiple image data sets and radiation therapy planning platforms that construct treatment plans to meet target dose limitations for both tumor and normal tissue volumes. Thus, both targeting, and outcome assessment are fully image driven and pre-therapy and outcome images provide invaluable information required for the application to AI techniques to improve patient care.

The quality of care will be greatly improved with the continued growth and development of both validated databases and tools for analysis. The databases need to be comprehensive and house patient-specific information with respect to pre-therapy outcome, anatomic and metabolic images to support target definition, and outcome images to support evaluation of treatment efficacy and normal tissue function. Tools to provide segmental analysis of normal tissue and apply them to dose volume analysis will greatly improve and optimize patient care. For example, cardiac structures are an indirect and unintentional target of radiation therapy for thoracic and upper abdominal malignancies. Correlating normal tissue segmental dose with outcome will require tool development with artificial intelligence platforms to provide contours to cardiac subsegments and correlate the dose volume to outcome. Often injury is identified through indirect mechanisms.

There is a growing need to optimize definitions of tumor dose and normal tissue tolerance in the era of targeted radiotherapies and immuno-oncology. Improved understanding of the dose required for tumor control and dose volume kinetics associated with normal tissue damage will greatly improve patient care. Increasingly these questions are being studied with advanced AI techniques, which require complex radiation therapy data sets for model development, testing, and validation.

2. AI in Radiation Therapy and Cancer Imaging

Machine learning (ML) has a relatively long history in quantitative image analysis beginning with early work in Computer Aided Detection and Diagnosis (Doi, 2007; Giger *et al.*, 2008; Sahiner *et al.*, 2019) in the 1990s. Although benefiting for advancements in ML-based segmentation, large-scale extension of these tools into Radiation Therapy (RT) began more recently (Sahiner *et al.*, 2019; Thompson *et al.*, 2018). Advanced ML techniques are rapidly gaining traction in most aspects of RT, including treatment planning, segmentation and auto-contouring, quality assurance, clinical decision support and adaptive therapy (Huynh *et al.*, 2020; Kiser *et al.*, 2019; Thompson *et al.*, 2018; Wang *et al.*, 2019). In all these areas of active ML research, a key limitation is the availability of data.

The accuracy of AI model outputs depends on the quality and quantity of data used for training. It is usually the training data rather than the details of the models that have the greatest impact on accuracy and generalizability (Kiser *et al.*, 2019). Data must be of sufficient quality and acquired with consistent parameters to be usable for training and validation of supervised ML models. For trained models to generalize, the data must appropriately represent the variance in the human population, the presentation of the target disease, therapy systems, protocols and treatment plans, and imaging systems and imaging protocols (Prior *et al.*, 2020). Much of the existing literature is based on data that do not accurately represent the human population due to limited geographic diversity and the lack of healthy controls.

Accumulating data on a sufficiently large scale poses a significant challenge. Two approaches exist for meeting this challenge: open access data repositories and distributed or federated machine learning.

3. Open Access Data Repositories

Vincente-Saez and Martinez-Fuentes define open science as "transparent and accessible knowledge that is shared and developed through collaborative networks" (Vicente-Saez & Martinez-Fuentes, 2018). A key component of open science is open access to data and analysis results that enable the creation of research communities and enhance research reproducibility (F. W. Prior, 2013). To be useful, open access repositories must comply with the FAIR principles for data management and stewardship to make data findable, accessible, interoperable, and reusable (Jacobsen *et al.*, 2020; Wilkinson *et al.*, 2016). To actually develop a research community, a repository must be reliable and sustainable, factors included in the TRUST principles for digital repositories: Transparency, Responsibility, User focus, Sustainability, and Technology (Lin *et al.*, 2020).

The National Cancer Institute (NCI) has been a historical leader in making DICOM images available for public use to support research and education. Since 2011, the Cancer Imaging Archive (TCIA) has supported open science and cancer research by acquiring, curating, hosting, and distributing collections of multi-modal information (Kenneth Clark *et al.*, 2013; Prior *et al.*, 2020, 2017; Prior, 2013). TCIA supports FAIR and TRUST compliant access to a growing number of radiation therapy data collections (23 collections comprising data from 4,284 research participants) derived from completed clinical trials and research projects. Unfortunately, existing repositories, including TCIA, tend to focus on data from patient populations but not healthy controls, and no single repository represents sufficient geographic diversity.

While a growing number of open access cancer image repositories have been deployed, particularly in the United States (Fedorov *et al.*, 2021; Giger, 2021; Grossberg *et al.*, 2018; Prior *et al.*, 2020), patient privacy concerns have led to restrictive regulatory environments, particularly in Europe (Minssen *et al.*, 2020). Such concerns have given rise to increased interest in distributed or federated approaches to machine learning that allow data to remain in the control of the institution that created it.

4. Distributed ML Without Data Sharing

US human subjects' regulations require patient consent to share data (Menikoff *et al.*, 2017). Patient privacy regulations require data to be used for research to be de-identified prior to leaving the covered entity that created them (Freymann *et al.*, 2012). The European Union expanded patient privacy rights with the creation of the General Data Protection Regulation (GDPR) (Minssen *et al.*, 2020) and in so doing made sharing of data related to a European person difficult or impossible to share for research purposes. Unlike the US privacy regulation Health Insurance Portability and Accountability Act (HIPAA) there is no standard for anonymization in GDPR and a requirement that a person can opt out of permitting the use of their data at any time. Such data privacy concerns have placed a premium on the use of analytic techniques that are applied at each data origination site (i.e., hospital or clinic) with only the parameter derived from that analysis being shared.

Distributed machine learning frameworks send the analysis software to the data and thus do not require data sharing (Field *et al.*, 2021). A variety of training techniques have been developed that either use a central service to collect and merge the parameters of the model based on training at each site, or pass the parameters from one site to the next such that the model accumulates what it learns from each site's data (Chang *et al.*, 2018). While these techniques have been successfully applied in a number of Radiation Therapy research applications, (e.g., Field *et al.*, 2021; Lustberg *et al.*, 2017), they suffer from two critical problems. The approach assumes consistent data quality and curation processes have been applied at each site and that each participating institution has appropriate computing resources to run the software. The lack of consistent curation and quality assurance processes have the greatest impact as they lead to greater variance in the training data.

5. Acquisition, Curation, and Quality

Information quality is defined by Talburt (2011) as creating value in the use of the data and meeting the user's requirements. While common quality measures can be extracted (e.g., MRQy (Sadri *et al.*, 2020)), image quality is difficult to generalize as it depends on the ever evolving and diverse needs of the user community and the rapid advance of cancer research. A base set of quality measures, nevertheless, can be identified:

(1) Completeness — minimize missing data elements and capture the full data set that represents a collection;
(2) Correctness — the data are in a standard format and syntactically correct relative to that standard;
(3) Artifact free — the existence and relative severity of image artifacts have been established, and low-quality data eliminated;
(4) Fit for use — quality metrics provided for a particular use case.

The data from clinical trials have typically undergone some type of quality assessment by a clinical trial QA office as part of data collection. The process varies by trial, but generally addresses basic data quality, image segmentation (and registration, if applicable), and dosimetric plan evaluation. Historically, QA of segmentation (contouring) has been performed by human experts (mostly physicians), but increasingly automated segmentation methods are being used for this purpose. The result of the assessment is sometimes reported as a score indicating that a particular subject's data are (a) per protocol, (b) acceptable variation, or (c) deviation from protocol.

Data that are captured for most clinical trials and patient registries may not fully reflect the dose delivered to the patient. The information about the actual delivery of treatments is often acquired by manual transcription from an oncology information system/treatment management system to case report forms. This is especially challenging in adaptive RT treatments, where multiple treatment plans are used. This leads to a significant quality problem: which plans were used, and which doses were delivered to the patient? There are always cases that fall outside of the treatment protocol and the ability to detect those would have value.

To accomplish this would require new tools for automatic scoring by evaluating dosimetric criteria with respect to protocol requirements (Kalet *et al.*, 2020).

DICOM is the international standard (ISO 12052:2017) for the exchange of digital images and related information (DICOM, 2022). Treatment planning data are exported as DICOM objects, in the form of CT Images, RT Structure Sets, RT Plans, and RT Doses, from a treatment planning system. The DICOM RT Treatment Record is ground truth for how a patient was treated, however, the information it contains is not generally available in a structured form from clinical trials.

Before data can be exported from a data origination site, the data are required to be de-identified (anonymized) in accordance with one of the two mechanisms specified in the HIPAA regulations. De-identification is a balance between data utility and patient privacy. DICOM Standard PS3.15 2016a — Security and System Management Profiles (DICOM, 2016) defines how to correctly de-identify DICOM objects. It contains confidentiality profiles and options that can be used to amend the profile for specific applications.

Data de-identification, completeness, and correctness have been the guiding principles of TCIA data curation for the past decade. In this time, the open-source Posda tools have supported a scalable workflow, based on the DICOM standard, for curation of DICOM objects prior to publication on TCIA (Bennett *et al.*, 2018). The TCIA process consists of multiple automated and manual steps to ensure the integrity of publicly available data without protected health information/personal identification information (PHI/PII) while preserving scientifically relevant data associated with the images. The TCIA curation team verifies completeness of the received collection, full removal of all PHI, proper labeling of all information to facilitate retrieval, and proper linkages among components of the collection (Bennett *et al.*, 2018; Clark, 2013; Moore *et al.*, 2015).

The Posda tools suite was originally developed to support RT data acquisition and QA (Bennett *et al.*, 2010), and Posda capabilities for acquisition and curation of RT data have continuously evolved to meet the needs of the cancer research community served by TCIA. Currently, Posda tools in combination with TCIA curation procedures support:

- De-identification.
- DICOM conformance verification,
- Data integrity checks of the completeness and consistency of RT data sets,
- Referential integrity of inter-object linkages, particularly for RT data,
- Spatial registration in multiple frames of reference,
- Calculation of dose-volume histograms.

While not a complete package for RT data de-identification, curation, and QA, Posda provides a standards-based, best-practices solution that is applicable both for data publication and use in clinical trials (e.g., Bekelman *et al.*, 2019).

6. Annotations and Labeled Data

Radiologists have used image annotation and markup (Channin *et al.*, 2010) to highlight significant features in an image since the introduction of picture archive and communication systems and digital imaging workstations. Supervised machine learning algorithms are trained and tested on data sets that have been augmented to contain a label or tag that identifies the class to which each datum belongs. These labels can be derived from image annotations, or they may come from a variety of other sources (Bera *et al.*, 2021; Willemink *et al.*, 2020).

Labels depend on the research question being addressed by the ML algorithm. Thus, an appropriate label may be a binary outcome (cancer/no cancer), a lesion location (bounding box), a lesion segmentation, or a complex combination of clinical parameters, pathology results, and image annotations. In some cases, the needed label for a new study might be the result of a previous radiomics or segmentation analysis.

Labeled data are created manually by human experts resulting in high cost and limited volume of high-quality training (and testing) data sets. Crowdsourcing can be used to both expand the pool of annotators and generate error estimates (Prior *et al.*, 2020). Because labeled data are both complex and expensive to produce, they need to be shared. While adherence to the FAIR principle is now common practice for images, associated labels are not always easily found or accessed.

7. Remaining Challenges

The changing international regulatory environment poses a major challenge for global data sharing to create open access data repositories that reflect the variance in the human population and in target diseases. Even when local and national repositories are created, the tools for querying across repositories in a manner that accounts for the differing regulatory requirements are largely missing. Cross-linkage and semantic integration of radiology/pathology/clinical/omics data on a sufficiently large scale is essential for addressing the needs of advanced AI applications. Such cross-linkage greatly exacerbates the problem of protecting patient privacy (Prosperi *et al.*, 2018).

There is a growing body of literature demonstrating that 3-Dimensional (3D) reconstructions of human faces rendered from MRI and CT images are equivalent to photographs for identifying the human being who was imaged (Prior *et al.*, 2008; Schwarz *et al.*, 2019). The advent of free software for 3D reconstruction and facial recognition coupled with the huge corpus of photographs available on the internet has made this a unique privacy issue. Image defacing algorithms that preserve essential scientific data without distortion exist in MRI-based neuroimaging (e.g., (Schwarz *et al.*, 2021)), but these do not generalize to other imaging modalities used in cancer diagnosis and therapy. For head/neck cancers, or radiation therapy planning, it is not possible with existing approaches to distort or hide the patient's face without destroying the scientific value of the data.

Standards and standard operating processes for data representation, curation, evaluation, and sharing of labeled data sets are in early stages of development. Mechanisms for identifying labeled data across repositories or determining which of several available annotations are best for a specific problem are largely non-existent. These limitations severely constrain our ability to create truly generalizable AI applications.

In RT, the relationship between Structured Reports, Segmentations, Presentations States, Key Value Objects, and Associated Image Sets are very complex. These relationships are not normally captured as part of standard clinical or research workflows. Presenting the relationships among these objects for rapid review by curators is a significant technical challenge. There is a fundamental difference between the kinds of visualization tools required for data curation versus the kinds of visualization required in clinical practice. Curation tools require simple, holistic visualizations of the full set of data either by patient or collection. These views have minimal controls for varying the presentation but allow a curator to easily separate those data which may require detailed attention from those which are good.

While there are an increasing number of anonymization tools for images and RT data (Robinson, 2014), data and procedures for validating that such tools meet regulatory requirements are still in development (Rutherford *et al.*, 2021). Approaches for automating the anonymization process, which today contains manual review to achieve a close approximation to zero defects required for regulatory compliance, are largely lacking. Similarly lacking are tools for data submitters to acquire, integrate, and properly anonymize clinical data, annotations, and other forms of labeled data. Quality standards and tools for measuring quality of annotations, labels, and image derived features are slowly evolving as are tools and standards for image quality.

8. Conclusions

Machine learning-based algorithms to enhance radiation therapy require large quantities of high-quality and associated data labels or tags for training and testing. For algorithms to generalize, they must train on a representative sample of the human population including both the varying presentations of the target disease and healthy controls. Open access information repositories and distributed machine learning approaches are attempting to address this problem but face substantial obstacles related to differing privacy regulations and tools for assuring consistent data quality. Acquisition, quality assurance, de-identification, and curation tools based on DICOM are key to the success of machine learning approaches as they facilitate data reuse and combining data from multiple sources.

References

Bekelman, J. E., Lu, H., Pugh, S., Baker, K., Berg, C. D., De Gonzalez, A. B., Braunstein, L. Z., Bosch, W., Chauhan, C., & Ellenberg, S. (2019). Pragmatic randomized clinical trial of proton versus photon therapy for patients with non-metastatic breast cancer: The Radiotherapy Comparative Effectiveness (RadComp) Consortium trial protocol. *BMJ Open*, *9*(10), e025556.

Bennett, W., Matthews, J., & Bosch, W. (2010). SU-GG-T-262: Open-source tool for assessing variability in DICOM data. *Medical Physics*, *37*(6Part19), 3245.

Bennett, W., Smith, K., Jarosz, Q., Nolan, T., & Bosch, W. (2018). Reengineering workflow for curation of DICOM datasets. *Journal of Digital Imaging*, *31*(6), 783–791.

Bera, K., Braman, N., Gupta, A., Velcheti, V., & Madabhushi, A. (2022). Predicting cancer outcomes with radiomics and artificial intelligence in radiology. *Nature Reviews Clinical Oncology*, *19*(2), 132–146.

Chang, K., Balachandar, N., Lam, C., Yi, D., Brown, J., Beers, A., Rosen, B., Rubin, D. L., & Kalpathy-Cramer, J. (2018). Distributed deep learning networks among institutions for medical imaging. *Journal of the American Medical Informatics Association*, *25*(8), 945–954. https://doi.org/10.1093/jamia/ocy017.

Channin, D. S., Mongkolwat, P., Kleper, V., Sepukar, K., & Rubin, D. L. (2010). The caBIG™ annotation and image markup project. *Journal of Digital Imaging*, *23*(2), 217–225.

Clark, K., Vendt, B., Smith, K., Freymann, J., Kirby, J., Koppel, P., Moore, S., Phillips, S., Maffitt, D., Pringle, M., Tarbox, L., & Prior, F. (2013). The Cancer Imaging Archive (TCIA): Maintaining and operating a public information repository. *Journal of Digital Imaging*, *26*(6), 1045–1057. https://doi.org/10.1007/s10278-013-9622-7.

DICOM. (2016). Digital Imaging and Communications in Medicine (DICOM). In *PS3.15 2016a — Security and System Management Profiles*. Rosslyn, VA: NEMA.

DICOM. (2022). Digital Imaging and Communications in Medicine (DICOM). In Rosslyn, VA: NEMA.

Doi, K. (2007). Computer-aided diagnosis in medical imaging: historical review, current status and future potential. *Computerized Medical Imaging and Graphics*, *31*(4–5), 198–211.

Fedorov, A., Longabaugh, W. J., Pot, D., Clunie, D. A., Pieper, S., Aerts, H. J., Homeyer, A., Lewis, R., Akbarzadeh, A., & Bontempi, D. (2021). NCI imaging data commons. *Cancer Research*, *81*(16), 4188–4193.

Field, M., Hardcastle, N., Jameson, M., Aherne, N., & Holloway, L. (2021). Machine learning applications in radiation oncology. *Physics and Imaging in Radiation Oncology*, *19*, 13–24.

Freymann, J. B., Kirby, J. S., Perry, J. H., Clunie, D. A., & Jaffe, C. C. (2012). Image data sharing for biomedical research — meeting HIPAA requirements for de-identification. *Journal of Digital Imaging*, *25*(1), 14–24.

Giger, M. (2021). Medical imaging of COVID-19. *Journal of Medical Imaging (Bellingham, Wash.)*, *8*(Suppl 1), 010101–010101. https://doi.org/10.1117/1.JMI.8.S1.010101.

Giger, M. L., Chan, H. P., & Boone, J. (2008). Anniversary paper: History and status of CAD and quantitative image analysis: The role of Medical Physics and AAPM. *Medical Physics*, *35*(12), 5799–5820.

Grossberg, A. J., Mohamed, A. S., Elhalawani, H., Bennett, W. C., Smith, K. E., Nolan, T. S., Williams, B., Chamchod, S., Heukelom, J., & Kantor, M. E. (2018). Imaging and clinical data archive for head and neck squamous cell carcinoma patients treated with radiotherapy. *Scientific Data*, *5*, 180173.

Huynh, E., Hosny, A., Guthier, C., Bitterman, D. S., Petit, S. F., Haas-Kogan, D. A., Kann, B., Aerts, H. J. W. L., & Mak, R. H. (2020). Artificial intelligence in radiation oncology. *Nature Reviews Clinical Oncology*, *17*(12), 771–781. https://doi.org/10.1038/s41571-020-0417-8.

Jacobsen, A., de Miranda Azevedo, R., Juty, N., Batista, D., Coles, S., Cornet, R., Courtot, M., Crosas, M., Dumontier, M., & Evelo, C. T. (2020). *FAIR Principles: Interpretations and Implementation Considerations*. Cambridge, MA: MIT Press.

Kalet, A. M., Luk, S. M., & Phillips, M. H. (2020). Radiation therapy quality assurance tasks and tools: The many roles of machine learning. *Medical Physics*, *47*(5), e168–e177.

Kiser, K. J., Fuller, C. D., & Reed, V. K. (2019). Artificial intelligence in radiation oncology treatment planning: A brief overview. *Journal of Medical Artificial Intelligence*, *2*(9).

Lin, D., Crabtree, J., Dillo, I., Downs, R. R., Edmunds, R., Giaretta, D., De Giusti, M., L'Hours, H., Hugo, W., & Jenkyns, R. (2020). The TRUST principles for digital repositories. *Scientific Data*, *7*(1), 1–5.

Lustberg, T., van Soest, J., Jochems, A., Deist, T., van Wijk, Y., Walsh, S., Lambin, P., & Dekker, A. (2017). Big Data in radiation therapy: Challenges and opportunities. *The British Journal of Radiology*, *90*(1069), 20160689.

Menikoff, J., Kaneshiro, J., & Pritchard, I. (2017). The common rule, updated. *The New England Journal of Medicine*, *376*(7), 613–615.

Minssen, T., Rajam, N., & Bogers, M. (2020). Clinical trial data transparency and GDPR compliance: Implications for data sharing and open innovation. *Science and Public Policy*, *47*(5), 616–626. https://doi.org/10.1093/scipol/scaa014.

Moore, S. M., Maffitt, D. R., Smith, K. E., Kirby, J. S., Clark, K. W., Freymann, J. B., Vendt, B. A., Tarbox, L. R., & Prior, F. W. (2015). De-identification of medical images with retention of scientific research value. *RadioGraphics*, *35*(3), 727–735. https://doi.org/10.1148/rg.2015140244.

Prior, F., Almeida, J., Kathiravelu, P., Kurc, T., Smith, K., Fitzgerald, T. J., & Saltz, J. (2020). Open access image repositories: High-quality data to enable machine learning research. *Clinical Radiology*, *75*(1), 7–12. https://doi.org/10.1016/j.crad.2019.04.002.

Prior, F., Smith, K., Sharma, A., Kirby, J., Tarbox, L., Clark, K., Bennett, W., Nolan, T., & Freymann, J. (2017). The public cancer radiology imaging collections of The Cancer Imaging Archive. *Scientific Data*, *4*, 170124. https://doi.org/10.1038/sdata.2017.124.

Prior, F. W., Brunsden, B., Hildebolt, C., Nolan, T. S., Pringle, M., Vaishnavi, S. N., & Larson-Prior, L. J. (2008). Facial recognition from volume-rendered magnetic resonance imaging data. *IEEE Transactions on Information Technology in Biomedicine, 13*(1), 5–9.

Prior, F. W., Clark, K., Commean, P., Freymann, J., Jaffe, C., Kirby, J., Moore, S., Smith, K., Tarbox, L., Vendt, B., & Marquez, G. (2013). TCIA: An information resource to enable open science. *Annual International Conference of the IEEE Engineering in Medicine and Biology Society. IEEE Engineering in Medicine and Biology Society. Annual International Conference*, pp. 1282–1285. https://doi.org/10.1109/EMBC.2013.6609742.

Prosperi, M., Min, J. S., Bian, J., & Modave, F. (2018). Big Data hurdles in precision medicine and precision public health. *BMC Medical Informatics and Decision Making*, *18*(1), 1–15.

Robinson, J. D. (2014). Beyond the DICOM header: Additional issues in deidentification. *American Journal of Roentgenology*, *203*(6), W658–W664. https://doi.org/10.2214/AJR.13.11789.

Rutherford, M., Mun, S. K., Levine, B., Bennett, W., Smith, K., Farmer, P., Jarosz, Q., Wagner, U., Freyman, J., Blake, G., Tarbox, L., Farahani, K., & Prior, F. (2021). A DICOM dataset for evaluation of medical image de-identification. *Scientific Data, 8*(1), 183. https://doi.org/10.1038/s41597-021-00967-y.

Sadri, A. R., Janowczyk, A., Zhou, R., Verma, R., Beig, N., Antunes, J., Madabhushi, A., Tiwari, P., & Viswanath, S. E. (2020). MRQy — An open-source tool for quality control of MR imaging data. *Medical Physics*, *47*(12), 6029–6038.

Sahiner, B., Pezeshk, A., Hadjiiski, L. M., Wang, X., Drukker, K., Cha, K. H., Summers, R. M., & Giger, M. L. (2019). Deep learning in medical imaging and radiation therapy. *Medical Physics*, *46*(1), e1–e36. https://doi.org/https://doi.org/10.1002/mp.13264.

Schwarz, C. G., Kremers, W. K., Therneau, T. M., Sharp, R. R., Gunter, J. L., Vemuri, P., Arani, A., Spychalla, A. J., Kantarci, K., & Knopman, D. S. (2019). Identification of anonymous MRI research participants with face-recognition software. *New England Journal of Medicine*, *381*(17), 1684–1686.

Schwarz, C. G., Kremers, W. K., Wiste, H. J., Gunter, J. L., Vemuri, P., Spychalla, A. J., Kantarci, K., Schultz, A. P., Sperling, R. A., Knopman, D. S., Petersen, R. C., & Jack, C. R. (2021). Changing the face of neuroimaging research: Comparing a new MRI de-facing technique with popular alternatives. *NeuroImage*, *231*, 117845. https://doi.org/https://doi.org/10.1016/j.neuroimage.2021.117845.

Talburt, J. R. (2011). *Entity Resolution and Information Quality*. Burlington: Elsevier.

Thompson, R. F., Valdes, G., Fuller, C. D., Carpenter, C. M., Morin, O., Aneja, S., Lindsay, W. D., Aerts, H. J. W. L., Agrimson, B., Deville, C., Rosenthal, S. A., Yu, J. B., & Thomas, C. R. (2018). Artificial intelligence in radiation oncology: A specialty-wide disruptive transformation? *Radiotherapy and Oncology*, *129*(3), 421–426. https://doi.org/https://doi.org/10.1016/j.radonc.2018.05.030.

Vicente-Saez, R. & Martinez-Fuentes, C. (2018). Open Science now: A systematic literature review for an integrated definition. *Journal of Business Research*, *88*, 428–436.

Wang, C., Zhu, X., Hong, J. C., & Zheng, D. (2019). Artificial intelligence in radiotherapy treatment planning: Present and future. *Technology in Cancer Research & Treatment*, *18*, 1533033819873922. https://doi.org/10.1177/1533033819873922.

Wilkinson, M. D., Dumontier, M., Aalbersberg, I. J., Appleton, G., Axton, M., Baak, A., Blomberg, N., Boiten, J.-W., da Silva Santos, L. B., & Bourne, P. E. (2016). The FAIR guiding principles for scientific data management and stewardship. *Scientific Data*, *3*(1), 1–9.

Willemink, M. J., Koszek, W. A., Hardell, C., Wu, J., Fleischmann, D., Harvey, H., Folio, L. R., Summers, R. M., Rubin, D. L., & Lungren, M. P. (2020). Preparing medical imaging data for machine learning. *Radiology*, *295*(1), 4–15. https://doi.org/10.1148/radiol.2020192224.

Part 3

AI Tools

Chapter 5

Science and Tools of Radiomics for Radiation Oncology

Christopher Wardell

Department of Biomedical Informatics, University of Arkansas for Medical Sciences, Little Rock AR, USA

Abstract

Radiomics is a catchall term used for the quantitative analysis of medical imaging data and is heavily dependent on machine learning. The central hypothesis of radiomics is that quantitative analysis of images can reveal correlations between radiomic features and molecular or clinical features that are otherwise invisible to normal visual inspection by humans. This field has experienced substantial advances in the first decades of the 21st century, formalizing and supplementing the qualitative analysis that is routinely performed by all users of imaging data. This chapter reviews the common inputs, outputs, methods, and software tools used in radiomic analyses.

1. Radiomics Definition and History

Radiology began as a qualitative rather than quantitative field for two reasons. Firstly, the images often speak for themselves; there are conditions that even laypeople with no training can identify such as a severely broken bone, or a large tumor. Secondly, it was qualitative out of necessity because the mathematical and computational tools required for quantitative analysis were yet to be invented.

Following the discovery and application of X-rays, throughout the 20th century new imaging modalities were established and quantitative methods to analyze images were steadily developed and refined. The term *radiomics* is potentially best understood as a catchall term for the quantitative analysis of medical imaging data.

This same pattern of development has been seen in adjacent disciplines. Molecular biology was fundamentally revolutionized by *bioinformatics*, which added statistical and machine learning methods to largely pre-existing fields. Sequencing the DNA of the tiny ~5000 base pair ΦX174 virus was readily achieved with little more than electrophoresis gels, time, and dedication in the late 1970s (Sanger *et al.*, 1977), but it took two more decades, serious computation, and billions of dollars to assemble a draft of the 3 billion base pairs of the human genome at the turn of the century (Craig Venter *et al.*, 2001; Lander *et al.*, 2001). Today, molecular biology has truly become a branch of data science and bioinformatics is a required part of almost any project.

A similar outcome is envisioned in the future of radiology. Radiologists will not be replaced by machine learning algorithms, but their work will be augmented by algorithms, and research will become ever more quantitative.

The term *radiomics* itself is a neologism coined in 2012 (Lambin *et al.*, 2012), part of the trend at the time to name all biological data sets with the *omics* suffix. The discipline was born surprisingly complete and much of the following decade of work has been in formalizing the field.

The central hypothesis of radiomics is that features in radiographic images can be used for diagnostic and prognostic purposes. The aim is to quantify these features and automate the process to improve the treatment and standard of care for patients. A defining characteristic of current radiomics is the use of engineered radiomic features that have been carefully selected and standardized, rather than feeding raw image data to machine learning algorithms. A common workflow for radiomics studies is shown in Fig. 1.

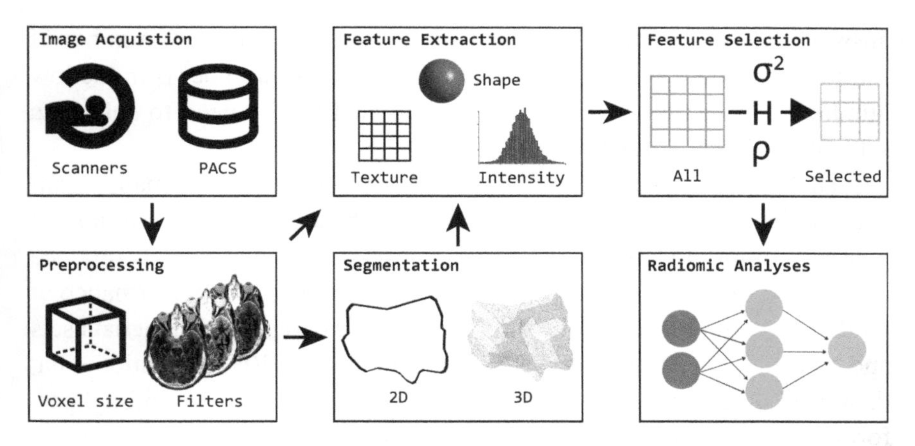

Fig. 1. A common radiomics workflow. Images are acquired using standard techniques either directly from patients or retrieved from a Picture Archiving and Communication Systems (PACS) database. Preprocessing is applied and the ROI segmented either manually or by AI. Radiomic features are then extracted from the ROI, selected based on their information content, and finally further analyses may be performed to link them with real-world variables and outcomes such as genetic mutations and prognosis.

Radiomics also usually refers to imaging data at the anatomical scale. The quantitative analysis of smaller structures in pathology slides and cell culture is a closely related sister discipline called *pathomics* or *computational pathology*.

2. Input Data and Preprocessing

Radiomics can be performed using any imaging modality as an input, but it is most commonly done using volumetric methods such as computed tomography (CT), positron emission tomography (PET), and magnetic resonance imaging (MRI) data rather than two-dimensional digital X-ray images such as computed radiography (CR).

A critical issue that is often only considered late in the process is how much input data are required, or how many samples to use. Many clinical trials have the benefit of power analyses performed in advance to answer this question. Biostatisticians can determine the optimal size of a clinical trial and ensure that it is adequately powered to reach statistical significance. Machine learning methods are harder to predict, and the short answer is that more data are better. In general, the minimum number of samples should be at least tens of samples and a fair number is in the low hundreds. Sample numbers are further inflated by the need to split data sets into training, validation, and testing sets.

The objective is to divide the totality of the data into smaller non-overlapping data sets for sequential steps in the analysis. The training set is used to train models, the validation set to confirm that models produce acceptable predictions, and finally the test set assesses the performance of models. A common protocol would be to gather two independent data sets and split the largest one into 70% training data and 30% validation data, then use the slightly smaller second data set as a test set. For optimal performance, it is vital that the composition of data sets is similar; it would be undesirable to group all disease cases into the training set, as the validation and test sets would be unlike the training data. An alternative approach is cross-validation, where a single data set is sampled multiple times to generate many overlapping data sets; this can be particularly useful when samples are scarce.

Consideration should also be given to the source of the data used. Most researchers only use data generated at their own institution. This is a potential problem, as it not only limits the potential size of a data set but may introduce bias. A better approach is to include data from multiple institutions, which also validates the findings and eliminates local biases within the data. A recent review of AI algorithms for diagnostic analysis of medical images found that only 6% of studies performed external validation (Kim *et al.*, 2019). Gathering multi-center data sets requires either collaboration between institutions or alternatively downloading additional samples from online repositories such as The Cancer Imaging Archive (TCIA) (Clark *et al.*, 2013). The benefits of gathering immense, multi-site data sets have been clearly illustrated by genome-wide association studies (GWAS), where studies with samples in the hundreds of thousands have the statistical power to dissect the inheritance of complex traits and diseases.

The hardware and software used to capture data have a substantial effect on the images produced. This includes everything from the manufacturer, model, software, and settings used. Medical scanning devices and software often offer a variety of preprocessing methods, including correcting for the motion caused by breathing and signal attenuation inherently caused by the size and density of patients. Only some of these factors can be influenced by an operator and if engaged in a large or multi-center study, these variables should be tracked, even if they cannot be controlled. The variability between data sets introduced by such non-biological factors is commonly known as batch effects.

If batch effects are observed in radiomic data sets, there are methods to help ameliorate them. The ComBat algorithm was initially developed to cope with the batch effects commonly seen in DNA expression micro-arrays and it has recently been modified specifically for radiomics (Da-ano *et al.*, 2020; Johnson *et al.*, 2007).

Once captured, there are file-type issues to contend with. Namely, choosing between Digital Imaging and Communications in Medicine (DICOM) or the Neuroimaging Informatics Technology Initiative (NIfTI) file format.

First introduced in 1985 and still evolving, the DICOM standard governs the communication and management of medical imaging data and associated metadata. In short, it can be thought of as the file type used to store the data created by medical imaging devices. More accurately, it's a container format with a header in which various metadata can be stored describing the patient, the data itself, and how it was created. DICOM is extremely flexible and mature, with decades of updates and extensions. However, its maturity and complexity can make it appear somewhat arcane to new users. For example, DICOM data sets usually store one file per two-dimensional plane, so a single data set can consist of hundreds of individual files in a single directory.

On the other hand, the NIfTI file format offers a more streamlined experience; NIfTI files pack everything into a single binary file containing a descriptive header and a three-dimensional matrix of data. However, the two formats are not completely interchangeable and there are subtleties and edge cases that cannot be handled by NIfTI. NIfTI was explicitly designed to handle MRI data for neuroimaging studies, whereas DICOM was intended for any digital imaging data.

After image acquisition and reconstruction, further preprocessing may be necessary. For example, it is standard to resample data so that all voxels are the same isotropic size; voxels become cubes with identical dimensions and spacing. It is typical for medical imaging data to have a higher resolution within the axial plane than between slices, so some interpolation may be necessary. Just like filetype conversions, this could be a source of error if data sets have used different interpolation methods.

There is another layer of image preprocessing that is commonly performed, known as filtering (Fig. 2). Image filters are commonly understood by anyone who has used photo editing software or even photo or video mobile applications. They apply a function to an image and alter it. In regular photography this is usually performed for a purely aesthetic effect, but it can also serve practical purposes such as blurring, smoothing, or sharpening images.

Radiomic filters can be very simple, such as taking the exponential, log, or square of the intensity values of voxels, but are commonly more involved and convolutional. A common convolutional filter is the Laplacian of Gaussian (LoG). LoG filters are effective at highlighting the coarseness of texture in a volume, which is inelegantly named *blob detection*. It should be noted that LoG filters require the user to specify the size of features they

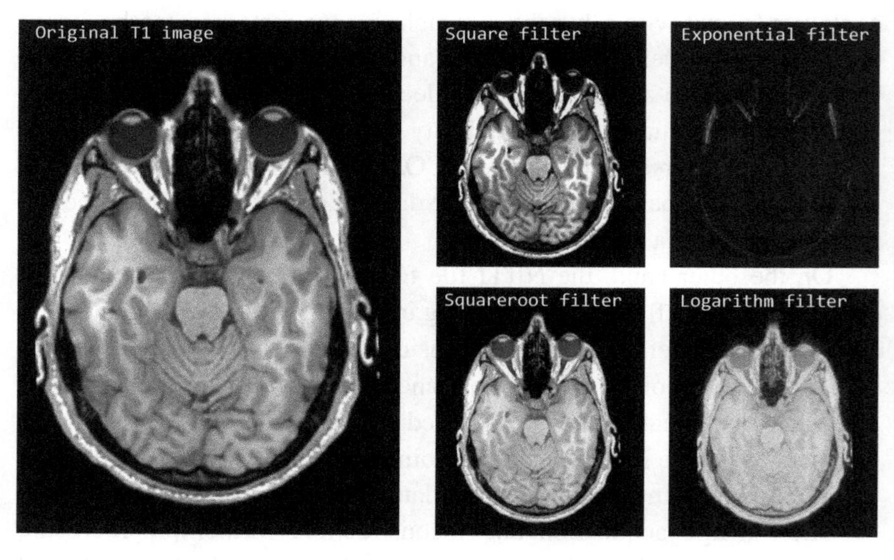

Fig. 2. Effects of filters on images. Original T1 MRI is on the left and a variety of common image filters are on the right.

are looking for, so it may be beneficial to apply several LoG filters independently. It has been demonstrated that image reconstruction settings including slice thickness, voxel size, and preprocessing steps affect radiomic features (Lu *et al.*, 2016; Shiri *et al.*, 2017).

3. Segmentation

Image segmentation is fundamental to radiomics and the concept is simple; regions of interest (ROIs) in images are identified and labeled. This can be performed in a slice-by-slice manner where pixels are labeled, or volumetrically where voxels are labeled. The purpose is to label large biological features such as bones, organs, or tumor tissue. Labeled data are essential for supervised machine learning methods.

In practice, segmentation can be extremely challenging and is often the bottleneck which limits and arrests further work. Creating these segmentations is a detailed and time-consuming task if performed manually and scales extremely poorly. A qualified radiologist can sift through and label data as required, but there are neither enough radiologists nor sufficient time available to segment the amount of data required for real-time analysis, let alone retrospective analyses. It is common to draft colleagues, researchers, and students to assist in segmentation tasks, but ultimately segmentations must be approved and verified by a qualified radiologist to prevent incorrect labels from polluting data sets.

Fortunately, we are living through a veritable Cambrian explosion in terms of artificial intelligence research. As detailed in other chapters and thanks to the researchers who have dedicated their careers to it, great progress has been made in automated segmentation. The two key advances in recent years have been moving from segmenting 2D images to directly segmenting 3D volumes and the invention of the U-Net and its derivatives (Ronneberger *et al.*, 2015). U-Nets are effective because they marry encoder and decoder networks that perform opposite tasks. The encoder down-samples and pools the input data using convolutional layers, then the decoder up-samples the data, resulting in an output segmentation map at the same resolution as the original data.

It is interesting to note that a development and testing ground for segmentation algorithms has been competitions such as the Brain Tumor

Segmentation (BraTS) Challenge. This yearly competition has been operating for a decade and now includes radiomics-specific challenges.

Recent automated segmentation methods are sufficiently accurate that it may be sufficient for radiologists to confirm the ROIs as correct, at least for research purposes. Current systems are analogous to the output of a skilled apprentice whose work requires some oversight and occasional manual correction, but segmentation remains far from trivial. The amount of time and effort consumed by this step should not be underestimated, especially in cases where researchers must first train and validate their own segmentation methods.

4. Radiomic Feature Extraction and Standardization

Radiomic features are simply numeric values calculated from the ROI of an image or volume. They can be split into several broad categories; shape-based, first-order and second (or higher)-order features. The first two groups are the most intuitively understood and refer to the base morphological and radiological features of an ROI. Morphological features are values describing the physical characteristics of an ROI, such as the volume, surface-to-volume ratio, and sphericity. First-order features describe the intensities of the observed voxels such as minimum and maximum values, as well as statistical descriptions such as the mean, range, and skewness of intensities.

Higher-order features are more complex and difficult to describe and interpret but are equally valid. The origin of these features comes from efforts to classify images based on texture in the 1970s (Haralick *et al.*, 1973). Starting with only 13 features, this class has grown considerably and numbers in the hundreds in current applications.

A further complication in higher-order texture feature calculation is the concept of discretization. Imaging data is numeric and the most common way to visualize it is in a grayscale format, where values are shades of gray, with only the most extreme values such as the background being close to black or white. The color gray is arbitrary, as any sequential color palette could be used, but the important point is that the value of each pixel is stored as a number with between 12 and 16 bits. This corresponds to 4,096 to 65,536 shades of gray. These thousands of gray levels are discretized by grouping or "binning" them into a smaller number of gray levels to reduce variability and increase interpretability of the data.

Radiomic features are calculated after gray-level discretization, therefore the choice to use either a fixed bin size or a fixed number of bins, as well as how many of these bins to use, will affect results. This has been demonstrated to affect radiomic feature values in modalities including PET (Leijenaar *et al.*, 2015), CT (Larue *et al.*, 2017; Shafiq-Ul-Hassan *et al.*, 2017), and MRI (Duron *et al.*, 2019).

The Image Biomarker Standardization Initiative (IBSI) has made significant headway into codifying radiomic features (Hatt *et al.*, 2018). This is an extremely important project because standards are the foundation of interoperability and robust, reproducible science and engineering. We must agree on the naming and implementation of radiomic features or we will endlessly reinvent the wheel.

There have been two major IBSI projects thus far. IBSI 1 was completed in 2020 and was dedicated to standardizing the methods for computing commonly used radiomic features (Zwanenburg *et al.*, 2020) in CT, PET, and T1-weighted MRI.

IBSI 1 was structured as a collaboration between many international groups and was split into three phases of increasing complexity. The first phase analyzed a data set created using a simple digital phantom, the second used CT data from a lung cancer patient. The third phase used CT, PET, and MRI data from 51 sarcoma patients to assess the reproducibility of features. The metric for success was consensus between the output of the participating groups.

In total, a set of 169 commonly used features was established by IBSI 1. These reference data were made available to developers to assist in designing and calibrating their own software. It is notable that because some radiomic software predate IBSI, they may deviate from IBSI definitions, and these deviations are noted in the software documentation.

IBSI 2 is dedicated to standardizing commonly used imaging filters (discussed above) and is ongoing. It is almost identically structured as a large collaboration with three phases; technical validation using digital phantoms, establishing reference values using CT lung cancer data, and finally the validation phase using sarcoma patients' data. Ultimately, IBSI 2 will result in a publication and publicly available standards for filter implementation.

There will be further chapters in IBSI that will likely be focused on reinforcing reproducibility in the various aspects of deep learning in radiomics. These include data preprocessing, splitting data into training, validation and test sets, and augmenting the data.

5. Software Tools for Radiomic Feature Extraction

Researchers aiming to extract radiomic features from an ROI have many software options open to them, as there are more than ten implementations of the IBSI 1 standards at the time of writing. Rather than engaging in an exhaustive and quickly outdated discussion on each of these implementations, we discuss general issues and spotlight some of the more popular software (Table 1).

Radiomics is a branch of academic research and this is reflected in the software available. The quality of the software is generally high and is fit for purpose, but they are not simple turnkey solutions. Users should be

Table 1. A selection of IBSI-1 compliant software which can be used to extract radiomic features from radiographic imaging data. Also noted is whether the software has a graphical user interface (GUI) or command line interface (CLI), the language it is written in, the software license covering it, and a link to the software.

Software	Type	Language	Software License	Link to Project
Pyradiomics	CLI	Python	BSD 3-clause	https://github.com/AIM-Harvard/pyradiomics
CaPTk	GUI/CLI	C++	Multiple	https://github.com/CBICA/CaPTk
MITK	GUI/CLI	C++	BSD 3-clause	https://github.com/MITK/MITK
CERR	GUI/CLI	MATLAB	LGPL-2.1	https://github.com/cerr/CERR
LIFEx	GUI	Java	CEA license (free for non-commercial research)	https://www.lifexsoft.org/
radiomics-develop	CLI	MATLAB	GPL-3.0	https://github.com/mvallieres/radiomics-develop
MIRP	CLI	Python	EUPL-1.2	https://github.com/oncoray/mirp
SERA	CLI	MATLAB	GPL-3.0	https://github.com/ashrafinia/SERA

prepared to do some command-line work, scripting, and data wrangling of their own, or at least collaborate with someone who can.

Standardization initiatives such as IBSI mean that many of the features extracted are named and calculated in the same way, but it is not guaranteed that the outputs will be identical between software.

The unifying characteristic of these software is that they have been produced by academic researchers and have grown directly out of the research interests of their authors. This approach often leads to software that is continuously developed, well-maintained, efficient, and well-tested, but can create usability issues in use cases which were not predicted or intended by the developers.

A second shared characteristic is they tend to be free and open-source software (OSS), often available via GitHub. This provides users with access to the original source code and a direct line of communication to the developers to ask questions, report potential bugs, and request additional features. Alternatively, users may directly modify the code themselves and submit these changes back to the project.

Language choice may be influenced by what has been used historically in a field or project, what is popular at the time when new software is developed, and what developers are comfortable using. MATLAB has been a popular language for image analysis, but Python's recent primacy in data science and machine learning has made anything else written in Python inherently attractive. C++ remains a perennial choice for developers aiming to write fast, highly optimized code. Again, there are parallels in other fields; early genomics tools were written in Perl, modern ones are typically written in Python, and tools requiring extreme speed such as sequence aligners are often written in C++.

While rich in imaging libraries and functionality, the proprietary nature of MATLAB is a potential concern, particularly for academic researchers. While the MATLAB Compiler Runtime (MCR) allows users to run MATLAB code without a paid license, the code must be compiled for distribution. Even if the source code is publicly available, it is impossible for end users without a MATLAB license to edit it.

Radiomics software have light hardware requirements and almost any modern computer should be capable of running them. The primary target operating systems are UNIX-derivatives such as Linux distributions and macOS. Although Windows is sometimes not directly supported, the Windows Subsystem for Linux (WSL) has effectively eliminated compatibility issues, as it allows UNIX-targeted code and binaries to run natively. It is also common for radiomics software to be command-line only and have no graphical user interface, but this is unlikely to faze the intended audience.

Radiomics software can broadly be divided into two categories: dedicated software packages and extensions to existing applications. Software packages provide a very specific set of radiomic functions and are intended for standalone use. Extensions are add-ons for existing applications for viewing and editing imaging data that have a graphical user interface (GUI) that provide tools for radiomics. Both types of software may provide a direct command-line interface (CLI) to allow scripting.

Each has advantages and disadvantages and users may benefit from utilizing both. GUI-enabled programs allow visual interaction and immediate feedback, so are an excellent way to explore data. However, human interaction is error prone and not scalable if studying more than a handful of samples. CLI access is required for automated processing of samples and performing reproducible research. Conversely, the raw text output from CLI programs does not lend itself to rapid and easy interpretation.

The most widely used CLI software package is Pyradiomics (Van Griethuysen *et al.*, 2017), but it is by no means the only option. It can be deployed as a command-line application, or alternatively imported into other software, so users can manage both feature extraction and analysis in one codebase.

6. Feature Selection and Dimensionality Reduction

Researchers face a significant hurdle once they have extracted radiomic features from an image. The combination of filters and features is multiplicative; if one extracts 100 features from an image and uses the original image and a dozen filters, then one can have over 1000 radiomic features to contend with. Multiple testing correction will quickly dilute statistical significance and render any analysis futile. Therefore, the number of features must be pared down. This process is termed feature selection and should use only the training data set.

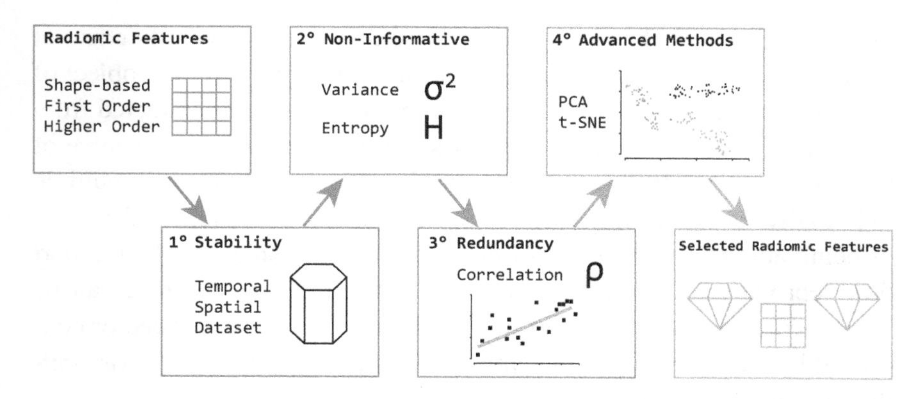

Fig. 3. Radiomic feature selection. A linear pipeline drastically pares down the number of features based on their stability, information content, and redundancy, aiming to retain the minimal number of features to aid statistical power.

The issues associated with large numbers of features are not unique to radiomics and are commonly known as the *curse of dimensionality*. Fortunately, decades of experience and problem solving have been gained in other fields which are directly applicable to mitigating this curse in radiomics (Fig. 3).

The first step in this process is to look for feature stability, which tests for radiomic features that are reproducible, with similar values when measured multiple times. Features with high stability are good candidates for biomarkers to correlate with genomic and clinical features, whereas low stability implies that a feature is either noisy or even potentially random and should be discarded. Many radiomic features frequently display a lack of robustness to perturbation and this remains an ongoing concern in the field (Reiazi *et al.*, 2021).

Stability can be defined and tested in multiple ways. Temporal stability can only be measured if one has access to series of images taken over a period of hours or days. However, most medical imaging data are created opportunistically during the routine diagnosis and treatment of patients. In this setting, testing for temporal stability would introduce significant additional cost, inefficiency, and inconvenience.

A more commonly tested definition is spatial stability. Individual radiologists or algorithms will produce subtly different segmentations of the same ROI from the same image. These differences generally occur at the edges of the ROI and the most clinically relevant part of the object of study is captured in all cases. Therefore, radiomic features extracted from these segmentations should be highly similar, regardless of the source of the segmentation. In practice, this can be achieved by having multiple radiologists or algorithms segment ROIs. This has the additional benefit of being able to generate inter-user variability assessments, which report how reproducible the segmentations are. Alternatively, the ROI can be jittered computationally. For example, the edges can be expanded or contracted by a few voxels, or the entire ROI shifted to simulate the variability introduced by humans.

Data set stability compares radiomic features between data sets; for example, the training and validation data sets. If data sets are reasonably sized and balanced in their sample composition, then one expects similar ranges of values detected in both.

Analogously, consider photographs of an iconic building. One might expect it to have similar features in different photographs taken days apart (temporal stability), if the images were segmented by different individuals (spatial stability), or in completely separate photographs (data set stability).

Whichever definition of stability is considered, the concepts for testing stability remain similar. Sets of radiomics features are computed from the two data sets in question and the correlation between them is assessed by examining a correlation coefficient. Spearman's rho may be preferred over Pearson's rho, as it is more forgiving of outliers when looking for a monotonic relationship.

A robust solution is to calculate the concordance correlation coefficient (CCC) (Lin, 1989), which also takes into account the mean and variance of the radiomic features. The resulting score ranges between 0 and 1 and although somewhat arbitrary, scores above 0.85 are considered acceptable (Peerlings *et al.*, 2019).

Counter-intuitively, there do not appear to be common radiomic features or classes of features that are inherently stable or unstable, with results varying substantially between studies. This may be driven by differences between imaging modalities, image acquisition parameters, or even the subjects of the images themselves. Whatever the causes, the best solution is that researchers test the stability of their radiomic features in every study.

The second step is to discard non-informative features which contain little meaningful information. Features that have very little or no change in their variance or entropy can be safely removed and this depends on the study. For example, the size of a tumor is a clinically important feature, but if a study were conducted with tumors of approximately the same size, then shape-based features such as volume would likely become non-informative.

The third step is to remove redundant features. If multiple features are highly correlated, then keeping them all only serves to dilute the statistical significance and important findings could be missed. When removing highly correlated features, it is often best to manually choose which to keep. A complex wavelet-based radiomic feature could potentially be acting as a proxy for something simpler to measure and more intuitive such as a shape feature.

Finally in feature selection, there are many more advanced methods that can be employed. The objective is to minimize the correlation between individual radiomic features and maximize the relevance of them to target features such as clinical features. As an example, the minimum redundancy maximum relevance (mRMR) method (Ding & Peng, 2005) does exactly this. However, there are other options available that only consider minimizing the correlation between radiomic features and are well known among machine learning practitioners, examples being classic principal components analysis (PCA) and t-distributed stochastic neighbor embedding (t-SNE).

7. Radiomic Analyses

Once researchers have finalized data sets of informative, non-redundant, and stable radiomic features, the radiomic hypothesis can be tested; are there associations between radiomic features and clinical, molecular, or genomic features?

This is a task of training, validating, and testing models using the data sets defined earlier. The only requirement is that researchers have a good understanding of machine learning methods. Researchers could potentially have very little knowledge of radiomics or the target variables they are correlating them with. However, as with all translational research, it is important to keep domain experts such as physicians in the loop to help interpret the findings. Without this sanity-check, researchers could report trivial or even incorrect findings.

A factor in choosing appropriate methods is whether the target clinical or genomic variables are continuous or discrete. The most common continuous variables in a clinical setting are time to disease progression and overall survival time, which require building a Cox proportional hazards model.

Radiomics tends to revolve around discrete variables such as the presence of specific mutations, rather than continuous variables such as the amounts of specific molecules or metabolites in the blood. Therefore, radiomics leans toward the domain of classification problems. These methods range from classifiers such as naïve Bayes, random forests, k-nearest neighbors, to support vector machines and neural networks (Fig. 4). However, modern machine learning methods such as neural networks can equally be used as regression models, so the same tools can be used in a variety of applications.

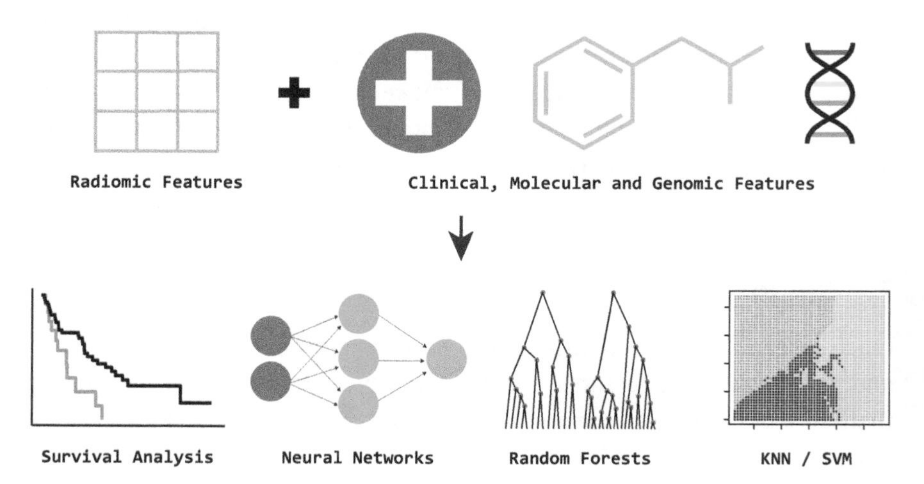

Fig. 4. Machine learning methods for radiomics. Using a variety of machine learning methods, radiomic features can be used to predict other variables including clinical, molecular, and genomic features.

Ensemble methods should be considered, which are combinations of the classifiers above. The results of multiple methods can be aggregated using something as simple as a majority voting rule or something more complex such as using bagging or boosting of multiple random forests.

After the first decade of research, there are examples that demonstrate the radiomic hypothesis to be true, or at the very least that we cannot reject it. Radiomic features in multiple cancer types across a range of imaging modalities have been associated with both clinical features, such as survival time, and genomic features, such as mutations of specific genes.

The most common cancer types studied have been those that are both common and have large amounts of imaging data, meaning that the literature is rich in lung cancer studies. It has been demonstrated that radiomic features have some prognostic value in lung cancer (Aerts *et al.*, 2014; Chong *et al.*, 2014; Coroller *et al.*, 2016; Fried *et al.*, 2014). Radiomic features may also predict the activity of specific transcriptional pathways (Grossmann *et al.*, 2017) or presence of EGFR mutations in lung cancer (Yip *et al.*, 2017). Similarly, the radiomic features of head and neck cancers have been shown to be prognostic (Aerts *et al.*, 2014; Vallières *et al.*, 2017). Radiomic features in CT imaging have also been linked to multiple RAS-pathway mutations in colorectal cancer (Yang *et al.*, 2018). BRAF mutations in melanoma are detectable using both PET imaging in the primary tissues (Saadani *et al.*, 2019) and MRI imaging of melanoma metastases to the brain (Shofty *et al.*, 2020). Additionally, IDH and EGFR mutations can be predicted in glioblastoma using MRI data (Verduin *et al.*, 2021).

Mutations are not the only genomic lesions that are detectable through radiomics; the co-deletion of 1p and 19q chromosomal arms has been found in low grade glioma (Casale *et al.*, 2021) and MGMT promoter methylation in glioblastoma (Verduin *et al.*, 2021). Physiological phenomena may also be predicted; radiomic signatures derived from PET and CT data can predict tumor hypoxia, which indicates poor prognosis (Sanduleanu *et al.*, 2020).

Most radiomics papers focus on data gathered at a single time point, but in recent years there have been studies that have analyzed the changes in radiomic features over time; so-called *delta radiomics* (Fave *et al.*,

2017). The concept is that changes in radiomic features may reflect disease progression or therapeutic response. For example, a higher-order radiomic feature could be used to stratify non-small cell lung cancer patients into high and low risk groups.

Course corrections have taken place as research has advanced. A study reexamined a prognostic radiomic signature in lung cancer and found that the prognostic feature was in fact tumor volume. The initially reported intensity and texture features themselves were acting as proxies, illustrating the importance of rigorous validation (Welch *et al.*, 2019).

There have been efforts to standardize and report the quality of entire radiomic studies. The most notable is the radiomics quality score (RQS) (Lambin *et al.*, 2017). This is a metric with 16 categories spanning the entire process from data collection through to model validation, with each category offering positive or negative points, up to a perfect score of 36. However, this is not in common use and there are acceptable reasons why researchers may not employ it. Researchers may not be aware of it and an imperfect score does not mean a careless piece of work; for example, seven points (~20% of the total) are lost if the work is not a prospective study in a trial database, which is not applicable in many cases. It remains a useful template for developing and assessing radiomic studies.

8. Conclusions

Invented in the 20th century under other names such as quantitative imaging analysis, the 21st century has seen radiomics exit infancy and enter adolescence. Radiomics is still very much in a developmental stage and the field continues on its rapid evolution driven by a variety of factors.

Machine learning is fundamental to radiomics, as the immense and formerly intractable scale of segmentation problems are beginning to be addressed through automated methods. Secondly, machine learning methods are vital for finding associations between clinical and molecular features and radiomic features, once they have been extracted and appropriately selected.

As capabilities increase and barriers to entry decrease, there are massive opportunities for further breakthroughs to be made in the next decade of radiomics research.

References

Aerts, H. J. W. L., Emmanuel Rios Velazquez, Ralph T. H. Leijenaar, Chintan Parmar, Patrick Grossmann, Sara Cavalho, Johan Bussink, René Monshouwer, Benjamin Haibe-Kains, Derek Rietveld, Frank Hoebers, Michelle M. Rietbergen, C. René Leemans, Andre Dekker, John Quackenbush, Robert J. Gillies, & Philippe Lambin. (2014). Decoding tumour phenotype by noninvasive imaging using a quantitative radiomics approach. *Nature Communications, 5*, 4006. https://doi.org/10.1038/ncomms5006.

Casale, Roberto, Elizaveta Lavrova, Sebastian Sanduleanu, Henry C. Woodruff, & Philippe Lambin. (2021). Development and external validation of a non-invasive molecular status predictor of chromosome 1p/19q co-deletion based on MRI radiomics analysis of low grade glioma patients. *European Journal of Radiology, 139*, 109678. https://doi.org/10.1016/j.ejrad.2021.109678.

Chong, Yousun, Jae Hun Kim, Ho Yun Lee, Yong Chan Ahn, Kyung Soo Lee, Myung Ju Ahn, Jhingook Kim, Young Mog Shim, Joungho Han, & Yoon La Choi. (2014). Quantitative CT variables enabling response prediction in neoadjuvant therapy with EGFR-TKIs: Are they different from those in neoadjuvant concurrent chemoradiotherapy? *PLoS ONE, 9*(2), e88598. https://doi.org/10.1371/journal.pone.0088598.

Clark, Kenneth, Bruce Vendt, Kirk Smith, John Freymann, Justin Kirby, Paul Koppel, Stephen Moore, Stanley Phillips, David Maffitt, Michael Pringle, Lawrence Tarbox, & Fred Prior. (2013). The Cancer Imaging Archive (TCIA): Maintaining and operating a public information repository. *Journal of Digital Imaging, 26*(6), 1045–1057. https://doi.org/10.1007/s10278-013-9622-7.

Coroller, Thibaud P., Vishesh Agrawal, Vivek Narayan, Ying Hou, Patrick Grossmann, Stephanie W. Lee, Raymond H. Mak, & Hugo J. W. L. Aerts. (2016). Radiomic phenotype features predict pathological response in non-small cell radiomic predicts pathological response lung cancer. *Radiotherapy and Oncology, 119*(3), 480–486. https://doi.org/10.1016/j.radonc.2016.04.004.

Craig Venter, J., M. D. Adams, E. W. Myers, P. W. Li, R. J. Mural, G. G. Sutton, H. O. Smith, M. Yandell, C. A. Evans, R. A. Holt, J. D. Gocayne, P. Amanatides, R. M. Ballew, D. H. Huson, J. R. Wortman, Q. Zhang, C. D. Kodira, X. H. Zheng, L. Chen, M. Skupski, G. Subramanian, P. D. Thomas, J. Zhang, G. L. Gabor Miklos, C. Nelson, S. Broder, A. G. Clark, J. Nadeau, V. A. McKusick, N. Zinder, A. J. Levine, R. J. Roberts, M. Simon, C. Slayman, M. Hunkapiller, R. Bolanos, A. Delcher, I. Dew, D. Fasulo, M. Flanigan, L. Florea, A. Halpern, S. Hannenhalli, S. Kravitz, S. Levy, C. Mobarry, K. Reinert, K. Remington, J. Abu-Threideh, E. Beasley, K. Biddick, V. Bonazzi, R. Brandon, M. Cargill, I. Chandramouliswaran, R. Charlab, K. Chaturvedi, Z. Deng, V. di Francesco, P. Dunn, K. Eilbeck, C. Evangelista, A. E. Gabrielian, W. Gan, W. Ge, F. Gong, Z. Gu, P. Guan, T. J. Heiman, M. E. Higgins, R. R. Ji, Z. Ke, K. A. Ketchum, Z. Lai, Y. Lei, Z. Li, J. Li, Y. Liang, X. Lin, F. Lu, G. V. Merkulov, N. Milshina, H. M. Moore, A. K. Naik, V. A. Narayan, B. Neelam, D.

Nusskern, D. B. Rusch, S. Salzberg, W. Shao, B. Shue, J. Sun, Z. Yuan Wang, A. Wang, X. Wang, J. Wang, M. H. Wei, R. Wides, C. Xiao, C. Yan, A. Yao, J. Ye, M. Zhan, W. Zhang, H. Zhang, Q. Zhao, L. Zheng, F. Zhong, W. Zhong, S. C. Zhu, S. Zhao, D. Gilbert, S. Baumhueter, G. Spier, C. Carter, A. Cravchik, T. Woodage, F. Ali, H. An, A. Awe, D. Baldwin, H. Baden, M. Barnstead, I. Barrow, K. Beeson, D. Busam, A. Carver, A. Center, M. Lai Cheng, L. Curry, S. Danaher, L. Davenport, R. Desilets, S. Dietz, K. Dodson, L. Doup, S. Ferriera, N. Garg, A. Gluecksmann, B. Hart, J. Haynes, C. Haynes, C. Heiner, S. Hladun, D. Hostin, J. Houck, T. Howland, C. Ibegwam, J. Johnson, F. Kalush, L. Kline, S. Koduru, A. Love, F. Mann, D. May, S. McCawley, T. McIntosh, I. McMullen, M. Moy, L. Moy, B. Murphy, K. Nelson, C. Pfannkoch, E. Pratts, V. Puri, H. Qureshi, M. Reardon, R. Rodriguez, Yu H. Rogers, D. Romblad, B. Ruhfel, R. Scott, C. Sitter, M. Smallwood, E. Stewart, R. Strong, E. Suh, R. Thomas, N. Ni Tint, S. Tse, C. Vech, G. Wang, J. Wetter, S. Williams, M. Williams, S. Windsor, E. Winn-Deen, K. Wolfe, J. Zaveri, K. Zaveri, J. F. Abril, R. Guigo, M. J. Campbell, K. V. Sjolander, B. Karlak, A. Kejariwal, H. Mi, B. Lazareva, T. Hatton, A. Narechania, K. Diemer, A. Muruganujan, N. Guo, S. Sato, V. Bafna, S. Istrail, R. Lippert, R. Schwartz, B. Walenz, S. Yooseph, D. Allen, A. Basu, J. Baxendale, L. Blick, M. Caminha, J. Carnes-Stine, P. Caulk, Y. H. Chiang, M. Coyne, C. Dahlke, A. Deslattes Mays, M. Dombroski, M. Donnelly, D. Ely, S. Esparham, C. Fosler, H. Gire, S. Glanowski, K. Glasser, A. Glodek, M. Gorokhov, K. Graham, B. Gropman, M. Harris, J. Heil, S. Henderson, J. Hoover, D. Jennings, C. Jordan, J. Jordan, J. Kasha, L. Kagan, C. Kraft, A. Levitsky, M. Lewis, X. Liu, J. Lopez, D. Ma, W. Majoros, J. McDaniel, S. Murphy, M. Newman, T. Nguyen, N. Nguyen, M. Nodell, S. Pan, J. Peck, M. Peterson, W. Rowe, R. Sanders, J. Scott, M. Simpson, T. Smith, A. Sprague, T. Stockwell, R. Turner, E. Venter, M. Wang, M. Wen, D. Wu, M. Wu, A. Xia, A. Zandieh, & X. Zhu. (2001). The sequence of the human genome. *Science, 291*(5507), 1304–1351. https://doi.org/10.1126/science.1058040.

Da-ano, R., I. Masson, F. Lucia, M. Doré, P. Robin, J. Alfieri, C. Rousseau, A. Mervoyer, C. Reinhold, J. Castelli, R. De Crevoisier, J. F. Rameé, O. Pradier, U. Schick, D. Visvikis, & M. Hatt. (2020). Performance comparison of modified ComBat for harmonization of radiomic features for multicenter studies. *Scientific Reports, 10*(1), 10248. https://doi.org/10.1038/s41598-020-66110-w.

Ding, Chris & Hanchuan Peng. (2005). Minimum redundancy feature selection from microarray gene expression data. *Journal of Bioinformatics and Computational Biology, 3*(2), 185–205. https://doi.org/10.1142/S0219720005001004.

Duron, Loïc, Daniel Balvay, Saskia Vande Perre, Afef Bouchouicha, Julien Savatovsky, Jean Claude Sadik, Isabelle Thomassin-Naggara, Laure Fournier, & Augustin Lecler. (2019). Gray-level discretization impacts reproducible MRI radiomics texture features. *PLoS ONE, 14*(3), e0213459. https://doi.org/10.1371/journal.pone.0213459.

Fave, Xenia, Lifei Zhang, Jinzhong Yang, Dennis MacKin, Peter Balter, Daniel Gomez, David Followill, Aaron Kyle Jones, Francesco Stingo, Zhongxing Liao, Radhe

Mohan, & Laurence Court. (2017). Delta-radiomics features for the prediction of patient outcomes in non-small cell lung cancer. *Scientific Reports, 7*(1), 588. https://doi.org/10.1038/s41598-017-00665-z.

Fried, David V., Susan L. Tucker, Shouhao Zhou, Zhongxing Liao, Osama Mawlawi, Geoffrey Ibbott, & Laurence E. Court. (2014). Prognostic value and reproducibility of pretreatment CT texture features in stage III non-small cell lung cancer. *International Journal of Radiation Oncology Biology Physics, 90*(4), 834–842. https://doi.org/10.1016/j.ijrobp.2014.07.020.

Van Griethuysen, Joost J. M., Andriy Fedorov, Chintan Parmar, Ahmed Hosny, Nicole Aucoin, Vivek Narayan, Regina G. H. Beets-Tan, Jean Christophe Fillion-Robin, Steve Pieper, & Hugo J. W. L. Aerts. (2017). Computational radiomics system to decode the radiographic phenotype. *Cancer Research, 77*(21), e104–7. https://doi.org/10.1158/0008-5472.CAN-17-0339.

Grossmann, Patrick, Olya Stringfield, Nehme El-Hachem, Marilyn M. Bui, Emmanuel Rios Velazquez, Chintan Parmar, Ralph T. H. Leijenaar, Benjamin Haibe-Kains, Philippe Lambin, Robert J. Gillies, & Hugo J. W. L. Aerts. (2017). Defining the biological basis of radiomic phenotypes in lung cancer. *ELife, 6*, e23421. https://doi.org/10.7554/eLife.23421.

Haralick, Robert M., Its'hak Dinstein, & K. Shanmugam. (1973). Textural features for image classification. *IEEE Transactions on Systems, Man and Cybernetics, SMC-3*(6), 610–621. https://doi.org/10.1109/TSMC.1973.4309314.

Hatt, Mathieu, Martin Vallieres, Dimitris Visvikis, & Alex Zwanenburg. (2018). IBSI: An international community radiomics standardization initiative. *Journal of Nuclear Medicine, 59*(supplement 1), 287.

Johnson, W. Evan, Cheng Li, & Ariel Rabinovic. (2007). Adjusting batch effects in microarray expression data using empirical Bayes methods. *Biostatistics, 8*(1), 118–127. https://doi.org/10.1093/biostatistics/kxj037.

Kim, Dong Wook, Hye Young Jang, Kyung Won Kim, Youngbin Shin, & Seong Ho Park. (2019). Design characteristics of studies reporting the performance of artificial intelligence algorithms for diagnostic analysis of medical images: Results from recently published papers. *Korean Journal of Radiology, 20*(3), 405–410. https://doi.org/10.3348/kjr.2019.0025.

Lambin, Philippe, Ralph T. H. Leijenaar, Timo M. Deist, Jurgen Peerlings, Evelyn E. C. De Jong, Janita Van Timmeren, Sebastian Sanduleanu, Ruben T. H. M. Larue, Aniek J. G. Even, Arthur Jochems, Yvonka Van Wijk, Henry Woodruff, Johan Van Soest, Tim Lustberg, Erik Roelofs, Wouter Van Elmpt, Andre Dekker, Felix M. Mottaghy, Joachim E. Wildberger, & Sean Walsh. (2017). Radiomics: The bridge between medical imaging and personalized medicine. *Nature Reviews Clinical Oncology, 14*(12), 749–762. https://doi.org/10.1038/nrclinonc.2017.141.

Lambin, Philippe, Emmanuel Rios-Velazquez, Ralph Leijenaar, Sara Carvalho, Ruud G. P. M. Van Stiphout, Patrick Granton, Catharina M. L. Zegers, Robert Gillies, Ronald

Boellard, André Dekker, & Hugo J. W. L. Aerts. (2012). Radiomics: Extracting more information from medical images using advanced feature analysis. *European Journal of Cancer, 48*(4), 441–446. https://doi.org/10.1016/j.ejca.2011.11.036.

Lander, Eric S., Lauren M. Linton, Bruce Birren, Chad Nusbaum, Michael C. Zody, Jennifer Baldwin, Keri Devon, Ken Dewar, Michael Doyle, William Fitzhugh, Roel Funke, Diane Gage, Katrina Harris, Andrew Heaford, John Howland, Lisa Kann, Jessica Lehoczky, Rosie Levine, Paul McEwan, Kevin McKernan, James Meldrim, Jill P. Mesirov, Cher Miranda, William Morris, Jerome Naylor, Christina Raymond, Mark Rosetti, Ralph Santos, Andrew Sheridan, Carrie Sougnez, Nicole Stange-Thomann, Nikola Stojanovic, Aravind Subramanian, Dudley Wyman, Jane Rogers, John Sulston, Rachael Ainscough, Stephan Beck, David Bentley, John Burton, Christopher Clee, Nigel Carter, Alan Coulson, Rebecca Deadman, Panos Deloukas, Andrew Dunham, Ian Dunham, Richard Durbin, Lisa French, Darren Grafham, Simon Gregory, Tim Hubbard, Sean Humphray, Adrienne Hunt, Matthew Jones, Christine Lloyd, Amanda McMurray, Lucy Matthews, Simon Mercer, Sarah Milne, James C. Mullikin, Andrew Mungall, Robert Plumb, Mark Ross, Ratna Shownkeen, Sarah Sims, Robert H. Waterston, Richard K. Wilson, Ladeana W. Hillier, John D. McPherson, Marco A. Marra, Elaine R. Mardis, Lucinda A. Fulton, Asif T. Chinwalla, Kymberlie H. Pepin, Warren R. Gish, Stephanie L. Chissoe, Michael C. Wendl, Kim D. Delehaunty, Tracie L. Miner, Andrew Delehaunty, Jason B. Kramer, Lisa L. Cook, Robert S. Fulton, Douglas L. Johnson, Patrick J. Minx, Sandra W. Clifton, Trevor Hawkins, Elbert Branscomb, Paul Predki, Paul Richardson, Sarah Wenning, Tom Slezak, Norman Doggett, Jan Fang Cheng, Anne Olsen, Susan Lucas, Christopher Elkin, Edward Uberbacher, Marvin Frazier, Richard A. Gibbs, Donna M. Muzny, Steven E. Scherer, John B. Bouck, Erica J. Sodergren, Kim C. Worley, Catherine M. Rives, James H. Gorrell, Michael L. Metzker, Susan L. Naylor, Raju S. Kucherlapati, David L. Nelson, George M. Weinstock, Yoshiyuki Sakaki, Asao Fujiyama, Masahira Hattori, Tetsushi Yada, Atsushi Toyoda, Takehiko Itoh, Chiharu Kawagoe, Hidemi Watanabe, Yasushi Totoki, Todd Taylor, Jean Weissenbach, Roland Heilig, William Saurin, Francois Artiguenave, Philippe Brottier, Thomas Bruls, Eric Pelletier, Catherine Robert, Patrick Wincker, André Rosenthal, Matthias Platzer, Gerald Nyakatura, Stefan Taudien, Andreas Rump, Douglas R. Smith, Lynn Doucette-Stamm, Marc Rubenfield, Keith Weinstock, Mei Lee Hong, Joann Dubois, Huanming Yang, Jun Yu, Jian Wang, Guyang Huang, Jun Gu, Leroy Hood, Lee Rowen, Anup Madan, Shizen Qin, Ronald W. Davis, Nancy A. Federspiel, A. Pia Abola, Michael J. Proctor, Bruce A. Roe, Feng Chen, Huaqin Pan, Juliane Ramser, Hans Lehrach, Richard Reinhardt, W. Richard McCombie, Melissa De La Bastide, Neilay Dedhia, Helmut Blöcker, Klaus Hornischer, Gabriele Nordsiek, Richa Agarwala, L. Aravind, Jeffrey A. Bailey, Alex Bateman, Serafim Batzoglou, Ewan Birney, Peer Bork, Daniel G. Brown, Christopher B. Burge, Lorenzo Cerutti, Hsiu Chuan Chen, Deanna Church, Michele Clamp, Richard R. Copley, Tobias Doerks,

Sean R. Eddy, Evan E. Eichler, Terrence S. Furey, James Galagan, James G. R. Gilbert, Cyrus Harmon, Yoshihide Hayashizaki, David Haussler, Henning Hermjakob, Karsten Hokamp, Wonhee Jang, L. Steven Johnson, Thomas A. Jones, Simon Kasif, Arek Kaspryzk, Scot Kennedy, W. James Kent, Paul Kitts, Eugene V. Koonin, Ian Korf, David Kulp, Doron Lancet, Todd M. Lowe, Aoife McLysaght, Tarjei Mikkelsen, John V. Moran, Nicola Mulder, Victor J. Pollara, Chris P. Ponting, Greg Schuler, Jörg Schultz, Guy Slater, Arian F. A. Smit, Elia Stupka, Joseph Szustakowki, Danielle Thierry-Mieg, Jean Thierry-Mieg, Lukas Wagner, John Wallis, Raymond Wheeler, Alan Williams, Yuri I. Wolf, Kenneth H. Wolfe, Shiaw Pyng Yang, Ru Fang Yeh, Francis Collins, Mark S. Guyer, Jane Peterson, Adam Felsenfeld, Kris A. Wetterstrand, Richard M. Myers, Jeremy Schmutz, Mark Dickson, Jane Grimwood, David R. Cox, Maynard V. Olson, Rajinder Kaul, Christopher Raymond, Nobuyoshi Shimizu, Kazuhiko Kawasaki, Shinsei Minoshima, Glen A. Evans, Maria Athanasiou, Roger Schultz, Aristides Patrinos, & Michael J. Morgan. (2001). Initial sequencing and analysis of the human genome. *Nature, 409*(6822), 860–921. https://doi.org/10.1038/35057062.

Larue, Ruben T. H. M., Lien Van De Voorde, Janna E. van Timmeren, Ralph T. H. Leijenaar, Maaike Berbée, Meindert N. Sosef, Wendy M. J. Schreurs, Wouter van Elmpt, & Philippe Lambin. (2017). 4DCT imaging to assess radiomics feature stability: An investigation for thoracic cancers. *Radiotherapy and Oncology, 125*(1), 147–153. https://doi.org/10.1016/j.radonc.2017.07.023.

Leijenaar, Ralph T. H., Georgi Nalbantov, Sara Carvalho, Wouter J. C. Van Elmpt, Esther G. C. Troost, Ronald Boellaard, Hugo J. W. L. Aerts, Robert J. Gillies, & Philippe Lambin. (2015). The effect of SUV discretization in quantitative FDG-PET radiomics: The need for standardized methodology in tumor texture analysis. *Scientific Reports, 5*, 11075. https://doi.org/10.1038/srep11075.

Lin, Lawrence I. Kuei. (1989). A concordance correlation coefficient to evaluate reproducibility. *Biometrics, 45*(1), 255. https://doi.org/10.2307/2532051.

Lu, Lin, Ross C. Ehmke, Lawrence H. Schwartz, & Binsheng Zhao. (2016). Assessing agreement between radiomic features computed for multiple CT imaging settings. *PLoS ONE, 11*(12), e0166550. https://doi.org/10.1371/journal.pone.0166550.

Peerlings, Jurgen, Henry C. Woodruff, Jessica M. Winfield, Abdalla Ibrahim, Bernard E. Van Beers, Arend Heerschap, Alan Jackson, Joachim E. Wildberger, Felix M. Mottaghy, Nandita M. DeSouza, & Philippe Lambin. (2019). Stability of radiomics features in apparent diffusion coefficient maps from a multi-centre test-retest trial. *Scientific Reports, 9*(1), 4800. https://doi.org/10.1038/s41598-019-41344-5.

Reiazi, Reza, Engy Abbas, Petra Famiyeh, Aria Rezaie, Jennifer Y. Y. Kwan, Tirth Patel, Scott V. Bratman, Tony Tadic, Fei Fei Liu, & Benjamin Haibe-Kains. (2021). The impact of the variation of imaging parameters on the robustness of computed tomography radiomic features: A review. *Computers in Biology and Medicine, 133*, 104400. https://doi.org/10.1016/j.compbiomed.2021.104400.

Ronneberger, Olaf, Philipp Fischer, and Thomas Brox. (2015). U-Net: Convolutional networks for biomedical image segmentation. *Lecture Notes in Computer Science (Including Subseries Lecture Notes in Artificial Intelligence and Lecture Notes in Bioinformatics), 9351*, 234–241. https://doi.org/10.1007/978-3-319-24574-4_28.

Saadani, Hanna, Bernies Van der Hiel, Else A. Aalbersberg, Ioannis Zavrakidis, John B. A. G. Haanen, Otto S. Hoekstra, Ronald Boellaard, & Marcel P. M. Stokkel. (2019). Metabolic biomarker–based BRAFV600 mutation association and prediction in melanoma. *Journal of Nuclear Medicine, 60*(11), 1545–1552. https://doi.org/10.2967/jnumed.119.228312.

Sanduleanu, Sebastian, Arthur Jochems, Taman Upadhaya, Aniek J. G. Even, Ralph T. H. Leijenaar, Frank J. W. M. Dankers, Remy Klaassen, Henry C. Woodruff, Mathieu Hatt, Hans J. A. M. Kaanders, Olga Hamming-Vrieze, Hanneke W. M. van Laarhoven, Rathan M. Subramiam, Shao Hui Huang, Brian O'Sullivan, Scott V. Bratman, Ludwig J. Dubois, Razvan L. Miclea, Dario Di Perri, Xavier Geets, Mireia Crispin-Ortuzar, Aditya Apte, Joseph O. Deasy, Jung Hun Oh, Nancy Y. Lee, John L. Humm, Heiko Schöder, Dirk De Ruysscher, Frank Hoebers, & Philippe Lambin. (2020). Non-invasive imaging prediction of tumor hypoxia: A novel developed and externally validated CT and FDG-PET-based radiomic signatures. *Radiotherapy and Oncology, 153*, 97–105. https://doi.org/10.1016/j.radonc.2020.10.016.

Sanger, F., G. M. Air, B. G. Barrell, N. L. Brown, A. R. Coulson, J. C. Fiddes, C. A. Hutchison, P. M. Slocombe, & M. Smith. (1977). Nucleotide sequence of bacteriophage Φx174 DNA. *Nature, 265*(5596), 687–695. https://doi.org/10.1038/265687a0.

Shafiq-Ul-Hassan, Muhammad, Geoffrey G. Zhang, Kujtim Latifi, Ghanim Ullah, Dylan C. Hunt, Yoganand Balagurunathan, Mahmoud Abrahem Abdalah, Matthew B. Schabath, Dmitry G. Goldgof, Dennis Mackin, Laurence Edward Court, Robert James Gillies, & Eduardo Gerardo Moros. (2017). Intrinsic dependencies of CT radiomic features on voxel size and number of gray levels. *Medical Physics, 44*(3), 1050–1062. https://doi.org/10.1002/mp.12123.

Shiri, Isaac, Arman Rahmim, Pardis Ghaffarian, Parham Geramifar, Hamid Abdollahi, & Ahmad Bitarafan-Rajabi. (2017). The impact of image reconstruction settings on 18F-FDG PET radiomic features: Multi-scanner phantom and patient studies. *European Radiology, 27*(11), 4498–4509. https://doi.org/10.1007/s00330-017-4859-z.

Shofty, Ben, Moran Artzi, Shai Shtrozberg, Claudia Fanizzi, Francesco DiMeco, Oz Haim, Shira Peleg Hason, Zvi Ram, Dafna Ben Bashat, & Rachel Grossman. (2020). Virtual biopsy using MRI radiomics for prediction of BRAF status in melanoma brain metastasis. *Scientific Reports, 10*(1), 6623. https://doi.org/10.1038/s41598-020-63821-y.

Vallières, Martin, Emily Kay-Rivest, Léo Jean Perrin, Xavier Liem, Christophe Furstoss, Hugo J. W. L. Aerts, Nader Khaouam, Phuc Felix Nguyen-Tan, Chang Shu Wang, Khalil Sultanem, Jan Seuntjens, & Issam El Naqa. (2017). Radiomics strategies for risk assessment of tumour failure in head-and-neck cancer. *Scientific Reports, 7*(1), 1–14. https://doi.org/10.1038/s41598-017-10371-5.

Verduin, Maikel, Sergey Primakov, Inge Compter, Henry C. Woodruff, Sander M. J. van Kuijk, Bram L. T. Ramaekers, Maarten Te Dorsthorst, Elles G. M. Revenich, Mark Ter Laan, Sjoert A. H. Pegge, Frederick J. A. Meijer, Jan Beckervordersandforth, Ernst Jan Speel, Benno Kusters, Wendy W. J. de Leng, Monique M. Anten, Martijn P. G. Broen, Linda Ackermans, Olaf E. M. G. Schijns, Onno Teernstra, Koos Hovinga, Marc A. Vooijs, Vivianne C. G. Tjan-heijnen, Danielle B. P. Eekers, Alida A. Postma, Philippe Lambin, & Ann Hoeben. (2021). Prognostic and predictive value of integrated qualitative and quantitative magnetic resonance imaging analysis in glioblastoma. *Cancers, 13*(4), 1–20. https://doi.org/10.3390/cancers13040722.

Welch, Mattea L., Chris McIntosh, Benjamin Haibe-Kains, Michael F. Milosevic, Leonard Wee, Andre Dekker, Shao Hui Huang, Thomas G. Purdie, Brian O'Sullivan, Hugo J. W. L. Aerts, & David A. Jaffray. (2019). Vulnerabilities of radiomic signature development: The need for safeguards. *Radiotherapy and Oncology, 130*, 2–9. https://doi.org/10.1016/j.radonc.2018.10.027.

Yang, Lei, Di Dong, Mengjie Fang, Yongbei Zhu, Yali Zang, Zhenyu Liu, Hongmei Zhang, Jianming Ying, Xinming Zhao, & Jie Tian. (2018). Can CT-based radiomics signature predict KRAS/NRAS/BRAF mutations in colorectal cancer? *European Radiology, 28*(5), 2058–2067. https://doi.org/10.1007/s00330-017-5146-8.

Yip, Stephen S. F., John Kim, Thibaud P. Coroller, Chintan Parmar, Emmanuel Rios Velazquez, Elizabeth Huynh, Raymond H. Mak, & Hugo J. W. L. Aerts. (2017). Associations between somatic mutations and metabolic imaging phenotypes in non-small cell lung cancer. *Journal of Nuclear Medicine, 58*(4), 569–576. https://doi.org/10.2967/jnumed.116.181826.

Zwanenburg, Alex, Martin Vallières, Mahmoud A. Abdalah, Hugo J. W. L. Aerts, Vincent Andrearczyk, Aditya Apte, Saeed Ashrafinia, Spyridon Bakas, Roelof J. Beukinga, Ronald Boellaard, Marta Bogowicz, Luca Boldrini, Irène Buvat, Gary J. R. Cook, Christos Davatzikos, Adrien Depeursinge, Marie Charlotte Desseroit, Nicola Dinapoli, Cuong Viet Dinh, Sebastian Echegaray, Issam El Naqa, Andriy Y. Fedorov, Roberto Gatta, Robert J. Gillies, Vicky Goh, Michael Götz, Matthias Guckenberger, Sung Min Ha, Mathieu Hatt, Fabian Isensee, Philippe Lambin, Stefan Leger, Ralph T. H. Leijenaar, Jacopo Lenkowicz, Fiona Lippert, Are Losnegård, Klaus H. Maier-Hein, Olivier Morin, Henning Müller, Sandy Napel, Christophe Nioche, Fanny Orlhac, Sarthak Pati, Elisabeth A. G. Pfaehler, Arman Rahmim, Arvind U. K. Rao, Jonas Scherer, Muhammad Musib Siddique, Nanna M. Sijtsema, Jairo Socarras Fernandez, Emiliano Spezi, Roel J. H. M. Steenbakkers, Stephanie Tanadini-Lang, Daniela Thorwarth, Esther G. C. Troost, Taman Upadhaya, Vincenzo Valentini, Lisanne V. van Dijk, Joost van Griethuysen, Floris H. P. van Velden, Philip Whybra, Christian Richter, & Steffen Löck. (2020). The image biomarker standardization initiative: Standardized quantitative radiomics for high-throughput image-based phenotyping. *Radiology, 295*(2), 328–338. https://doi.org/10.1148/radiol.2020191145.

Chapter 6

Artificial Intelligence for Image Segmentation in Radiation Oncology

Xue Feng* and Quan Chen†

**Carina Medical LLC, 145 Graham Ave, A168, Lexington, KY 40506, USA*

†*Radiation Oncology, City of Hope Comprehensive Cancer Center, 1500 E Duarte Rd, Duarte, CA 91010, USA*

Abstract

Image segmentation is an important task in radiation oncology. For example, radiation therapy requires accurate organ and tumor contours to design the treatment plan. In addition, outcome prediction using radiomics also needs structures of interest to be accurately segmented in order to obtain intensity, texture, and statistical information. Recently, artificial intelligence (AI), represented by the deep-learning approaches, has shown great performance improvements in medical image segmentation compared to traditional approaches. However, while the deep-learning approach showed great promise in clinical adoption, issues on robustness of the AI model arise. In this chapter, the AI techniques will be first introduced, followed by the advantages and limitations of the AI segmentation models, finally, strategies for clinical adoption will be recommended.

1. Importance of Segmentation in Radiation Oncology

Radiation Oncology primarily relies on ionizing radiation to treat cancer, a process called radiation therapy. In radiation therapy, the ability of local control increases with the administrated dose (Hara *et al.*, 2002; Rusthoven *et al.*, 2009). However, as higher doses are applied, the organs-at-risk (OARs) around the tumor may receive high enough doses to affect their functions, which in turn can increase morbidity and reduce overall survival (Stam *et al.*, 2017; Timmerman *et al.*, 2006; Wu *et al.*, 2014). As radiation therapy techniques have improved, both in treatment delivery and in treatment planning, it is possible to create sharp dose fall-offs around the tumor and trade-off between tumor coverage and OAR sparing. In order for the optimizer to make appropriate adjustments, both tumor and OARs have to be accurately segmented. Errors in tumor or OAR segmentation could lead to over- or under-coverage of the tumor or damage to critical organs. Therefore, accurate segmentation is very important for radiation therapy treatment planning.

Conventionally, the tumor and OARs are segmented manually by radiation oncologists or dosimetrists. However, as manual contouring is a tedious task, it often suffers from human fatigue. Contouring error has been identified as one of the most critical in the treatment planning process (Broggi *et al.*, 2013; Chen *et al.*, 2015; Ford *et al.*, 2020; Hui *et al.*, 2018). In addition, there can be fairly large inter- and intra-observer variability even among expert radiation oncologists. Li *et. al.* compared target and normal structure delineation by nine expert radiation oncologists from eight institutions (Li *et al.*, 2009). They found that the variability in contouring the targets and OARs was substantial, with overlaps as low as 10% and standard deviation in volume as high as 60% for target structures, and overlaps as low as 35.8% and standard deviation in volume as high as 18.3% for the heart. This created variation in target coverage (range of 85–95%) and OAR dose (Lung V20 from 5% to 25%, Heart V10 from 2% to 20%) (Li *et al.*, 2009). An analysis of prostate contouring by five well-trained radiation oncologist showed that the inter-observer variability for prostate is the largest at the anterior side with a standard deviation of 7.1 mm and between 2–3 mm at other sides (Fiorino *et al.*, 1998). Due to this uncertainty, often-used larger margins increase dose to surrounding OARs. The inaccuracy and inconsistency in organ contouring impede obtaining accurate data to model normal tissue toxicity, especially in national clinical trials. Researchers from Memorial Sloan-Kettering Cancer Center examined the treatment plans submitted to the Radiation Therapy Oncology Group (RTOG) 0617 dose escalation trial. Using a coherent heart definition, they found that the heart dose in RTOG 0617 is significantly higher than reported using the contouring in the original treatment plan (Thor *et al.*, 2021). In this case, the inaccuracy of the clinical contour leads to higher toxicity to patients and could affect the determination of the radiation toxicity to the heart.

In addition to accuracy and consistency, another concern for manual contouring is the cost of time and labor. It can take several hours to contour a head and neck case (Hong *et al.*, 2012; Vorwerk *et al.*, 2014). This presents a barrier for wider adoption of adaptive radiation therapy (ART) (Yan *et al.*, 1997, 1998). In ART, the treatment plan is adjusted during the course of treatment to account for the anatomical changes in the patient (e.g. weight loss, bladder filling, tumor response) or the patient's response to the current treatment (e.g. normal tissue toxicity). The end result is an improved tumor control and/or reduction in normal tissue toxicity. Studies have demonstrated improved loco-regional control in nasopharyngeal and oropharyngeal cancers (Schwartz *et al.*, 2012; Yang *et al.*, 2013), improvements in both normal tissue toxicity and tumor control in prostate cancers (Brabbins *et al.*, 2005), 20% improvement in two-year tumor controls in non-small-cell lung cancer (Kong *et al.*, 2017). In order to perform adaptive re-planning, organ segmentation has to be performed on the new planning imaging. This dramatically increases the workload for radiation oncologists and dosimetrists. Recently, the online-ART approach (Lim-Reinders *et al.*, 2017), which involves adjusting treatment plan based on the daily imaging of patient anatomy, demonstrates great promise in improving treatment outcome. It has produced 60% improvement in two-year overall survival in pancreatic cancer cases (Rudra *et al.*, 2019). In online-ART, the treatment plan adjustment is performed while the patient is lying on the table waiting for the treatment to start.

Thus, the speed for segmentation is very important for online-ART (Byrne *et al.*, 2021).

The conventional cancer treatment is a "one-size-fits-all" approach, where the patients who have the same cancer and staging receive the same standardized treatment. Multiple evidences have shown the heterogeneity of the tumor and the patient response (Li *et al.*, 2018; Nardone *et al.*, 2018; Paul *et al.*, 2017). In particular, information about tumor genotypes and patients' responses can be mined from medical images. This approach was termed as "radiomics" (Lambin *et al.*, 2012). Personalized treatment based on radiomics has gained a lot of interest. Radiomics features have shown good performance in predicting the treatment response (Li *et al.*, 2018; Nardone *et al.*, 2018; Paul *et al.*, 2017). This information can help oncologists select a better treatment plan based on the expected response. Radiomics features include shape-based, intensity-based, and texture-based features. The first step in the calculation of the radiomics feature is the segmentation of the region of interest (ROI), usually the tumor itself. Conventionally, the ROI were outlined manually by expert oncologists or radiologists. Similar to the treatment planning, the accuracy and consistency of manual contouring will affect the validity of the radiomic features identified and negatively impact the interpretation of the radiomics study.

2. Review of Deep Learning Technologies in Medical Image Segmentation

Tremendous effort has been invested into the development of auto-segmentation solutions. The atlas-based auto-segmentation showed a promising result and multiple commercial software were developed based on that technology, including Varian Smart Segmentation, Elekta ABAS, Pinnacle SPICE, Raystation, VelocityAI, and MIM Maestro. However, a survey showed that while 70% of the clinics have one of these tools, only 30% of them used these tools in clinical practice (Sharp *et al.*, 2014). The major issue cited for underutilization of these tools was poor segmentation quality. Studies has have shown that substantial manual editing times are still required after the auto-segmentation (Caria *et al.*, 2013; Gambacorta *et al.*, 2013; Gooding *et al.*, 2013; La Macchia *et al.*, 2012; Teguh *et al.*, 2011; Walker *et al.*, 2014). In some cases, the operator prefers to perform manual contours from scratch rather than edit existing contours (Thomson *et al.*, 2014).

Deep learning — a recently developed technique that applies artificial intelligence techniques to image classification, detection, and segmentation — has demonstrated superior performance over that of humans alone (Krizhevsky *et al.*, 2012; Long *et al.*, 2015; Ren *et al.*, 2015). Early adoptions in medical imaging applications, including segmentation, have shown great promise (Çiçek *et al.*, 2016; Havaei *et al.*, 2017; Ronneberger *et al.*, 2015). Different from traditional atlas-, edge-, or shape-based segmentation methods, which mainly rely on pre-defined rules or priors, deep learning mainly uses a convolutional neural network (CNN) structure that contains many convolution, pooling, and/or upsampling layers and the network is trained from a given dataset with ground-truth to optimize itself toward a specific task with few, if at all, prior information. Many neural network architectures have been proposed in order for the deep learning model to better learn the segmentation task from the limited training data. It is not the purpose of this chapter to perform a comprehensive literature review. Instead, only a few core network architectures will be briefly introduced.

2.1. *Fully Convolution Network (FCN)*

Fully convolution network (FCN) is one of the earliest network architectures developed for segmentation tasks (Long *et al.*, 2015). It converts fully connected layers in classification network architectures, which throw away spatial coordinates and produce only predictions, into convolution layers, which preserves spatial information. In order to produce pixel-by-pixel segmentation, backwards strided convolution was used to up-sample the result. Figure 1 illustrates the basic FCN architecture. The FCN was

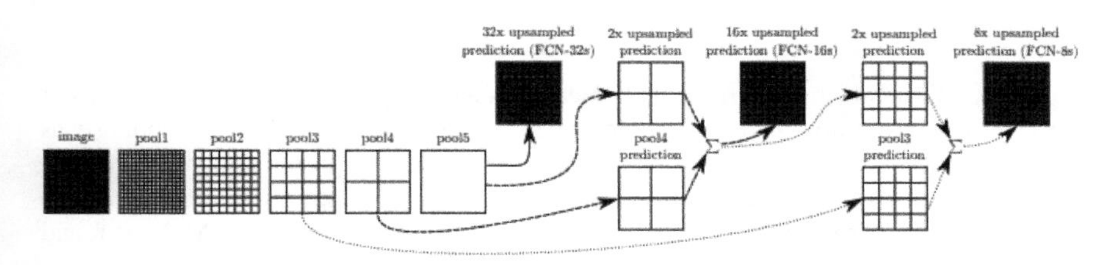

Fig. 1. FCN architecture (Long *et al.*, 2015).

adapted for different segmentation problems and demonstrated good performance, including the segmentation of infant brain image during the isotense phase on MRI images (Nie *et al.*, 2018), multi-organ segmentation on abdominal CT (Roth *et al.*, 2018), and intervertebral disk segmentation on multi-modality MRI (Li *et al.*, 2018).

2.2. *U-Net*

U-Net architecture is an extension of the FCN architecture. The general structure of the U-Net is shown in Fig. 2. In essence, it is can be considered as an encoder–decoder with skip connections between different feature scales of the encoder and decoder. On the encoder side, the image feature information is extracted while the spatial information is reduced. Similar to the FCN network, the spatial information was recovered through the up-sampling with the decoder. At the same time, the skip connection brings high-resolution features from the encoder side to help with

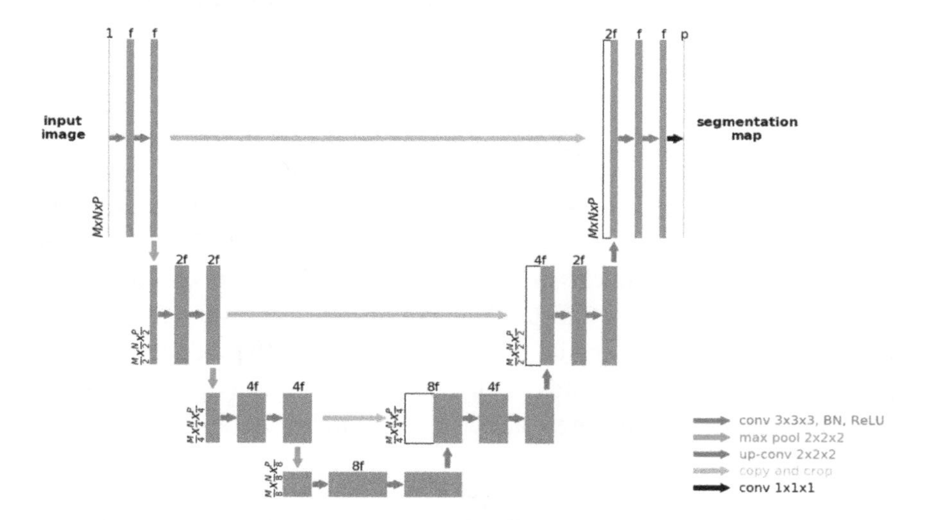

Figure 2. General structure for a 3D U-Net. Each encoding block consists of two sets of consecutive convolution, batch norm, and rectifier linear activation layers. Padding was used to maintain the spatial dimension during convolution. Number of features were doubled after each pooling layer. Long range connections were used by concatenating the outputs from the corresponding encoding blocks with the decoding blocks. M, N, P, f, and p are parameters that are unique for each network.

the spatial information recover. This innovative design improves the segmentation performance dramatically (Ronneberger *et al.*, 2015).

Since the introduction of the original U-Net concept, multiple adjustments have been attempted. The original U-Net was implemented for 2D images. To better utilize the 3D spatial information carried by most medical imaging modalities for volumetric segmentation, the U-Net architecture was simply extended to accommodate 3D volumetric data and become 3D U-Nets (Çiçek *et al.*, 2016; Feng *et al.*, 2019; Yang *et al.*, 2018) (shown in Fig. 2). On the other hand, 3D U-Net requires large amount of GPU memory and incurs much higher computational cost. To address these issues, a 2.5D approach was tested (Angermann & Haltmeier, 2019; Hu *et al.*, 2018).

To better accommodate the 3D volumetric images, V-Net was developed based on the U-Net architecture (Milletari *et al.*, 2016). The V-Net also has the encoder–decoder design and the skip connections between them. The major difference is that the V-Net introduces residual blocks at each stage. The introduction of residual blocks allows the information flows to deep layers of the network, allowing more accurate and faster convergence. Also, the pooling layer is replaced by convolution. One variant of the V-Net architecture, Dense V-Net, achieved significantly better results on abdominal CT segmentation than other methods (Gibson *et al.*, 2018).

In the U-Net design, the skip connection is designed to bring in spatial information from the encoder side. However, this also brings across redundant low-level feature extractions that can degrade the segmentation performance. To suppress activation in irrelevant regions, "soft attention" is implemented which weights the skip-connected images from the encoder side based on the relevance. The resulting attention U-Net has shown to improve the segmentation of the pancreas in the abdominal CT (Oktay *et al.*, 2018).

U-Net++ (Zhou *et al.*, 2018, 2019) is another attempt to improve upon U-Net by using the dense block ideas from the DenseNet (Iandola *et al.*, 2014). The key innovations in U-Net++ include the use of dense skip connections to improve gradient flow, perform convolution on skip pathways to bridge the semantic gap between the encoder and decoder feature maps, and perform deep supervision to improve the model performance.

The U-Net++ has demonstrated better performance than baseline models on multiple imaging modalities such as CT and MRI (Zhou *et al.*, 2019).

2.3. *Generative Adversarial Network (GAN)*

GAN is originally designed for generative modeling. The basic GAN consists of a discriminator and a generator. The generator learns to create "fakes" that can fool the discriminator and the discriminator learns to catch those "fakes". While the initial application was in image enhancement, it quickly finds application in a variety of applications, including segmentation. To train GAN for segmentation, the generator becomes a segmentor, which takes in images and produces a segmentation. The segmentor can use any existing architectures for segmentation, such as FCN, U-Net, etc. The discrimator needs to read the segmentation and the original images and determine whether the segmentation is good or bad. The architectures used for the discrimator can be a classifier network such as FCN. During the training process, both the discrimator and the segmentor try to defeat each other. Any improvement for one network would prompt the other to learn. The end result of this adversarial learning process is that the segmentor learns to produce accurate segmentation. Using MICCAI brain tumor segmentation challenge data, a SegAN network with multi-scale loss was trained with this adversarial learning process and demonstrated better performance than the state-of-the-art U-net segmentation method (Xue *et al.*, 2018).

Since the GAN is very successful in generating realistic images, another use of GAN for segmentation is to perform data augmentation. The training of deep learning models requires a large amount of training data for the massive neural network to properly train. However, this is often difficult to satisfy. Data augmentation is one of the basic strategies to increase the training data by performing simple translation, rotation. However, these simple strategies are limited in the variations they can create. A GAN can produce variations in the training data, which can help reducing overfitting and improving model generalization. This method had been applied to brain tumor segmentation tasks and demonstrated improvement in segmentation accuracy (Bowles *et al.*, 2018). In another study, the U-Net trained on contrast enhanced CT images generalized poorly on non-contrast CTs. With a cycleGAN model that was trained on a separate image database to transform contrast CT images into non-contrast images, non-contrast CTs were created from the contrast CTs in the training data. The U-Net re-trained on both original and synthetic non-contrast images demonstrated dramatic improvement in kidney segmentation on non-contrast CTs (*DSC* improves from 0.09 to 0.94) (Sandfort *et al.*, 2019).

3. Evaluation of Auto-segmentation Performance

The simplest method for evaluating auto-segmentation performance is to compare the contours created with a ground truth contour. Various indexes can be computed to reflect the geometric similarity with the ground truth. These indexes include dice similarity coefficient (*DSC*), *recall*, *precision*, Hausdorff distance (*HD*) (including maximum and different percentile), and mean surface distance (*MSD*). *DSC* is calculated as follows:

$$DSC = \frac{2|X \cap Y|}{|X| + |Y|} \tag{1}$$

where *X* and *Y* are the ground truth and the tested contours, respectively.

Alternatively, we can consider the part of ground truth contour *X* covered by the tested contour *Y* as true-positive (*TP*). Similarly, we can define false-negative (*FN*) and false-positive (*FP*) as Fig. 3 illustrated. *Recall*, or true positive rate, can be calculated as follows:

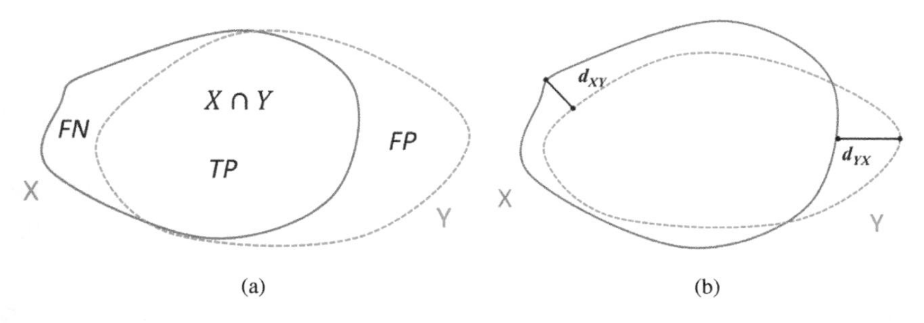

Fig. 3. Illustration for (a) *DSC, Recall, Precision* and (b) *HD*.

$$Recall = \frac{|X \cap Y|}{|X|}. \tag{2}$$

Precision, or positive predictive value can be calculated as follows:

$$Precision = \frac{|X \cap Y|}{|Y|}. \tag{3}$$

The directed *HD* from contour *X* to *Y* is defined as

$$\vec{d}_{X,Y} = max_{x \in X}(min_{y \in Y} d(x, y)), \tag{4}$$

where $d(x,y)$ is the distance between point x in X and point y in Y.

The maximum bidirectional *HD* between contour *X* and *Y* is then

$$HD = max\left(\vec{d}_{X,Y}, \vec{d}_{Y,X}\right). \tag{5}$$

The percentile *HD* can be similarly defined by switching the max function in Eq. (4) into percentile function, and turn the max function in Eq. (5) into mean.

The directed average Hausdorff measure is the average distance of a point in *X* to its closest point in *Y*, given as

$$\vec{d}_{H,avg}(X, Y) = \frac{1}{|X|} \sum_{x \in X} min_{y \in Y} d(x, y). \tag{6}$$

The mean surface distance (*MSD*) is then defined as the average of the two directed average Hausdorff measures, as follows:

$$MSD = \frac{\vec{d}_{H,avg}(X, Y) + \vec{d}_{H,avg}(Y, X)}{2}. \tag{7}$$

DSC, *precision*, and *recall* are unitless quantities between [0, 1], with higher value indicating better agreement. *HD* (maximum and percentile) and *MSD* have the unit of distance with smaller value indicating better agreement. While the general properties of each of the metrics are clear, it is difficult to tell directly whether a contour is "good" based on the value of those metrics alone. Due to the limited imaging resolution, as well as the instability of the human hand when drawing contours, it is expected that manual contours contain deviations from the underlying anatomical structures. In addition, structures lacking contrast along their borders would also pose challenges for the interpretation of the true boundaries. It has been well documented that the inter-observer and intra-observer variability remains high even among expert radiation oncologists (Joskowicz *et al.*, 2019; Loo *et al.*, 2012; Tao *et al.*, 2015). However, the same amount of deviation in distance would produce different impact on the *DSC*, *recall*, *precision* scores on structures of different sizes. Smaller structures will experience a bigger drop in these metrics than larger structures. As a result, a *DSC* score of 0.95 may not be considered good enough for lungs, while a *DSC* score of 0.6 for optic chiasm is considered very good.

Inter-observer variability (IOV) for each structure under evaluation is often characterized when evaluating auto-segmentation performance. Multiple human experts would independently contour the same group of cases. The disagreement between the human experts' contours would be measured using the geometric evaluation metrics such as *DSC*, *HD*. These measures of IOV will serve as benchmarks. If an auto-segmentation algorithm achieves the geometric evaluation metrics better than the IOV, it is usually considered to achieve "similar or better than human expert performance". In multiple studies, the deep learning-based segmentation algorithms have demonstrated similar or better performance than human experts based on one or multiple metrics (Feng *et al.*, 2019; Wong *et al.*, 2020; Yang *et al.*, 2018).

The choice of contours used as "ground truth" also requires attention. Often, the contours used clinically were taken as the "ground truth". However, the quality of such a contour depends on how rigorously the contouring was created and its quality controlled. Therefore, those contours need to be carefully reviewed and, in many cases, edited before they can be regarded as good quality contours. Still, this contouring only reflects the judgment of one observer. A "consensus" contour could be created from multiple observers through a simultaneous truth and performance level estimation (STAPLE) algorithm (Kosmin *et al.*, 2019;

Liu *et al.*, 2019; Warfield *et al.*, 2004). This consensus contour would be more robust to random errors from individual observers. This may lead to better agreement with a segmentation that is also unbiased, as Liu *et al.*'s study (Liu *et al.*, 2019) demonstrated.

The geometric indexes had been widely adopted in the evaluation of the segmentation performance. They provide an objective measure of the contour agreement and are very convenient to compare different algorithms or adjustments on the same reference. IOV studies can be used to establish relevant benchmarks for these indexes. However, there are still limitations on these indexes. *DSC*, *recall*, *precision*, and *MSD* are indexes that assess the overall agreement of the entire structure. As a result, good agreement on the majority of the contours could mask out large deviations on a small section of the contour. Figure 4 illustrates this scenario. *DSC*, *recall*, *precision* would be very close to a perfect score of 1.0, and the *MSD* would also be nearly perfect, even though the contour *Y* contained a mis-contouring and likely significantly impacts the maximum dose evaluation of this structure. The percentile *HD* may also fail to detect this except for the maximum bidirectional *HD*. This example shows that passing certainty threshold for one or several geometric indexes does not necessary guarantee the clinical acceptability of a contour.

In radiation therapy treatment planning workflow, the contouring for target and organs created by resident oncologists or dosimetrists needs to be reviewed and approved by the attending radiation oncologist. For deep learning-based auto-segmentation used in clinical practice, the contours created have to also pass the scrutiny of the attending radiation oncologist.

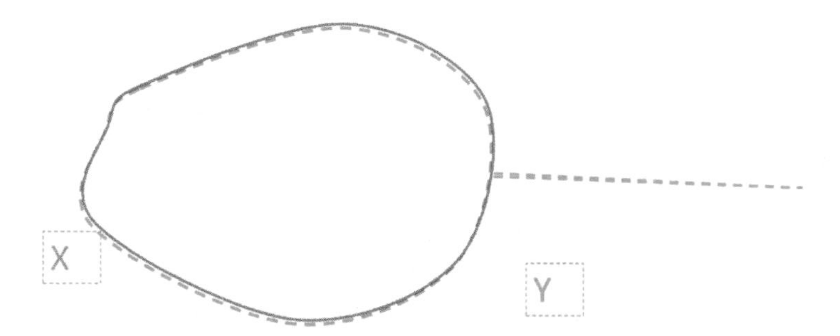

Fig. 4. An example illustrating the limitation of geometric indexes.

In the case that contour editing may be needed, the time taken for the editing should also be recorded to evaluate whether the auto-contouring can indeed improve the efficiency in the clinical workflow. A "Turing Test" was designed for eight clinical observers to evaluate the clinical acceptability of auto-contouring in a blinded study design (Gooding *et al.*, 2018). The manual editing time was also recorded. It was found that a significant portion of the deep learning-based auto-contour was deemed indistinguishable from the manual contour and therefore provides a great time saving option. One interesting finding is that the *DSC* scores are less correlated with the time saved as compared to the observer's assessment. This again highlights the importance of performing observer assessment of the contouring performance when evaluating the clinical utility of auto-segmentation methods. The time and workload saving of one deep-learning auto-contouring software were evaluated and compared against manual contouring and atlas-based auto-contouring of bladder and rectum (Zabel *et al.*, 2021). It was found that the deep-learning auto-contouring software requires similar radiation oncologist review and editing time compared with manual contours and much less than atlas-based methods.

The review by an expert radiation oncologist can identify clinically unacceptable contour deviations. However, this could be a time-consuming process if a thorough review is required. The clinically unacceptable designation is also subjective. Some may apply stricter criteria while others may be laxer. Even for the same oncologist, the criteria can be inconsistent and could be affected by other factors like the time of the day or the amount of clinical workload outstanding. The ultimate evaluation of the clinical acceptability of the auto-contours is to evaluate the clinical acceptability of the treatment plan created with the auto-contours. It should be noted that the ground truth contour should be used to evaluate the dosimetry of plans created with the auto-contour, otherwise it becomes a self-fulfilling prophecy. The dose volume histogram achieved by the plan can be compared against the tolerance tables adopted locally to determine if the auto-contour can be safely used to create treatment plans. This is an objective evaluation and the standards are consistent. Therefore, it is another important method for auto-segmentation evaluation.

4. Challenges in Adopting AI Segmentation in Clinical Practice

While superb performance metrics were reported in the literature or by vendors that use AI segmentation techniques, it should not be taken for granted that the same performance will be achieved in individual clinical practice. It has been well-documented that a well-trained deep learning model on data from one institution would produce worse results if tested on data from different institutions (AlBadawy *et al.*, 2018; Alis *et al.*, 2021). Factors that may contribute to this performance loss include generalization error and different contouring guidelines used.

4.1. *Generalization error*

Generalization error is a common issue that plagues the machine learning models (Advani *et al.*, 2020). Generalization error describes the loss of performance of a well-trained machine learning model due to overtraining on a distributationally shifted data set. There can be many sources contributing to the generalization error of a given neural network, such as imaging protocol, patient pose, contrast administration, implants, abnormal patient anatomy (collapsed lung, resection of organs). It has been shown that even simple transformations (Azulay & Weiss, 2018; Engstrom *et al.*, 2017; Pei *et al.*, 2017) can pose challenges to the neural network.

A study by Feng *et al.* (2020) showed that even a state-of-the-art model trained on data from three institutions and having achieved top finishes in a public challenge (Feng *et al.*, 2019; Yang *et al.*, 2018) had trouble with data from a different institution. The root cause was identified as the use of abdomen compression technique during the CT which changed the locations of organs relative to the bony anatomy, as illustrated in Fig. 5. Since the model was trained with data from institutions that do not adopt this practice, the model mishandled this anatomy and produced a completely wrong heart segmentation illustrated in Fig. 6(a). It was only after including the data with abdomen compression into the training data that the model learned how to correctly handle this anatomy, as illustrated in Fig. 6(b).

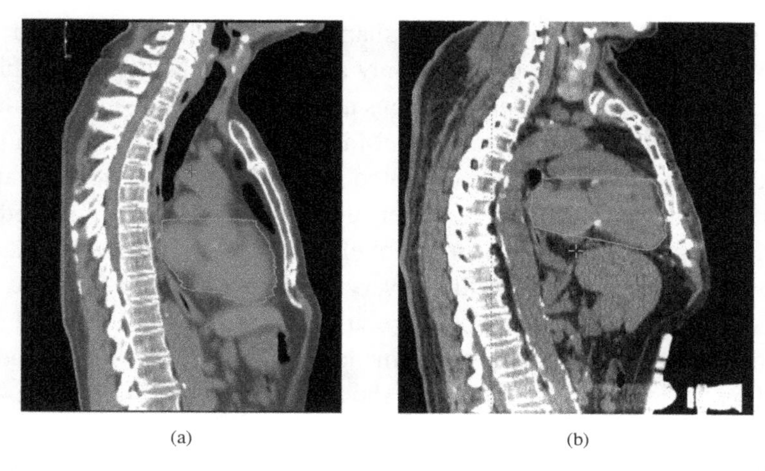

(a) (b)

Fig. 5. Difference between data used in model training (a) and the data from test institution (b). Due to the use of abdomen compression technique in the test institution (the compressor is visible at the bottom), internal organs such as liver and heart were pushed superiorly. The ground truth heart contour was overlaid on each image.

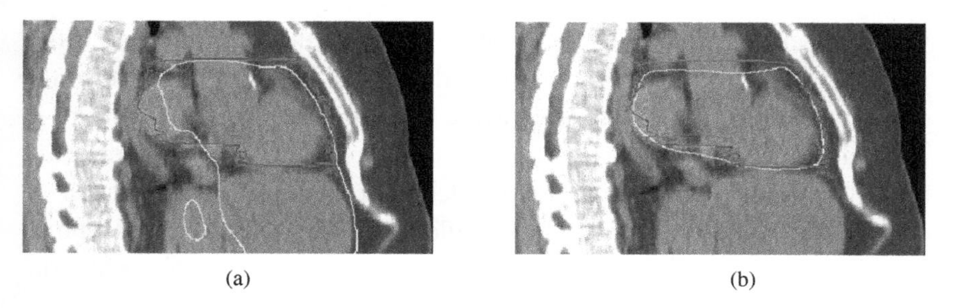

(a) (b)

Fig. 6. Example of (a) mis-segmentation of heart with the original model and (b) correct segmentation after the inclusion of data with abdomen compression in the training data. Blue contour shows the ground truth manual contour. Light green contour shows the auto-segmentation.

As this example shows, the most direct way to address the generalization issue of a deep learning model is to train the model with a great variety of data that can be seen in clinical practice. However, the effort involved in data collection and training can be prohibitive. Especially due to data privacy and data ownership concerns, institutions are reluctant to provide data to third-party vendors. While the Cancer Imaging Archive

(TCIA) provides a platform for sharing anonymized data, and the uploaded collections are growing, only a small percentage include high-quality contouring. Technical solutions attempting to bypass those limitations, such as federated learning (McMahan *et al.*, 2017), have been proposed and the feasibility demonstrated on medical image segmentation tasks (Sheller *et al.*, 2018). However, these approaches can only reduce the chance of generalization error, not eliminate them, as it is technically impossible to exhaustively collect every possible variety of data that can be seen in clinical practice. Therefore, it is expected that AI may fail during the clinical practice. It is recommended that users who wish to adopt an AI model into their local practice should rigorously test the model with the local data to ensure the generalization error is small.

Another issue in the generalization error for AI models is that it tends to fail in an unpredictable and unrealistic manner. As shown in Fig. 6(a), when the heart segmentation failed, it yielded a result that is very far away from the expected heart shape so that the impact to dose calculation may be higher if left uncorrected. This is because most AI models perform a voxel-by-voxel prediction instead of considering the overall shape information; while in atlas-based methods, the output shape is confined to the orthogonal space of the chosen atlases. Incorporating shape constraint in AI is a promising area for research, as summarized in Bohlender *et al.* (2021), however, one challenge is deciding when and how much to enforce the shape constraint. As the failed cases are usually a small number, or related to different imaging protocols, it may negatively affect the performance of the majority cases if the constraint is applied to every case. Further studies, such as automatic quality check for the output contours so that the shape constraint can be applied more aggressively to the failed cases, may provide a good solution for this problem.

4.2. *Variation in contouring standard*

In clinical practice, the contouring of the same organ can vary between physicians and clinics (Allen Li *et al.*, 2009; Nelms *et al.*, 2012; van der Veen *et al.*, 2019, 2021). Although contouring guidelines are developed to create consistent contouring across different institutions (Brouwer *et al.*, 2015; Jabbour *et al.*, 2014), the various guidelines themselves can become the source of confusion and inconsistent contouring. For example, in NRG-BR001{Oncology NRG, #134}, RTOG-0618{Timmerman, 2006 #135} and RTOG-0236{Timmerman, 2006 #136}, the heart is contoured with the superior aspect beginning at the level of the inferior aspect of the aortic arch. However, in RTOG-1106{Kong, 2012 #137}, the heart is contoured with the superior aspect beginning at the level of the inferior aspect of the pulmonary artery passing the midline. In another example, the parotid is defined to have superior boundary at external auditory canal and in mastoid process in a 2009 guideline{Van de Water, 2009 #139}. However, in a 2013 guideline, the superior border is defined as a zygomatic arch{Hoebers, 2013 #138}. It is expected that with the accumulation of more normal tissue complication cases, guidelines for contouring those normal tissues as avoidance can be updated accordingly (Caglar *et al.*, 2008; Christianen *et al.*, 2011, 2012; Barbara Stam *et al.*, 2017). Physicians following different studies may adopt different contouring guidelines, which can lead to inconsistent contouring (Brouwer *et al.*, 2014). While there are efforts from multiple organizations to create a unified contour guideline (Brouwer *et al.*, 2015; Grégoire *et al.*, 2018), with the most recent being initiated by NRG{Mir, 2020 #140}, new clinical evidence may prompt the change in guidelines again, such as the most recent update of the prostate and prostate bed contouring guideline (Grégoire *et al.*, 2018; Robin *et al.*, 2021). Therefore, an AI segmentation model trained with data following one contouring guideline may face resistance from clinics that follow a different contouring guideline. Also, the AI segmentation model trained to follow the current contouring guideline may become obsolete a few years later. In those cases, either the vendor needs to provide the new model, or the clinic has to train their own model. However, collecting enough data, training, and tuning the AI model will require a lot of effort and expertise that are beyond most clinical users. Therefore, this can be another challenge to the universal adoption of AI segmentation. Users who wish to adopt an AI model should evaluate the contour and determine if it follows their clinical practice as part of their commissioning process. Subsequently, routine QA should be established to check if the performance of an AI model is still satisfactory as clinically adopted contouring guidelines change.

5. Summary

In this chapter, we reviewed the use of AI segmentation in radiation oncology. The primary application of the segmentation is to delineate the OAR and determine accurate treatment plans. The AI segmentation relieves humans from repetitive tasks so that they can focus their attention on more important tasks. In addition, the speediness of AI segmentation can facilitate the online-ART process to produce better treatment for patients. A few popular neural network architectures and approaches have been briefly introduced, along with literature that reports good results using these networks and approaches. Various metrics that were frequently used to evaluate AI segmentation performance have been described. Pros and Cons of each metrics in the performance evaluation have been discussed. While geometric indexes such as DSC have been widely adopted, these values are insufficient to determine the clinical acceptability of a given contour. It is recommended to include the expert's evaluation as well as dosimetric analysis for the assessment of the clinical acceptability of AI contours. Finally, the challenges of the clinical adoption of AI contours have been discussed. Due to the limitation of AI segmentation models, before adopting a given model into clinical practice, it is highly recommended that the model's performance is evaluated on the local data set to ensure that the generalization error is small, and the contouring conforms to the guideline adopted by the local clinic.

References

Advani, M. S., Saxe, A. M., & Sompolinsky, H. (2020). High-dimensional dynamics of generalization error in neural networks. *Neural Networks, 132*, 428–446.

AlBadawy, E. A., Saha, A., & Mazurowski, M. A. (2018). Deep learning for segmentation of brain tumors: Impact of cross-institutional training and testing. *Medical Physics, 45*(3), 1150–1158.

Alis, D., Yergin, M., Alis, C., Topel, C., Asmakutlu, O., Bagcilar, O., ... Dogan, S. N. (2021). Inter-vendor performance of deep learning in segmenting acute ischemic lesions on diffusion-weighted imaging: A multicenter study. *Scientific Reports, 11*(1), 1–10.

Angermann, C. & Haltmeier, M. (2019). Random 2.5 d u-net for fully 3d segmentation. In *Machine Learning and Medical Engineering for Cardiovascular Health and Intravascular Imaging and Computer Assisted Stenting* (pp. 158–166). Springer.

Azulay, A. & Weiss, Y. (2018). Why do deep convolutional networks generalize so poorly to small image transformations? *arXiv preprint arXiv:1805.12177.*

Bohlender, S., Oksuz, I., & Mukhopadhyay, A. (2021). A survey on shape-constraint deep learning for medical image segmentation. *arXiv preprint arXiv:2101.07721.*

Bowles, C., Chen, L., Guerrero, R., Bentley, P., Gunn, R., Hammers, A., ... Rueckert, D. (2018). Gan augmentation: Augmenting training data using generative adversarial networks. *arXiv preprint arXiv:1810.10863.*

Brabbins, D., Martinez, A., Yan, D., Lockman, D., Wallace, M., Gustafson, G., ... Wong, J. (2005). A dose-escalation trial with the adaptive radiotherapy process as a delivery system in localized prostate cancer: Analysis of chronic toxicity. *International Journal of Radiation Oncology — Biology — Physics, 61*(2), 400–408. https://doi.org/10.1016/j.ijrobp.2004.06.001.

Broggi, S., Cantone, M. C., Chiara, A., Di Muzio, N., Longobardi, B., Mangili, P., & Veronese, I. (2013). Application of failure mode and effects analysis (FMEA) to pretreatment phases in tomotherapy. *Journal of Applied Clinical Medical Physics, 14*(5), 265–277. https://doi.org/10.1120/jacmp.v14i5.4329.

Brouwer, C. L., Steenbakkers, R. J., Bourhis, J., Budach, W., Grau, C., Grégoire, V., ... Nutting, C. (2015). CT-based delineation of organs at risk in the head and neck region: DAHANCA, EORTC, GORTEC, HKNPCSG, NCIC CTG, NCRI, NRG Oncology and TROG consensus guidelines. *Radiotherapy and Oncology, 117*(1), 83–90.

Brouwer, C. L., Steenbakkers, R. J., Gort, E., Kamphuis, M. E., Van Der Laan, H. P., van't Veld, A. A., ... Langendijk, J. A. (2014). Differences in delineation guidelines for head and neck cancer result in inconsistent reported dose and corresponding NTCP. *Radiotherapy and Oncology, 111*(1), 148–152.

Byrne, M., Archibald-Heeren, B., Hu, Y., Teh, A., Beserminji, R., Cai, E., ... Collett, N. (2021). Varian ethos online adaptive radiotherapy for prostate cancer: Early results of contouring accuracy, treatment plan quality, and treatment time. *Journal of Applied Clinical Medical Physics, 23*(1), e13479.

Caglar, H. B., Tishler, R. B., Othus, M., Burke, E., Li, Y., Goguen, L., ... Court, L. E. (2008). Dose to larynx predicts for swallowing complications after intensity-modulated radiotherapy. *International Journal of Radiation Oncology* Biology* Physics, 72*(4), 1110–1118.

Caria, N., Engels, B., Bral, S., Hung, V. V., Doornaert, P., Muraglia, A., ... Morgas, T. (2013). VARIAN SMARTSEGMENTATION® KNOWLEDGE-BASED CONTOURING Clinical Evaluation of an Automated Segmentation Module. In *Varian Medical Systems*, Palo Alto, CA USA.

Chen, H. C., Tan, J., Dolly, S., Kavanaugh, J., Anastasio, M. A., Low, D. A., ... Li, H. (2015). Automated contouring error detection based on supervised geometric attribute distribution models for radiation therapy: A general strategy. *Medical Physics, 42*(2), 1048–1059. https://doi.org/10.1118/1.4906197.

Christianen, M. E., Langendijk, J. A., Westerlaan, H. E., van de Water, T. A., & Bijl, H. P. (2011). Delineation of organs at risk involved in swallowing for radiotherapy treatment planning. *Radiotherapy and Oncology, 101*(3), 394–402.

Christianen, M. E., Schilstra, C., Beetz, I., Muijs, C. T., Chouvalova, O., Burlage, F. R., ... Rinkel, R. N. (2012). Predictive modelling for swallowing dysfunction after primary (chemo) radiation: Results of a prospective observational study. *Radiotherapy and Oncology, 105*(1), 107–114.

Çiçek, Ö., Abdulkadir, A., Lienkamp, S. S., Brox, T., & Ronneberger, O. (2016). *3D U-Net: Learning dense volumetric segmentation from sparse annotation.* Paper presented at the International Conference on Medical Image Computing and Computer-Assisted Intervention.

Engstrom, L., Tran, B., Tsipras, D., Schmidt, L., & Madry, A. (2017). A rotation and a translation suffice: Fooling cnns with simple transformations. *arXiv preprint arXiv:1712.02779.*

Feng, X., Bernard, M. E., Hunter, T., & Chen, Q. (2020). Improving accuracy and robustness of deep convolutional neural network based thoracic OAR segmentation. *Physics in Medicine & Biology, 65*(7), 07NT01.

Feng, X., Qing, K., Tustison, N. J., Meyer, C. H., & Chen, Q. (2019). Deep convolutional neural network for segmentation of thoracic organs-at-risk using cropped 3D images. *Medical Physics, 46*(5), 2169–2180.

Fiorino, C., Reni, M., Bolognesi, A., Cattaneo, G. M., & Calandrino, R. (1998). Intra- and inter-observer variability in contouring prostate and seminal vesicles: Implications for conformal treatment planning. *Radiotherapy Oncology, 47*(3), 285–292. https://doi.org/10.1016/s0167-8140(98)00021-8.

Ford, E., Conroy, L., Dong, L., de Los Santos, L. F., Greener, A., Gwe-Ya Kim, G., ... Wells, M. (2020). Strategies for effective physics plan and chart review in radiation therapy: Report of AAPM Task Group 275. *Medical Physics, 47*(6), e236–e272. https://doi.org/10.1002/mp.14030.

Gambacorta, M. A., Valentini, C., Dinapoli, N., Boldrini, L., Caria, N., Barba, M. C., ... Valentini, V. (2013). Clinical validation of atlas-based auto-segmentation of pelvic volumes and normal tissue in rectal tumors using auto-segmentation computed system. *Acta Oncology, 52*(8), 1676–1681. https://doi.org/10.3109/0284186X.2012.754989.

Gibson, E., Giganti, F., Hu, Y., Bonmati, E., Bandula, S., Gurusamy, K., ... Barratt, D. C. (2018). Automatic multi-organ segmentation on abdominal CT with dense V-Networks. *IEEE Transactions on Medical Imaging, 37*(8), 1822–1834. https://doi.org/10.1109/TMI.2018.2806309.

Gooding, M., Chu, K., Conibear, J., Dilling, T., Durrant, L., Fuss, M., ... Kadir, T. (2013). Multicenter clinical assessment of DIR atlas-based autocontouring. *International Journal of Radiation Oncology, Biology, Physics, 87*(2), S714–S715.

Gooding, M. J., Smith, A. J., Tariq, M., Aljabar, P., Peressutti, D., van der Stoep, J., ... van Elmpt, W. (2018). Comparative evaluation of autocontouring in clinical practice: A practical method using the Turing test. *Medical Physics, 45*(11), 5105–5115. https://doi.org/10.1002/mp.13200.

Grégoire, V., Evans, M., Le, Q.-T., Bourhis, J., Budach, V., Chen, A., ... Gupta, T. (2018). Delineation of the primary tumour clinical target volumes (ctv-p) in laryngeal, hypopharyngeal, oropharyngeal and oral cavity squamous cell carcinoma: Airo, caca, dahanca, eortc, georcc, gortec, hknpcsg, hncig, iag-kht, lprhht, ncic ctg, ncri, nrg oncology, phns, sbrt, somera, sro, sshno, trog consensus guidelines. *Radiotherapy and Oncology, 126*(1), 3–24.

Hara, R., Itami, J., Kondo, T., Aruga, T., Abe, Y., Ito, M., ... Kobiki, T. (2002). Stereotactic single high dose irradiation of lung tumors under respiratory gating. *Radiotherapy Oncology, 63*(2), 159–163. https://doi.org/10.1016/s0167-8140(02)00063-4.

Havaei, M., Davy, A., Warde-Farley, D., Biard, A., Courville, A., Bengio, Y., ... Larochelle, H. (2017). Brain tumor segmentation with deep neural networks. *Medical Image Analysis, 35*, 18–31.

Hong, T. S., Tome, W. A., & Harari, P. M. (2012). Heterogeneity in head and neck IMRT target design and clinical practice. *Radiotherapy Oncology, 103*(1), 92–98. https://doi.org/10.1016/j.radonc.2012.02.010.

Hu, K., Liu, C., Yu, X., Zhang, J., He, Y., & Zhu, H. (2018). *A 2.5 d cancer segmentation for mri images based on u-net.* Paper presented at the 2018 5th International Conference on Information Science and Control Engineering (ICISCE).

Hui, C. B., Nourzadeh, H., Watkins, W. T., Trifiletti, D. M., Alonso, C. E., Dutta, S. W., & Siebers, J. V. (2018). Quality assurance tool for organ at risk delineation in radiation therapy using a parametric statistical approach. *Medical Physics, 45*(5), 2089–2096.

Iandola, F., Moskewicz, M., Karayev, S., Girshick, R., Darrell, T., & Keutzer, K. (2014). Densenet: Implementing efficient convnet descriptor pyramids. *arXiv preprint arXiv:1404.1869.*

Jabbour, S. K., Hashem, S. A., Bosch, W., Kim, T. K., Finkelstein, S. E., Anderson, B. M., ... Haddock, M. G. (2014). Upper abdominal normal organ contouring guidelines and atlas: A Radiation Therapy Oncology Group consensus. *Practical Radiation Oncology, 4*(2), 82–89.

Joskowicz, L., Cohen, D., Caplan, N., & Sosna, J. (2019). Inter-observer variability of manual contour delineation of structures in CT. *European Radiology, 29*(3), 1391–1399. https://doi.org/10.1007/s00330-018-5695-5.

Kong, F. M., Ten Haken, R. K., Schipper, M., Frey, K. A., Hayman, J., Gross, M., ... Kalemkerian, G. P. (2017). Effect of midtreatment PET/CT-adapted radiation therapy with concurrent chemotherapy in patients with locally advanced non-small-cell lung cancer: A Phase 2 clinical trial. *JAMA Oncology, 3*(10), 1358–1365. https://doi.org/10.1001/jamaoncol.2017.0982.

Kosmin, M., Ledsam, J., Romera-Paredes, B., Mendes, R., Moinuddin, S., de Souza, D., ... Sharma, R. A. (2019). Rapid advances in auto-segmentation of organs at risk and target volumes in head and neck cancer. *Radiotherapy Oncology, 135*, 130–140. https://doi.org/10.1016/j.radonc.2019.03.004.

Krizhevsky, A., Sutskever, I., & Hinton, G. E. (2012). *Imagenet classification with deep convolutional neural networks.* Paper presented at the Advances in neural information processing systems.

La Macchia, M., Fellin, F., Amichetti, M., Cianchetti, M., Gianolini, S., Paola, V., ... Widesott, L. (2012). Systematic evaluation of three different commercial software solutions for automatic segmentation for adaptive therapy in head-and-neck, prostate and pleural cancer. *Radiation Oncology, 7*(1), 160.

Lambin, P., Rios-Velazquez, E., Leijenaar, R., Carvalho, S., Van Stiphout, R. G., Granton, P., ... Dekker, A. (2012). Radiomics: Extracting more information from medical images using advanced feature analysis. *European Journal of Cancer, 48*(4), 441–446.

Li, H., Galperin-Aizenberg, M., Pryma, D., Simone II, C. B., & Fan, Y. (2018). Unsupervised machine learning of radiomic features for predicting treatment response and overall survival of early stage non-small cell lung cancer patients treated with stereotactic body radiation therapy. *Radiotherapy and Oncology, 129*(2), 218–226.

Li, X., Dou, Q., Chen, H., Fu, C. W., Qi, X., Belavy, D. L., ... Heng, P. A. (2018). 3D multi-scale FCN with random modality voxel dropout learning for Intervertebral Disc Localization and Segmentation from Multi-modality MR Images. *Medical Image Analysis, 45*, 41–54. https://doi.org/10.1016/j.media.2018.01.004.

Li, X. A., Tai, A., Arthur, D. W., Buchholz, T. A., Macdonald, S., Marks, L. B., ... Taghian, A. (2009). Variability of target and normal structure delineation for breast cancer radiotherapy: An RTOG Multi-Institutional and Multiobserver Study. *International Journal of Radiation Oncology* Biology* Physics, 73*(3), 944–951.

Li, X. A., Tai, A., Arthur, D. W., Buchholz, T. A., Macdonald, S., Marks, L. B., ... Multiobserver, S. (2009). Variability of target and normal structure delineation for breast cancer radiotherapy: An RTOG Multi-Institutional and Multiobserver Study. *International Journal of Radiation Oncology, Biology, Physics, 73*(3), 944–951. https://doi.org/10.1016/j.ijrobp.2008.10.034.

Lim-Reinders, S., Keller, B. M., Al-Ward, S., Sahgal, A., & Kim, A. (2017). Online adaptive radiation therapy. *International Journal of Radiation Oncology, Biology, Physics, 99*(4), 994–1003. https://doi.org/10.1016/j.ijrobp.2017.04.023.

Liu, C., Gardner, S. J., Wen, N., Elshaikh, M. A., Siddiqui, F., Movsas, B., & Chetty, I. J. (2019). Automatic segmentation of the prostate on CT images using Deep Neural Networks (DNN). *International Journal of Radiation Oncology, Biology, Physics, 104*(4), 924–932. https://doi.org/10.1016/j.ijrobp.2019.03.017.

Long, J., Shelhamer, E., & Darrell, T. (2015). *Fully convolutional networks for semantic segmentation.* Paper presented at the Proceedings of the IEEE conference on computer vision and pattern recognition.

Loo, S. W., Martin, W. M., Smith, P., Cherian, S., & Roques, T. W. (2012). Interobserver variation in parotid gland delineation: A study of its impact on intensity-modulated radiotherapy solutions with a systematic review of the literature. *British Journal of Radiology, 85*(1016), 1070–1077. https://doi.org/10.1259/bjr/32038456.

McMahan, B., Moore, E., Ramage, D., Hampson, S., & y Arcas, B. A. (2017). *Communication-efficient learning of deep networks from decentralized data.* Paper presented at the Artificial intelligence and statistics.

Milletari, F., Navab, N., & Ahmadi, S.-A. (2016). *V-net: Fully convolutional neural networks for volumetric medical image segmentation.* Paper presented at the 2016 fourth international conference on 3D vision (3DV).

Nardone, V., Tini, P., Nioche, C., Mazzei, M. A., Carfagno, T., Battaglia, G., ... Pirtoli, L. (2018). Texture analysis as a predictor of radiation-induced xerostomia in head and neck patients undergoing IMRT. *La Radiologia Medica, 123*(6), 415–423.

Nelms, B. E., Tomé, W. A., Robinson, G., & Wheeler, J. (2012). Variations in the contouring of organs at risk: Test case from a patient with oropharyngeal cancer. *International Journal of Radiation Oncology* Biology* Physics, 82*(1), 368–378.

Nie, D., Wang, L., Adeli, E., Lao, C., Lin, W., & Shen, D. (2018). 3-D fully convolutional networks for multimodal isointense infant brain image segmentation. *IEEE Transactions on Cybernetics, 49*(3), 1123–1136.

Oktay, O., Schlemper, J., Folgoc, L. L., Lee, M., Heinrich, M., Misawa, K., ... Kainz, B. (2018). Attention u-net: Learning where to look for the pancreas. *arXiv preprint arXiv:1804.03999.*

Paul, J., Yang, C., Wu, H., Tai, A., Dalah, E., Zheng, C., ... Li, X. A. (2017). Early assessment of treatment responses during radiation therapy for lung cancer using quantitative analysis of daily computed tomography. *International Journal of Radiation Oncology* Biology* Physics, 98*(2), 463–472.

Pei, K., Cao, Y., Yang, J., & Jana, S. (2017). Towards practical verification of machine learning: The case of computer vision systems. *arXiv preprint arXiv:1712.01785.*

Ren, S., He, K., Girshick, R., & Sun, J. (2015). *Faster r-cnn: Towards real-time object detection with region proposal networks.* Paper presented at the Advances in neural information processing systems.

Robin, S., Jolicoeur, M., Palumbo, S., Zilli, T., Crehange, G., De Hertogh, O., ... Supiot, S. (2021). Prostate bed delineation guidelines for postoperative radiation therapy: On behalf of the francophone group of urological radiation therapy. *International Journal of Radiation Oncology* Biology* Physics, 109*(5), 1243–1253.

Ronneberger, O., Fischer, P., & Brox, T. (2015). *U-net: Convolutional networks for biomedical image segmentation.* Paper presented at the International Conference on Medical image computing and computer-assisted intervention.

Roth, H. R., Oda, H., Zhou, X., Shimizu, N., Yang, Y., Hayashi, Y., ... Mori, K. (2018). An application of cascaded 3D fully convolutional networks for medical image segmentation. *Computerized Medical Imaging and Graphics, 66*, 90–99. https://doi.org/10.1016/j.compmedimag.2018.03.001.

Rudra, S., Jiang, N., Rosenberg, S. A., Olsen, J. R., Roach, M. C., Wan, L., ... Lee, P. P. (2019). Using adaptive magnetic resonance image-guided radiation therapy for treatment of inoperable pancreatic cancer. *Cancer Medicine, 8*(5), 2123–2132. https://doi.org/10.1002/cam4.2100.

Rusthoven, K. E., Kavanagh, B. D., Burri, S. H., Chen, C., Cardenes, H., Chidel, M. A., ... Schefter, T. E. (2009). Multi-institutional phase I/II trial of stereotactic body radiation therapy for lung metastases. *Journal of Clinical Oncology, 27*(10), 1579–1584. https://doi.org/10.1200/JCO.2008.19.6386.

Sandfort, V., Yan, K., Pickhardt, P. J., & Summers, R. M. (2019). Data augmentation using generative adversarial networks (CycleGAN) to improve generalizability in CT segmentation tasks. *Scientific Reports, 9*(1), 1–9.

Schwartz, D. L., Garden, A. S., Thomas, J., Chen, Y., Zhang, Y., Lewin, J., ... Dong, L. (2012). Adaptive radiotherapy for head-and-neck cancer: initial clinical outcomes from a prospective trial. *International Journal of Radiation Oncology, Biology, Physics, 83*(3), 986–993. https://doi.org/10.1016/j.ijrobp.2011.08.017.

Sharp, G., Fritscher, K. D., Pekar, V., Peroni, M., Shusharina, N., Veeraraghavan, H., & Yang, J. (2014). Vision 20/20: Perspectives on automated image segmentation for radiotherapy. *Medical Physics, 41*(5), 050902.

Sheller, M. J., Reina, G. A., Edwards, B., Martin, J., & Bakas, S. (2018). *Multi-institutional deep learning modeling without sharing patient data: A feasibility study on brain tumor segmentation.* Paper presented at the International MICCAI Brainlesion Workshop.

Stam, B., Peulen, H., Guckenberger, M., Mantel, F., Hope, A., Werner-Wasik, M., ... Sonke, J.-J. (2017). Dose to heart substructures is associated with non-cancer death after SBRT in stage I–II NSCLC patients. *Radiotherapy and Oncology, 123*(3), 370–375.

Stam, B., Peulen, H., Guckenberger, M., Mantel, F., Hope, A., Werner-Wasik, M., ... Sonke, J. J. (2017). Dose to heart substructures is associated with non-cancer death after SBRT in stage I-II NSCLC patients. *Radiotherapy and Oncology, 123*(3), 370–375. https://doi.org/10.1016/j.radonc.2017.04.017.

Tao, C. J., Yi, J. L., Chen, N. Y., Ren, W., Cheng, J., Tung, S., ... Sun, Y. (2015). Multi-subject atlas-based auto-segmentation reduces interobserver variation and improves dosimetric parameter consistency for organs at risk in nasopharyngeal carcinoma: A multi-institution clinical study. *Radiotherapy and Oncology, 115*(3), 407–411. https://doi.org/10.1016/j.radonc.2015.05.012.

Teguh, D. N., Levendag, P. C., Voet, P. W., Al-Mamgani, A., Han, X., Wolf, T. K., ... Hoogeman, M. S. (2011). Clinical validation of atlas-based auto-segmentation of multiple target volumes and normal tissue (swallowing/mastication) structures in the head and neck. *International Journal of Radiation Oncology, Biology, Physics, 81*(4), 950–957. https://doi.org/10.1016/j.ijrobp.2010.07.009.

Thomson, D., Boylan, C., Liptrot, T., Aitkenhead, A., Lee, L., Yap, B., ... Slevin, N. (2014). Evaluation of an automatic segmentation algorithm for definition of head and neck organs at risk. *Radiotherapy and Oncology, 9*, 173. https://doi.org/10.1186/1748-717X-9-173.

Thor, M., Apte, A., Haq, R., Iyer, A., LoCastro, E., & Deasy, J. O. (2021). Using auto-segmentation to reduce contouring and dose inconsistency in clinical trials: The simulated impact on RTOG 0617. *International Journal of Radiation Oncology, Biology, Physics, 109*(5), 1619–1626. https://doi.org/10.1016/j.ijrobp.2020.11.011.

Timmerman, R., McGarry, R., Yiannoutsos, C., Papiez, L., Tudor, K., DeLuca, J., ... Fletcher, J. (2006). Excessive toxicity when treating central tumors in a phase II study of stereotactic body radiation therapy for medically inoperable early-stage lung cancer. *Journal of Clinical Oncology, 24*(30), 4833–4839. https://doi.org/10.1200/JCO.2006.07.5937.

van der Veen, J., Gulyban, A., & Nuyts, S. (2019). Interobserver variability in delineation of target volumes in head and neck cancer. *Radiotherapy and Oncology, 137*, 9–15.

van der Veen, J., Gulyban, A., Willems, S., Maes, F., & Nuyts, S. (2021). Interobserver variability in organ at risk delineation in head and neck cancer. *Radiation Oncology, 16*(1), 1–11.

Vorwerk, H., Zink, K., Schiller, R., Budach, V., Bohmer, D., Kampfer, S., ... Engenhart-Cabillic, R. (2014). Protection of quality and innovation in radiation oncology: the prospective multicenter trial the German Society of Radiation Oncology (DEGRO-QUIRO study). Evaluation of time, attendance of medical staff, and resources during radiotherapy with IMRT. *Strahlenther Onkol, 190*(5), 433–443. https://doi.org/10.1007/s00066-014-0634-0.

Walker, G. V., Awan, M., Tao, R., Koay, E. J., Boehling, N. S., Grant, J. D., ... Fuller, C. D. (2014). Prospective randomized double-blind study of atlas-based organ-at-risk autosegmentation-assisted radiation planning in head and neck cancer. *Radiotherapy and Oncology, 112*(3), 321–325. https://doi.org/10.1016/j.radonc.2014.08.028.

Warfield, S. K., Zou, K. H., & Wells, W. M. (2004). Simultaneous truth and performance level estimation (STAPLE): An algorithm for the validation of image segmentation. *IEEE Transactions on Medical Imaging, 23*(7), 903–921. https://doi.org/10.1109/TMI.2004.828354.

Wong, J., Fong, A., McVicar, N., Smith, S., Giambattista, J., Wells, D., ... Alexander, A. (2020). Comparing deep learning-based auto-segmentation of organs at risk and clinical target volumes to expert inter-observer variability in radiotherapy planning. *Radiotherapy and Oncology, 144*, 152–158. https://doi.org/10.1016/j.radonc.2019.10.019.

Wu, A. J., Williams, E., Modh, A., Foster, A., Yorke, E., Rimner, A., & Jackson, A. (2014). Dosimetric predictors of esophageal toxicity after stereotactic body radiotherapy for central lung tumors. *Radiotherapy and Oncology, 112*(2), 267–271. https://doi.org/10.1016/j.radonc.2014.07.001.

Xue, Y., Xu, T., Zhang, H., Long, L. R., & Huang, X. (2018). SegAN: Adversarial network with multi-scale L1 loss for medical image segmentation. *Neuroinformatics, 16*(3–4), 383–392. https://doi.org/10.1007/s12021-018-9377-x.

Yan, D., Vicini, F., Wong, J., & Martinez, A. (1997). Adaptive radiation therapy. *Physics in Medicine and Biology, 42*(1), 123–132. https://doi.org/10.1088/0031-9155/42/1/008.

Yan, D., Ziaja, E., Jaffray, D., Wong, J., Brabbins, D., Vicini, F., & Martinez, A. (1998). The use of adaptive radiation therapy to reduce setup error: A prospective clinical study. *International Journal of Radiation Oncology, Biology, Physics, 41*(3), 715–720. https://doi.org/10.1016/s0360-3016(97)00567-1.

Yang, H., Hu, W., Wang, W., Chen, P., Ding, W., & Luo, W. (2013). Replanning during intensity modulated radiation therapy improved quality of life in patients with nasopharyngeal carcinoma. *International Journal of Radiation Oncology, Biology, Physics, 85*(1), e47–54. https://doi.org/10.1016/j.ijrobp.2012.09.033.

Yang, J., Veeraraghavan, H., Armato III, S. G., Farahani, K., Kirby, J. S., Kalpathy-Kramer, J., ... Feng, X. (2018). Autosegmentation for thoracic radiation treatment planning: A grand challenge at AAPM 2017. *Medical Physics, 45*(10), 4568–4581.

Zabel, W. J., Conway, J. L., Gladwish, A., Skliarenko, J., Didiodato, G., Goorts-Matthews, L., ... McVicar, N. (2021). Clinical evaluation of deep learning and atlas-based auto-contouring of bladder and rectum for prostate radiation therapy. *Practical Radiation Oncology, 11*(1), e80–e89. https://doi.org/10.1016/j.prro.2020.05.013.

Zhou, Z., Siddiquee, M. M. R., Tajbakhsh, N., & Liang, J. (2018). Unet++: A nested u-net architecture for medical image segmentation. In *Deep Learning in Medical Image Analysis and Multimodal Learning for Clinical Decision Support* (pp. 3–11). Springer.

Zhou, Z., Siddiquee, M. M. R., Tajbakhsh, N., & Liang, J. (2019). Unet++: Redesigning skip connections to exploit multiscale features in image segmentation. *IEEE Transactions on Medical Imaging, 39*(6), 1856–1867.

Chapter 7

Knowledge Representation for Radiation Oncology

Dongyang Zhang and Andrew Wilson

Oncology Informatics Solutions, Elekta, Inc., Sunnyvale CA, USA

Abstract

The term artificial intelligence (AI) has been nearly synonymous with machine learning (ML) in recent times. However, there's a lesser-discussed field within AI, knowledge representation (KR), that will be a big driver of the future of medical AI, ML, and intelligent oncology software in general. In this chapter, we will define and describe what KR is at a level that radiation oncologists and medical physicists should be familiar with, how it can help our field, and how it interacts with other medical AI technologies. Along the way, we'll describe how it can enhance efficiency of clinical workflows, reduce cognitive burden for physicians, and help to mature the vision of precision medicine.

1. Introduction

As we enter the era of precision medicine, there's a need to consider the patient in an increasingly holistic manner and with a finer level of detail.

This is needed to discover the ever-increasing array of variables that may impact patient care and outcomes. The fields of radiomics, pathomics, and genomics are currently leading this charge. In some instances, they are helping to augment traditional tumor characterizations with entirely new worldviews of how to describe tumors and are bringing increasingly quantitative measurements and frameworks into the analysis-fold. Clinical phenotyping of electronic health record (EHR) data is just as crucial to precision medicine. One example is the capture of adverse events and other short-term and long-term outcomes data, and then standardizing these data across all patients, hospitals, and clinics for analysis. Quantifying co-morbidities is another example. We can all probably think of a cancer patient with a relatively early-stage diagnosis on a straightforward treatment protocol but due to poorly controlled co-morbidities, their care can quickly devolve into complex management. The same logic extends to the rest of the patient history. Co-morbidities are important, but so are social determinants of health (SDoH). In fact, many predictive algorithms have shown that SDoH can sometimes be a better predictor of outcomes than clinical factors in the medical record. As a simple, but edge-case illustration, just think of the possible effects of homelessness on cancer prognosis.

All of this is to say that our consideration of the patient must be multifactorial and holistic if the goal is continued improvement in cancer care. With such a diversity and breadth of patient data, our analytics must increase in sophistication to keep pace. Most of the patient data are stored in textual format. Even non-text-based diagnostic testing results such as imaging and immunohistochemistry have accompanying reports, which are arguably more important from a multidisciplinary point of view as they contain a summary and interpretation of findings. Therefore, much of the sophistication for better clinical phenotyping and quantitation has been aimed at textual analysis. The main focus of this chapter will be accordingly aimed here as well.

Machine Learning (ML) represents a significant step toward sophistication with regard to pattern recognition, but as it's applied to medical text, most ML studies in the published literature are relatively rudimentary, treating for example words in a pathology or radiology report just as symbols (symbolic manipulation), unable to see the simple connection between the words "cancer" and "cancers". Natural Language Processing (NLP) adds an important layer of sophistication on top of this by modeling, for instance, the syntax of the English language, understanding parts of speech, differentiating between singular/plural via stemming and lemmatization techniques.

On top of these layers of symbolics and syntactics, knowledge representation (KR) adds semantics: the meaning behind the language. It's a layer of sophistication with an inherent understanding of medical concepts, whether they're represented by a single word or a descriptive phrasing that spans across multiple words. There's a framework for understanding synonyms and related concepts. On top of this, there is an interconnected web of relationships among all of these concepts. Taken together, all of the above constitute a semantic layer of information that adds crucial contextual background knowledge to any recorded description of a patient. Think of the conciseness of the "one-liner" in a written assessment and plan section of the medical record and the background knowledge to fully appreciate the depth of what's written. For medical students, it can take years of training to gain a sufficient level of understanding of just the "one-liner". For machines, we are now starting this journey of semantic understanding with the assistance of KR to help machines understand the same.

The implications of this added knowledge are vast (Fig. 1). Quantitating and contextualizing patient data for precision medicine is just one of many uses. For clinical workflows, this added contextual knowledge enables building smarter software with added automation, which in turn can enhance clinical efficiency, help alleviate cognitive fatigue, and reduce burn-out. For clinical research, data capture can be more automated and more comprehensive in their scope. Study results contextualized with KR may surface deeper insights with less manual effort involved.

In this chapter, we'll explore all of these topics and more in greater detail starting with a discussion of what KR is and technical details that practitioners should at least have some exposure to, followed by a discussion of potential applications.

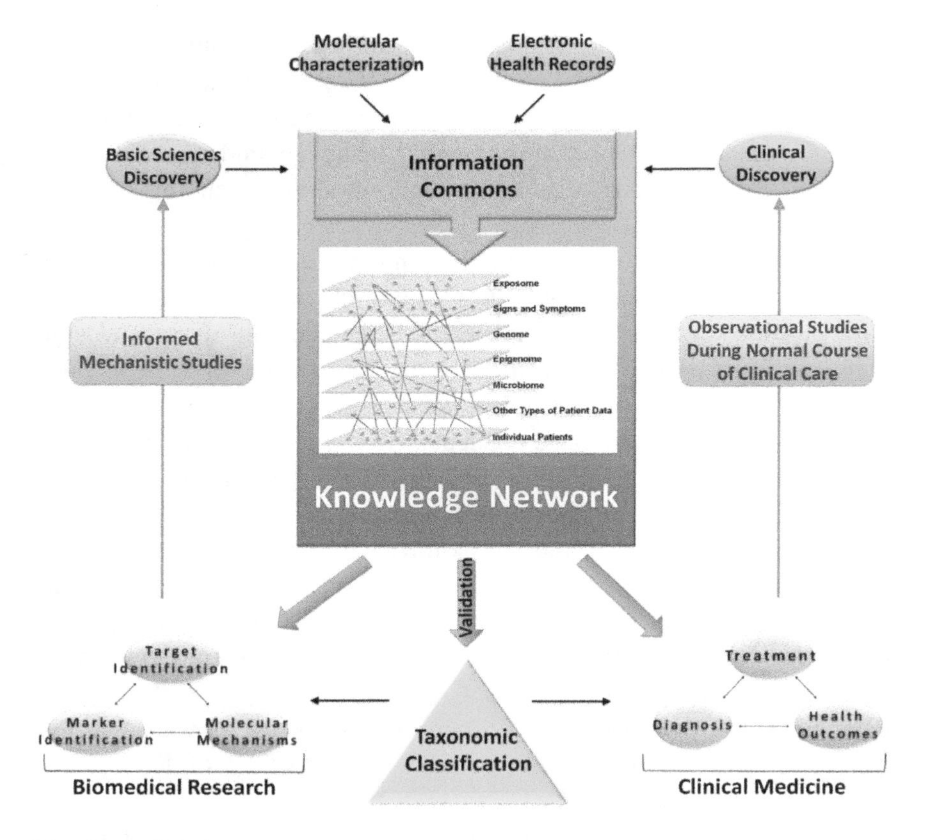

Fig. 1. Building a machine interpretable network of standardized knowledge that enhances clinical medicine and biomedical research. Reprinted with permission from (National Research Council (US) Committee on A Framework for Developing a New Taxonomy of Disease, 2011).

2. Knowledge Representation

The history and evolution of how humankind has sought to represent the knowledge existent in their heads is rich and vast and the theoretical constructs devised are multitudinous and varied. Thus, knowledge representation is a field of AI unto itself. A comprehensive and in-depth description of the field is beyond the scope of the current chapter. What we focus on here is a simplified description that is geared for practicality of usage in medicine and radiation oncology.

In this context, the purpose of knowledge representation can be simply stated as a way for machines to understand the world in a similar way to how we understand the world. Once the machine has some understanding of this world, the world of medicine, it can begin to reason for itself. Being able to reason independent of a human chaperone — to think, in a way — enables so many possibilities. If the reader stops to think about this, they can probably logically extrapolate on a few of these possibilities. Later on, we'll discuss this in more detail.

Next, let's look at some KR designs and implementations. We're going to focus on the areas of KR where most of the progress has been made, especially with regard to biomedical informatics. The scope is cast wider here than just radiation oncology because we would like the machine to have a holistic understanding of the patient including their medical problems — malignancies and otherwise — as well as a basic understanding of relevant biology including genes and small molecules which are increasing pertinent to cancer care and FDA approved therapies. First and foremost, the KR systems of interest to us here are designed to be intuitive. That's why at their core they deal with concepts that we as human beings and domain experts typically think about as important in medicine, from roots in basic science to implementations in clinical practice — concepts such as genes, proteins, cells, organs, body systems, pathophysiologic mechanisms, diseases/syndromes, signs/symptoms, tests, procedures, drugs, chemotherapies, biologics, radiotherapy techniques, and the more granular concepts within these (overlapping) categories. For each concept, the machine assigns a code to it that is used to uniquely identify and efficiently store that concept within the machine.

These concepts/facts in KR systems don't live in a vacuum. Instead, they are only meaningful when compared and contrasted with one another. This brings us to the second important component of KR systems: relations among concepts. One key relation is the type–subtype (also called the class–subclass) relation. For example: "NSCLC" (non-small-cell lung cancer) *is-a* type of "lung cancer"; and "lung cancer" *is-a* type of "cancer". This is analogous to what we learn as children on the taxonomic classification of animals and other kingdoms of life. This type of relation is intuitively called the *is-a* relation because e.g. NSCLC is a type of lung cancer. There are many other types of relations that match with the training and expertise in the reader's mind, connecting relevant concepts. "Procedure A" or "Drug B" *treats* "disease C"; "disease C" *manifests* as "symptoms D, E, F".

Concepts and relations are the basics of what makes an ontology, an important type of KR system we'll reference again and again. You may have heard of the term ontology before, and we'll talk more about a specific implementation that's highly pertinent to our space later on. An ontology, in the information sciences sense as opposed to ontology in the philosophical sense, is a formal system for capturing and representing the knowledge in a domain. It starts with what we just described: a vocabulary with standardized concepts plus relations among these concepts, but this is only the start. The architecture of knowledge can be as complex, detailed, and intricate as the best of human thought — seemingly infinite from our perspective. Therefore, many ontologies try to capture the most practically useful aspects of such complex knowledge, layering the architecture of these complexities on top of the core ideas of concepts and relations. One such layer of knowledge is specifying different types of relations, for example the *is-a*, *treats*, and *manifests* relations mentioned earlier. Similar to concepts, relations can also have synonyms and can be compared and contrasted with one another.

There are numerous other layers of knowledge that are practically useful and routinely captured in ontologies. For example, some relations have special properties. If we know that "NSCLC" *is-a* type of "lung cancer" and that "lung cancer" *is-a* type of "cancer", we as human beings can infer almost reflexively that "NSCLC" *is-a* type of "cancer". The property at play here is called transitivity and can be formalized as a knowledge representation structure to be used by a machine. The *is-a* relation is transitive. The general form of the reasoning is: if "X" *is-a* type of "Y", and "Y" *is-a* type of "Z", then "X" *is-a* type of "Z". Additionally, in a correctly constructed ontology, subtypes also inherit all the properties of the supertype. Thus, NSCLC inherits properties that all cancers have in common, including a neoplastic process. Ideally, we can use this knowledge to build a machine that performs the above reasoning in an automated way without human expertise or intervention.

When transitivity is correctly applied to medical ontologies, it gives us a very powerful tool set for reasoning. Here's a motivating clinical scenario: a patient has a newly discovered tumor with high clinical suspicion for malignancy. One question that every oncologist has as a next step is: has the patient ever had cancer before? Patient self-reporting is error-prone with mistakes and omissions and shouldn't be relied upon as the sole source of information. Thus, the medical record should be scanned. As every physician knows, due to substantial time constraints this task must be balanced with other parts of patient care. Every effort is made to find the most relevant documents as quickly as possible and mentally store as many relevant facts as possible. A complete review of the entire patient record is impossible so there's always a risk that a clinically important piece of information could be overlooked. This is where technology should come into play and relieve the majority of the burden and cognitive load away from the physician. Using ontologies and transitive *is-a* relations, a machine can find all subtypes of "cancer", then subtypes of subtypes, repeating this recursively until completion — to materialize the entire cancer taxonomic tree. Then it can search in all patient notes in the medical record for each cancer subtype and all the synonyms/abbreviations for each subtype. It can do this automatically, exhaustively, and if implemented correctly, finishes the search in a fraction of a second. The oncologist gets an answer right away, and armed with this knowledge, can more confidently prescribe the appropriate next steps of care.

A typical clinical workday is filled with countless similar situations that machine intelligence like the above can help expedite. What protocols were tried in the past; what were previously experienced adverse events; etc. All of these questions answered in an automated way saves the radiation oncologist valuable time and energy, and reduces cognitive burden in an era where these demands are ever increasing and in a specialty that requires providing complex care management for one of the sickest population of patients — elderly, with multiple co-morbidities, in the setting of a cancer diagnosis — and in the end ultimately should improve the lives of patients as well as their caregivers.

The machine intelligence described above requires many moving pieces to implement but are all feasible to build these days including a medical NLP engine, a search engine, and question answering capabilities. But the heart of this implementation requires something that is still very difficult to do accurately and reliably even with today's technological advancements in machine learning: reasoning capabilities. It is this part that knowledge representation, especially medical ontologies, can help with. That is why medical knowledge representation will be at the heart of the future of intelligent medical software.

3. Unified Medical Language System and Constituents

Multiple knowledge representation systems have been developed in the fields of medicine and biology over the decades. Some are as simple as a set of shared terms or a vocabulary for uses such as standardizing data collection for research studies and medical administration. Other KR systems are structured more like ontologies with relations connecting related concepts, transitive properties, etc. Each system has its own set of strengths and weaknesses. Some may cover one area of medicine more comprehensively than others. Some may have relations others don't have. Many systems have some overlap with each other in terms of the knowledge covered and represented. If one could merge concepts from different KR systems where there is overlap, then we can combine the knowledge of these various KR systems into one unified knowledge-base and create a radically more comprehensive knowledge source that everyone can benefit from. This is exactly what the Unified Medical Language System (UMLS) has done, as the name implies (Bodenreider, 2004). As of now, there are over 200 KR systems that are a part of what UMLS calls its Metathesaurus. Some are familiar: ICD-10 (International Classification of Diseases) (World Health Organization (WHO), 2003) and SNOMED CT (Systematized Nomenclature of Medicine-Clinical Terms) (SNOMED International, n.d.). The individual KR systems in UMLS are called source vocabularies because the vocabulary is the common denominator among all these KR systems even though many contain more than just a vocabulary. For example, SNOMED CT contains *is-a* relations that are poly-hierarchical in structure and is built on ontological foundations. For simplicity of nomenclature, we will follow similar conventions to UMLS and describe KR systems used in UMLS as vocabularies. In other texts, a vocabulary is also sometimes called a lexicon or terminology.

As a start to exploring UMLS, let's look at some vocabularies relevant to radiation oncology. ICD in its various versions and modifications has to be mentioned because of its prevalence in many countries for reimbursement and for attributing morbidity and mortality in population statistics. However, it's a poor vocabulary to use for capturing the clinically important nuances of a patient encounter (which was never its intended purpose). For example, there is no concept specifically for NSCLC. Therefore, we couldn't build, for example, a database containing only NSCLC patients if our starting point solely consisted of ICD-10 codes. It takes more than ICD to capture clinical details at a level that is appropriately granular to be useful in the everyday clinic. The finer the level of granularity we can represent and capture, the more useful this information would be to us and to the machine for downstream analytics. For this task, SNOMED CT is a much more preferred alternative to ICD.

SNOMED CT in its current state of development is designed to have broad coverage of many concepts important to medicine and radiation oncology such as neoplasms and most other diseases, signs/symptoms/adverse events, anatomy, many drugs and procedures, etc. From a practical perspective, there should be a SNOMED CT term for the vast majority of these medical concepts that physicians use to communicate and document in clinic.

Next, let's look at relations. As we mentioned earlier, SNOMED CT contains *is-a* relations. If we trace *is-a* relations consecutively for a concept like "lung cancer", we find that its lineage contains ancestors such as "neoplastic disease", which provides some information on the pathophysiologic process. The *is-a* relation then traces back to the concept of "disease" which tells us the high-level category that this concept falls under (as opposed to "drugs", "procedures", etc). "Lung cancer" also contains *is-a* ancestors to "respirator finding" and "disorder of trunk", which provides anatomical descriptors to compare and contrast with anatomy in other diseases. Remember, this knowledge is common sense to us, but for a machine to have this type of background knowledge to reason over is far beyond the reasoning found in medical software that we encounter in the typical clinic. In general, SNOMED CT contains many useful relations for various diseases that inform on pathophysiology and anatomy. However, one should not rely on these relations to convey for example the same breadth and depth of information on pathophysiology as a pathology textbook. Many other relations (non-*is-a* relations) exist in SNOMED CT such as "X disease" *has causative agent* "Y organism" or "Z substance", but these relations are much sparser in coverage and are therefore of limited utility as they exist today. If anything, they are more of a placeholder that guides future knowledge engineering (adding to the ontology).

Moving forward, let's look at some other important vocabularies included in UMLS. As much as SNOMED CT strives for broad coverage of medical concepts, no vocabulary is all-inclusive. For classification of neoplasms there is vast coverage in SNOMED CT, but there is even more coverage and more detailed subtype classifications of tumors in NCIt (National Cancer Institute Thesaurus) (Fragoso *et al.*, 2004). Similarly, SNOMED CT's coverage of drugs is vast, but RxNorm's (Nelson *et al.*, 2011) is better. RxNorm also contains many useful relations that, for example, can be used to convert between brand names and generic ingredients, and between combination drugs and their individual ingredients. This may be important in situations such as cataloging chemotherapy that is given as part of chemoradiation. For anatomical descriptions, SNOMED CT has decent coverage, but FMA (Foundational Model of Anatomy) (Rosse & Mejino, 2008) provides a richer framework for describing anatomy, with relations that describe the "part-of" hierarchy, arterial supply and venous drainage, adjacency, among others. For adverse events, most concepts can be captured as SNOMED CT signs/symptoms/diseases, but there is also a formal vocabulary dedicated to adverse events called CTCAE (Common Terminology Criteria for Adverse Events) (National Cancer Institute, n.d.) that is used as a reporting standard in contemporary clinical trials. Again, where there is overlap in coverage among vocabularies, UMLS can be used as a Rosetta Stone to translate across vocabularies. Where the overlap ends, one vocabulary can then be used to extend the knowledge of another vocabulary.

For coverage of different types of radiotherapy techniques, NCIt is preferred. NCIt also includes *is-a* relations that attempt to group radiotherapy techniques into a reasonable hierarchy. Similarly, oncogenes, tumor suppressor genes, as well as gene products have coverage as NCIt concepts. The Gene Ontology (GO) (Ashburner *et al.*, 2000) vocabulary takes this a step further and aims to comprehensively catalog genes as they relate to discovered molecular functions, biological processes, and cellular components. For example, with respect to oncology, GO has a listing of genes associated with the biological process of cell population proliferation, along with annotations and pointers to source references. This knowledge can be used in studies such as pathway analyses to discover cancer driver genes (Colaprico *et al.*, 2020).

4. UMLS Limitations

When trying to combine over 200 vocabularies with an aggregate of over 4.5 million concepts, mistakes are unavoidable. One of the biggest challenges is determining whether to merge concepts from different vocabularies into one concept in UMLS. It may be better to err more on the side of caution and not make the mistake of merging two similar but distinct concepts. However, this strategy can lead to more unintended redundancy. Also, in some instances it can be highly debatable where to draw the line between similar vs equivalent, and this can shift depending on the context of the usage and the intention of the author.

One other major class of UMLS limitations is with regard to relations. The coverage of concepts vs relations we described earlier in SNOMED CT is reflected more broadly in UMLS and many of its constituent vocabularies. The primary aim is for broad coverage of medical concepts. Representing relations is a secondary aim, with *is-a* relations many times prioritized over other types of relations. Given the stage of development of UMLS and its vocabularies, this is justifiably necessary: without first articulating the necessary concepts, one cannot begin to talk about relations with other concepts.

It should be noted that UMLS attempts to address this gap in relations with what it calls the Semantic Network (McCray, 2003). It assigns broad subject categories (semantic types) to every UMLS concept, then overlays relations on top of these broad categories; for example, "injury or poisoning" *disrupts* "physiologic function". These are "some–some" relations i.e. [some] injuries or poisonings disrupt [some types of] physiologic function, which can be useful at a high level, but at the level of granularity of clinical documentation the Semantic Network is of limited practical utility and informativeness for relation-building algorithms in many instances.

Due to a lack of detailed coverage of many important relations within any *one* vocabulary (even *is-a* relations), one can utilize UMLS to combine relations across vocabularies to greatly enhance, for example, the classification of diseases by pathophysiology and anatomy. Care should be taken during this procedure, as many vocabularies are not amenable to a simple merger of this kind. Curation at the level of ontologies and sub-ontologies using biomedical informatics domain expertise may be required. One prominent example is ICD, which was not constructed with this use case in mind and is typically excluded as a source vocabulary in order to preserve the accuracy of this type of semantic expansion across vocabularies.

Many other classes of errors exist, but for the most part UMLS and their source vocabularies do a commendable job given the scale and challenges of the tasks involved. UMLS has demonstrated proven practical utility in countless projects involving biomedical information retrieval, data standardization, and interoperability. There are continuous efforts at improvement through manual vetting and automated error detection algorithms. UMLS's current stage of development and limitations gives us a sense of its evolutionary path and future stages of advancements.

It should be noted that machines with reasoning algorithms built on top of ontologies are able to behave as if they understand the layer of knowledge that exists in the ontologies, but this is not to say there is an equivalence of reasoning or understanding capabilities similar to what we possess as human beings. Thus, more correctly, when we say that the machine performs reasoning we mean to say that the machine mimics some types of reasoning powers that we have, and it does so only to the extent and the level of complexity that is designed into the structure of the ontology and reasoning algorithms.

5. KR Outside UMLS

There are some prominent vocabularies not in UMLS but pertinent to radiation oncology. RadLex (Langlotz, 2006) is built to be a unified vocabulary for radiology terms with a classification hierarchy that mirrors the important conceptual categories in radiology reports. International Classification of Diseases for Oncology (ICD-O) is an extension to ICD used in cancer registries and oncology information systems (OIS). Its design is superior to ICD-10 alone because it explicitly recognizes there are multiple orthogonal categories of information that are clinically important to more accurately describing a tumor. It structures cancer descriptions according to tumor site (adapted from ICD-10's malignant neoplasm section), histologic cell type, differentiation and grade, as well as a range of behaviors from benign to malignant metastatic. These categories can be thought of as slots to be filled in for a tumor description. By design, one slot is independent of another slot so many permutations are possible when filling in these slots, which leads to a rich and flexible way to describe many clinically important features of tumors.

OncoTree (Kundra *et al.*, 2021) is a cancer classification system originally developed by Memorial Sloan Kettering. There is large overlap with NCIt and SNOMED CT classifications. Similar to ICD-O, it recognizes the importance of classifications independent of tumor site. Unique to OncoTree, there are genomic subclassifications that are today pertinent to diagnostics, prognostics, and therapeutics such as representing "BCR-ABL1-fusion positive chronic myeloid leukemia".

The Radiation Oncology Ontology (ROO) (Traverso *et al.*, 2018) purposefully reuses concepts from other vocabularies such as NCIt, FMA, ICD-10 and adds radiation oncology terms such as *target volume, organ at risk, nonuniform margin* that are infrequently or not at all covered by other vocabularies. The Radiation Oncology Structures ontology (ROS) contains a subset of anatomical and treatment planning structures relevant to radiation oncology delineation (Bibault *et al.*, 2018).

As the reader can see, it is together with this mosaic of vocabularies, each with their own strengths in representing a subdomain of knowledge, that we are able to build a more comprehensive source of knowledge for machines to use — one that begins to parallel our own knowledge. There are undoubtedly other vocabularies/ontologies useful to radiation oncology that are not exhaustively covered here. What we have described are the broad strokes and should represent a good first foray for exploring the world of knowledge representation as it applies to our field. There isn't one single ontology that fits every radiation oncology need and it's unlikely this will ever be the case. Therefore, more ongoing work will be needed to create a universal standard that is fit-for-purpose: which vocabularies should be used for which categories of concepts and relations important to radiation oncology (Hayman *et al.*, 2019; Mayo *et al.*, 2018; Phillips *et al.*, 2020).

Further exploration of vocabularies and ontologies is recommended within UMLS and beyond. UMLS Metathesaurus Browser (National Library of Medicine, n.d.) (free registration required) and BioPortal (Noy *et al.*, 2009) are two popular websites for browsing biomedical vocabularies.

6. Medical NLP Backed by KR

Data standardization is the primary reason many biomedical vocabularies were created. Traditionally and even today, standardizing data is performed predominantly by manual human data entry, whether it's medical coders assigning ICD-10 codes for billing purposes, or oncologists selecting SNOMED CT codes in an EHR/OIS, or a clinical data abstractor entering ICD-O codes in a cancer registry. The vast majority of this work can and should be (semi-)automated. There are no hard-stop technical barriers to doing so today.

Natural language processing (NLP; sometimes also called NLU for natural language understanding) is the preferred solution for this task. The promise of NLP is automated extraction of relevant information directly from the sentences, paragraphs in a patient record — information that may not exist elsewhere in a more organized and structured form — and standardizes that information for easier retrieval, analysis, and interoperability. An NLP engine reading through the entire EHR data set can theoretically be more thorough and accurate in extracting codes compared with a human being, while taking a fraction of the time required. Looking under the hood of NLP, it is heavily dependent on a KR system. Many medical NLP systems rely on a vocabulary to tell them which words or phrases are synonymous with one another. Vocabularies also represent different senses of the same word as separate concepts. As examples, *cold* could refer to temperature or illness; the abbreviation *SOB* has a very different meaning within and outside of medicine (shortness of breath in medicine).

Knowing the senses of a word helps the NLP choose the correct one in a process aptly named word sense disambiguation. A few vocabularies in UMLS have multilingual components: a medical concept is translated into multiple languages with the same ID code assigned to it across languages. NLP can use this feature to standardize patient data across multiple languages to enable interoperability across countries. Lastly, medical NLP systems designed for information extraction almost invariably produce output in the form of codes that are concept identifiers from a shared vocabulary (in order to standardize these medical concepts to a common knowledge space). This is true whether the NLP algorithm uses a vocabulary as an integral part of the pipeline from the very start in dictionary-based methods or whether the NLP is a transformer-based bidirectional encoder neural network in which the vocabulary codes are generated in a step termed entity linkage toward the end of the NLP pipeline.

One should be aware that a generic NLP software package is not well-suited to the above task. Instead, a specialized NLP system is usually designed with biomedical applications in mind from the start. This is due to the particular needs of the field such as the expanded dictionary of terms and abbreviations used in medicine, idiosyncrasies in the language model for patient records including those for negation and conveying uncertainty of findings (Chapman *et al.*, 2001), differences in document templates, lemmatization geared specifically toward the biomedical domain (Lu *et al.*, 2020), need for temporal processing to e.g. construct a patient timeline, and numerous other designs, features, and fine tunings involved. Thus, when we refer to NLP here, it is really a specialized medical NLP system that we have in mind and that the reader should be aware of. Some popular and freely available medical NLP systems in use today are cTAKES (Savova *et al.*, 2010) and MetaMap (Aronson & Lang, 2010). Promising future-facing NLP systems include BERT-based models such as BioBERT (Lee *et al.*, 2020).

7. Applications of Knowledge Representation

NLP is one of the most promising technical applications for KR, with the potential for mass adoption in select use cases in the near future. Therefore, there is a large overlap in current and potential use cases between NLP and KR in medicine. By combining the two, we can enable a wide gamut of radiation oncology end-user applications (Bitterman *et al.*, 2021) in clinical practice, academia, industry, and the payer space. Here, we'll focus on applications as they pertain to direct patient care and clinical research.

Standardization/curation of medical data remains one of the primary roadblocks to analytics for providers, academia, and industry support for these institutions. The way in which NLP + KR can help this process should be thought of as a stepwise process analogous to the six levels of autonomous driving capabilities in cars. Self-driving technology will advance in a stepwise manner from the first level of no automation to the last level of full automation. Fully autonomous driving on all open roads with human-level accuracy is currently impossible, but advanced driver assist technology currently is achievable, beneficial, and used on the road today. Similarly, NLP + KR is able to extract many types of medical information from unstructured/unorganized data, with accuracies that are undoubtedly clinically useful today (it's useful to remind ourselves that manually curated human data entry isn't 100% accurate). This type of AI-assist may not be fully autonomous but can still reduce the amount of traditional manual work by upwards of 90%, which could easily tip the balance between an infeasible, time- and resource-intensive project to one that is feasible, scalable, and sustainable.

Semi-automation could work in the following way in a two-step process: the NLP + KR machine would do the first pass analytics of information extraction and standardization to a vocabulary. Then, subsequently, a human domain expert would always be involved to vet the results to make sure they are correct before being used in downstream analytics. This is analogous to the two-step process of performing a screening test then diagnostic test when necessary, taking advantage of higher sensitivity then higher specificity. In our case the machine can filter out the vast majority of non-relevant documents as much as possible while aiming to not exclude relevant information (aiming for higher recall/sensitivity). This filtered set of documents, paragraphs, and snippets of text is much smaller than the full medical record, takes less time to read through, and contains a much higher percentage of relevant information that the domain expert then can more easily vet through to find the correct answers, with the aim of higher precision (positive predictive value) in the machine learning world (vs. specificity). The vetting process would be AI-assisted as well, with the machine highlighting snippets of possibly relevant text along with recommended matching codes from a vocabulary, thus saving additional time in the text search and codification process. AI-assist plus manual vetting (sometimes described as "human-in-the-loop" or intelligence amplification) is feasible and advantageous for a variety of applications including cancer registry abstraction, standardizing target volume labels, clinical trial recruitment, adverse events monitoring, semantic (intelligent) search of the medical record, and clinical quality measures capture.

For cancer registries, the primary task would be semi-automating coding into a North American Association of Central Cancer Registries (NAACCR) format (in the US). Ontological reasoning can be important. For example, NLP may pick up the concept "Herceptin" in the medical record. Ontological relations can be used to infer that "Herceptin" *has ingredient* "trastuzumab" and that "trastuzumab" *is-a* "anti-HER2 monoclonal antibody" which in turn *is-a* "antineoplastic biological agent" which now can be matched at the same level of granularity to a cancer registry's NAACCR formatted field of "biological response modifiers". In general, this type of ontological reasoning is a powerful tool to increase the degree of automation, although it should be noted that any depth of reasoning more advanced than what's described here becomes exponentially harder for current technologies to perform in a consistently accurate way for clinical use. NLP also relies on upfront iteration and optimization steps to adapt to verbiage, abbreviations, and document templates that are idiosyncratic to a particular institution.

Semi-automation of ICD-O coding is another clear goal for AI-assist in cancer registries. On top of this goal, NLP can supplement ICD-O descriptions by utilizing other, more detailed and expressive vocabularies compared with ICD-O, such as SNOMED CT. By doing so, we can extract multiple SNOMED CT medical concepts that when combined can better express a more complete, accurate, and granular clinical description. This would, for example, include genomic characterization. Depending on the level of manual vetting required, this process could exponentially expand the breadth and depth of clinical information captured in registries in a scalable way.

An analogous situation applies to adverse events monitoring. CTCAE is a well-established vocabulary for this task, but there are well-known limits to the granularity of the vocabulary. We can use other vocabularies to supplement CTCAE and capture a more detailed clinical description. The end result is a semi-automated adverse events capture pipeline that is applicable to treatment monitoring, research studies, clinical trials, and "real-world" postmarketing surveillance. Adverse events can be correlated with clinical phenotypes extracted by NLP. Ontological relations again can be used to "connect-the-dots". Statistical insights generated from such analyses may lead to immediately correctable actions in clinic if the cause were of a logistical nature in the delivery of medical care. Other categories of insights may serve as hypothesis generation for more rigorous studies of biological mechanistic causes that can subsequently translate from bench to bedside.

Radiation treatment summaries can also benefit from KR. A consensus recommendation was recently proposed for a treatment summary template (Christodouleas *et al.*, 2020). Further standardization using vocabularies would lead to greater machine readability that can be used for more automated clinical decision support and cross-institution analytics. Useful vocabularies include CTCAE, SNOMED CT for adverse events; RxNorm for systemic therapy; ICD-O, SNOMED CT, NCIt for tumor characterization; FMA, SNOMED CT for anatomy; and NCIt for radiotherapy techniques, with useful overlap in coverage of conceptual entities among these vocabularies. NLP can be reasonably expected to achieve clinically useful accuracy for a subset of the above vocabulary extractions with minimal vetting needed, which should offset the majority of the added burden of including these vocabulary codes in the radiation treatment summary. Furthermore, if a standardized treatment summary template is the starting point for NLP extraction, accuracy is expected to increase compared with NLP extraction on more unstructured data — non-relevant information is already filtered out from the summary. A bonus increase to accuracy can be achieved with ontological relations used to filter NLP results to specific categories of information pertinent to the section of the summary. This technique is analogous to what has been done outside of the radiation oncology space e.g. in NLP extractions of problem lists, we can reasonably confine our results to only concepts that descend from the ontological ancestors of diseases, syndromes, symptoms.

8. Machine Learning Backed by KR

ML has demonstrated usefulness for many potential applications in the clinical space. One application is in patient stratification: predicting patient subpopulations at highest risk of negative outcomes and introducing appropriate interventions such as ones aimed at early detection, reducing adverse events, reducing hospitalization time and urgent care visits — in an effort to ultimately increase quality of life and survival. Purely symbolic pattern detection efforts have already shown usefulness in estimating risk. Even more recently, strides in artificial neural network (ANN)-based ML development have shown that highly complex features can be learned by the network without *a priori* assumptions, for example functionally reproducing the fusiform face area in the inferior temporal cortex of our brains used for facial recognition. However, the data sets used to train these networks are usually massive — many orders of magnitude larger than data sets currently available in patient record databases. Therefore, today in medicine, augmentation using KR remains an important addition for increasing accuracy of ML models whether for ANNs (Michalopoulos *et al.*, 2021) or for more traditional methods such as feature generation for support vectors machines and random forests.

Historically, the richest ML features have been generated by human domain experts using their own knowledge and experience to shape these features. With ontological reasoning, we can automate feature generation to a useful degree and include complex and relevant features that were not previously possible to automate. This process would be similar to what was outlined earlier: using ontological relations to create a web of relevant background knowledge that surrounds the raw input data. This KR-enriched data set would then serve as the new input to ML. Recent precedents of analogous approaches exist and have been successfully applied in many areas of ML and ANN research. As a canonical example, convolutional neural networks (CNNs, a type of ANN) that are meant to classify images usually develop near-to-input network layers that recognize line orientations, similar to orientation columns in the primary visual cortex of our brains. This is a grossly reproducible finding for many CNNs trained from scratch for computer vision applications. Therefore, rather than reinventing the wheel each time, we can re-use what are functionally orientation columns as one useful set of features, thereby significantly reducing the time and cost of ML training. More generally, this type of approach is an example of transfer learning.

Another consideration is that there's no guarantee that a neural network can learn all the knowledge contained within an ontology. There are multiple variables of relevance here including data size, common vs rare findings, repeatability of training results, stability of representation with noisy input, the high non-linearity of many ontological relations compared with the limits of gradient descent on a finite data set. It is far more practical to use the ontological representations rather than try to reinvent the wheel. Of course, there are boundless features not contained in ontologies that should and need to be learned via ML training, but these two methods are complementary and shouldn't be thought of as mutually exclusive. Much can be achieved already in ML with just symbolic processing. KR backing can potentially take this to the next level of accuracy.

KR-backed feature enrichment can be equally useful for non-supervised methods/clustering to provide early insights to hidden undiscovered structures, relationships, and correlations in the data. All the usual caveats apply for use in supervised or unsupervised ML, including considerations of overfitting.

9. ANNs, Knowledge Representation, and Explainability

One important point of consideration that's worthy of discussion is the general topic ANNs. An ANN is able to retain a representation of the data that it's trained on, but the form of this representation is in stark contrast to the form in ontological representations. ANNs, at their core, represent knowledge and processes as very large mathematical matrices of artificial "synaptic" weights with varying high-level architectures. Gaining a detailed conceptual understanding of the representations within neural networks can be highly challenging even for their creators. Exceptions always apply, but this is the general rule especially for the ever more complex and exponentially large networks trained these days for state-of-the-art accuracy.

In contrast, ontologies are intuitive by nature, fitting with our preconceived notions of what are the important concepts/relations in medicine and radiation oncology. This intuitive design has a very important inherent advantage. It's easily explainable. There is a recently popularized term called "explainable AI", which is a phrase defined more by what it excludes rather than what it includes. Its usage was popularized specifically by the need to have a contrast against traditional ANNs which are typically described as "black boxes" i.e. it is hard to decipher how they work. Thus, any AI technology that is less of a "black box" is more "explainable AI". Ontologies fit well within an explainable AI framework. The concepts represented make sense to us and if we use ontologies to build algorithmic reasoners, we can easily trace back the steps in logic for how our machine arrived at a conclusion. If the conclusion is incorrect, there are straightforward ways to make changes to either the reasoner or the ontology as appropriate. Making corrections to ANNs with certain guarantees of correctness is a much harder task. In fact, trying to change the output of an ANN for a given input could very well change its output in unpredictable ways for *different/unrelated* inputs. ANNs can also be "brittle" in their output. Subtle differences in input data format compared with data that it was trained on — differences that would not stump a human being — can sometimes lead to highly unpredictable and incorrect results for an ANN.

It's this uncertainty and lack of easy explainability/provability that is a major hindrance for trust and adoption of ANNs for many uses in medicine. When an ANN makes an error in other fields — say a shopping recommendation engine — the error doesn't typically result in risk to human lives. Explainable AI is not a guarantee against bad outcomes but should be thought of as an important layer of protection against such outcomes.

The above considerations may make it seem that there is no role for ANNs. Quite the opposite, we believe some form of ANN will be key to the future of knowledge representation universally, in medicine and elsewhere. However, there is no predictable timeline for this future. ANNs are rapidly evolving and have many uses outside of KR, but within KR there's still a significant gap for usage in pure medical knowledge representation as a replacement for ontologies — thus the considerations and cautionary language elaborated above. Some state-of-the-art NLP engines use ANNs. Their trained models have an internal representation of semantic elements from the original text corpus used to train it and contain structural elements that are functionally analogous to many ontological concepts and relations. However, transparency and sufficient understanding into the details of how knowledge is represented in these ANNs is again hard to come by. Near-term practical challenges include efficiently updating knowledge contained within an ANN with new information such as adding the names and contextual knowledge of new drugs that are introduced with regular cadence to the market, and more easily correcting mistakes in ANN model representation in more stable and predictable ways.

10. The Future of KR in Medicine

The sheer size and number of biomedical informatics ontologies that one can pick and choose from is a pleasant surprise to many who first venture into knowledge representation in medicine. There are already significant challenges that KR can help tackle, but it still represents a drop in the ocean of the totality of medical knowledge in existence. Here's a peek at what the future of medical KR may hold.

As mentioned earlier, relationships other than *is-a* taxonomic hierarchy relationships will be represented more widely. Today, for example, causative agents linked to their respective diseases are sparsely represented. If they *are* represented, it's mostly in the form of subject–predicate–object triples at the level of e.g. some "viruses" *can cause* some "cancers". It's at a very high level of abstraction; there little nuances; therefore, not that useful as a piece of knowledge to reason on. A more granular statement that fills in the blanks a bit better is "Heliobacter pylori" *can cause* "gastric cancer". If one were to build a machine reasoner on top of this statement, it would be much more useful. For example, in clinics, for every gastric cancer patient seen, the machine will automatically search for a history of H. pylori infection and if it exists in the medical record, will present this fact to the physician. As another example, if a patient reports diarrhea after treatment, the machine should be able to use enhanced ontological relations to flag recent radiotherapy as well as recent antibiotic use, if present. There's little doubt representations of this kind will be more complete in the future.

Subject–predicate–object triples are how most biomedical KR systems store relations. They are also the mainstays at the top tech companies in the world. However, even for moderately complex medical information there is a need to improve the underlying KR architecture in various ways to match that complexity. We need to represent probabilistic relationships (and with more nuance) for machines to use e.g. "the relative risk of gastric non-cardia adenocarcinoma in individuals with H. pylori infection compared with no infection is six-fold". As another example, the collection and pattern of symptoms offers clues to a diagnosis. Therefore, representation of a *collection* of symptoms associated with a disease is warranted. Hypergraph representations may be a more efficient representation of this information, a more general form of the subject–predicate–object triple expressed as a graph, and compatible with the greater range of flexible expressions that are basic properties of set theory. Still, this is only the beginning of a generalized knowledge framework for reasoning on diagnoses: it must also include dimensions such as pertinent negatives, time course, severity, relevant past medical, family, and social history, active medications, physical exam findings to begin to have a firmer grasp on the clinical situation.

In the future, much of this knowledge engineering — creating new and increasingly complex knowledge — may not need to be done manually but instead could be extracted from "real-world" data such as patient records as well as scientific literature. Relations can be weighted to represent the strength of statistical associations and co-occurrences (versus a binary one that only expresses a relation/no relation representation). For example, patient record search could become even smarter. Given a seed concept of "cancer", a search engine should be able to pull up relevant past CT and PET scans and reports, pathology reports, referral notes, neoadjuvant chemotherapy regimen and automatically present this information to the radiation oncologist before his first consult with the patient. Current simple attempts at defining these relations, many in the form of co-occurrence databases, have been of limited value and usefulness due to the high level of noise in these databases. Near future attempts would require more domain knowledge to more properly design analytics for much higher accuracies.

Furthermore, it's exciting to ponder the largely undiscovered possibilities of what neural networks can bring to pure knowledge representation. For example, what are the best methods to interrogate, understand, manipulate, refine, extract, and utilize the vector representations latent within large-scale neural networks and the richness of the information learned in a self-supervised way on a large medical text corpus? What depth of reasoning powers can we achieve with the knowledge that resides in these ANNs? Disassembling, understanding, and utilizing the core representations of simpler neural networks such as word2vec implementations give us a glimpse of what might be possible with more complex and advanced ANN embeddings such as those based on shared convolution, attention, and beyond.

11. Conclusion

The geometry and dimensionality of knowledge representation architectures can be as complex as the best of human thought. That's the challenge, the opportunity, and the creativity of it — to flexibly, efficiently, and scalably represent the best and brightest ideas that humanity has discovered and created. Radiation oncology care is one of the most complex fields in medicine with foundational underpinnings in multiple scientific domains. Developing and applying KR-based AI for radiation oncology will not only advance our specialty and benefit patient care but also advance the basic science of artificial intelligence.

References

Aronson, A. R. & Lang, F. M. (2010). An overview of MetaMap: Historical perspective and recent advances. *Journal of the American Medical Informatics Association, 17*(3), 229–236. https://doi.org/10.1136/jamia.2009.002733.

Ashburner, M., Ball, C. A., Blake, J. A., Botstein, D., Butler, H., Cherry, J. M., Davis, A. P., Dolinski, K., Dwight, S. S., Eppig, J. T., Harris, M. A., Hill, D. P., Issel-Tarver, L., Kasarskis, A., Lewis, S., Matese, J. C., Richardson, J. E., Ringwald, M., Rubin, G. M., & Sherlock, G. (2000). Gene ontology: Tool for the unification of biology. *Nature Genetics, 25*(1), 25–29. https://doi.org/10.1038/75556.

Bibault, J. E., Zapletal, E., Rance, B., Giraud, P., & Burgun, A. (2018). Labeling for Big Data in radiation oncology: The radiation oncology structures ontology. *PLoS ONE, 13*(1). https://doi.org/10.1371/journal.pone.0191263.

Bitterman, D. S., Miller, T. A., Mak, R. H., & Savova, G. K. (2021). Clinical NLP for radiation oncology: A review and practical primer. *International Journal of Radiation Oncology Biology Physics, 110*(3), 641–655. https://doi.org/10.1016/j.ijrobp.2021.01.044.

Bodenreider, O. (2004). The Unified Medical Language System (UMLS): Integrating biomedical terminology. *Nucleic Acids Research, 32*(DATABASE ISS.). https://doi.org/10.1093/nar/gkh061.

Chapman, W. W., Bridewell, W., Hanbury, P., Cooper, G. F., & Buchanan, B. G. (2001). A simple algorithm for identifying negated findings and diseases in discharge summaries. *Journal of Biomedical Informatics, 34*(5), 301–310. https://doi.org/10.1006/jbin.2001.1029.

Christodouleas, J. P., Anderson, N., Gabriel, P., Greene, R., Hahn, C., Kessler, S., Mayo, C. S., McNutt, T., Shulman, L. N., Smith, B. D., West, J., & Williamson, T. (2020). A multidisciplinary consensus recommendation on a synoptic radiation treatment summary: A commission on cancer workgroup report. *Practical Radiation Oncology, 10*(6), 389–401. https://doi.org/10.1016/j.prro.2020.01.002.

Colaprico, A., Olsen, C., Bailey, M. H., Odom, G. J., Terkelsen, T., Silva, T. C., Olsen, A. V., Cantini, L., Zinovyev, A., Barillot, E., Noushmehr, H., Bertoli, G., Castiglioni, I., Cava, C., Bontempi, G., Chen, X. S., & Papaleo, E. (2020). Interpreting pathways to discover cancer driver genes with Moonlight. *Nature Communications, 11*(1). https://doi.org/10.1038/s41467-019-13803-0.

Fragoso, G., de Coronado, S., Haber, M., Hartel, F., & Wright, L. (2004). Overview and utilization of the NCI Thesaurus. *Comparative and Functional Genomics, 5*(8), 648–654. https://doi.org/10.1002/cfg.445.

Hayman, J. A., Dekker, A., Feng, M., Keole, S. R., McNutt, T. R., Machtay, M., Martin, N. E., Mayo, C. S., Pawlicki, T., Smith, B. D., Kudner, R., Dawes, S., & Yu, J. B. (2019). Minimum data elements for radiation oncology: An American Society for Radiation Oncology consensus paper. *Practical Radiation Oncology, 9*(6), 395–401. https://doi.org/10.1016/j.prro.2019.07.017.

Kundra, R., Zhang, H., Sheridan, R., Sirintrapun, S. J., Wang, A., Ochoa, A., Wilson, M., Gross, B., Sun, Y., Madupuri, R., Satravada, B. A., Reales, D., Vakiani, E., Al-Ahmadie, H. A., Dogan, A., Arcila, M., Zehir, A., Maron, S., Berger, M. F., … Schultz, N. (2021). OncoTree: A cancer classification system for precision oncology. *JCO Clinical Cancer Informatics, 5*, 221–230. https://doi.org/10.1200/cci.20.00108.

Langlotz, C. P. (2006). RadLex: A new method for indexing online educational materials. *Radiographics, 26*(6), 1595–1597. https://doi.org/10.1148/rg.266065168.

Lee, J., Yoon, W., Kim, S., Kim, D., Kim, S., So, C. H., & Kang, J. (2020). BioBERT: A pre-trained biomedical language representation model for biomedical text mining. *Bioinformatics, 36*(4), 1234–1240. https://doi.org/10.1093/bioinformatics/btz682.

Lu, C. J., Payne, A., & Mork, J. G. (2020). The unified medical language system specialist lexicon and lexical tools: Development and applications. *Journal of the American*

Medical Informatics Association, *27*(10), 1600–1605. https://doi.org/10.1093/JAMIA/OCAA056.

Mayo, C. S., Moran, J. M., Bosch, W., Xiao, Y., McNutt, T., Popple, R., Michalski, J., Feng, M., Marks, L. B., Fuller, C. D., Yorke, E., Palta, J., Gabriel, P. E., Molineu, A., Matuszak, M. M., Covington, E., Masi, K., Richardson, S. L., Ritter, T., … Yock, T. I. (2018). American association of physicists in medicine task group 263: Standardizing nomenclatures in radiation oncology. *International Journal of Radiation Oncology Biology Physics, 100*(4), 1057–1066. https://doi.org/10.1016/j.ijrobp.2017.12.013.

McCray, A. T. (2003). An upper-level ontology for the biomedical domain. *Comparative and Functional Genomics, 4*(1), 80–84. https://doi.org/10.1002/cfg.255.

Michalopoulos, G., Wang, Y., Kaka, H., Chen, H., & Wong, A. (2021). *UmlsBERT: Clinical Domain Knowledge Augmentation of Contextual Embeddings Using the Unified Medical Language System Metathesaurus*, 1744–1753. https://doi.org/10.18653/v1/2021.naacl-main.139.

National Cancer Institute. (n.d.). *Common Terminology Criteria for Adverse Events (CTCAE)*. February 21, 2022. https://ctep.cancer.gov/protocoldevelopment/electronic_applications/ctc.htm.

National Library of Medicine. (n.d.). *UMLS Metathesaurus Browser*. February 21, 2022. https://uts.nlm.nih.gov/uts/umls/home.

National Research Council (US) Committee on A Framework for Developing a New Taxonomy of Disease. (2011). Toward precision medicine. In *Toward Precision Medicine: Building a Knowledge Network for Biomedical Research and a New Taxonomy of Disease*. National Academies Press. https://doi.org/10.17226/13284.

Nelson, S. J., Zeng, K., Kilbourne, J., Powell, T., & Moore, R. (2011). Normalized names for clinical drugs: RxNorm at six years. *Journal of the American Medical Informatics Association*, *18*(4), 441–448. https://doi.org/10.1136/amiajnl-2011-000116.

Noy, N. F., Shah, N. H., Whetzel, P. L., Dai, B., Dorf, M., Griffith, N., Jonquet, C., Rubin, D. L., Storey, M. A., Chute, C. G., & Musen, M. A. (2009). BioPortal: Ontologies and integrated data resources at the click of a mouse. *Nucleic Acids Research*, *37*(Suppl. 2). https://doi.org/10.1093/nar/gkp440.

Phillips, M. H., Serra, L. M., Dekker, A., Ghosh, P., Luk, S. M. H., Kalet, A., & Mayo, C. (2020). Ontologies in radiation oncology. *Physica Medica, 72*, 103–113. https://doi.org/10.1016/j.ejmp.2020.03.017.

Rosse, C. & Mejino, J. L. V. (2008). *The Foundational Model of Anatomy Ontology*, 59–117. https://doi.org/10.1007/978-1-84628-885-2_4.

Savova, G. K., Masanz, J. J., Ogren, P. V., Zheng, J., Sohn, S., Kipper-Schuler, K. C., & Chute, C. G. (2010). Mayo clinical Text Analysis and Knowledge Extraction System (cTAKES): Architecture, component evaluation and applications. *Journal of the American Medical Informatics Association*, *17*(5), 507–513. https://doi.org/10.1136/jamia.2009.001560.

SNOMED International. (n.d.). *SNOMED International*. February 21, 2022. https://www.snomed.org/.

Traverso, A., van Soest, J., Wee, L., & Dekker, A. (2018). The radiation oncology ontology (ROO): Publishing linked data in radiation oncology using semantic web and ontology techniques. *Medical Physics, 45*(10), e854–e862. https://doi.org/10.1002/mp.12879.

World Health Organization (WHO). (2003). ICD-10, International Statistical Classification of Diseases-10. *International Statistical Classification of Diseases, 10.*

Chapter 8

Natural Language Processing for Radiation Oncology

Lisa Ni*, Christina Phuong* and Julian Hong

University of California San Francisco Department of Radiation Oncology, San Francisco CA, USA

Abstract

The bulk of clinical information in electronic medical records (EMR) is in narrative form. Unlike structured data, while free text is effective and convenient for communication and documentation, it is not easily translatable for research, quality improvement, or clinical decision support. Recently, there has been increasing interest in the use of natural language processing (NLP) to extract the valuable clinical information from free-text narratives available within EMRs. This chapter aims to provide an overview of NLP technologies, applications in medicine and oncology in particular, and future directions that will facilitate advances in the field of radiation oncology.

*These authors contributed equally to this work.

1. Introduction

Free narrative text is a convenient and commonly used form of communication in medicine. However, this type of text is difficult to search, summarize, and analyze for research or quality improvement purposes. Because of this, there has been increasing interest in using natural language processing (NLP) in the field of medicine across a wide variety of applications. In this chapter, our aim is to provide an overview of NLP, applications in medicine and oncology in particular, current work within radiation oncology, and future directions that will facilitate advances in our field.

2. What Is NLP?

NLP is an area of research in artificial intelligence (AI) at the intersection of computer science, linguistics, and psychology. NLP involves the use of a range of computational techniques to analyze and represent naturally occurring text to be used for a variety of tasks and applications. Because NLP involves such a wide range of disciplines, it is important for those interested in working in NLP to have a good knowledge base of concepts prior to proceeding. There are generally two overarching goals: language processing and language generation.

2.1. *The history of NLP*

Research into NLP has been ongoing for several decades, dating back to the late 1940s. One of the oldest applications of NLP is machine translation, which is the task of translating a text from a source language to a target language (Koehn, 2009). Later on, more sophisticated rule-based methods rooted in linguistic principles were developed, but due to natural language's vast size and unrestrictive nature, problems arose such as rules becoming unmanageably numerous and interacting unpredictably, or difficulty in handling ungrammatical prose that was comprehensible by humans but not with handwritten rules. Thus, since the 1980s, the trend has moved toward data-driven methods for machine translation, including statistical and neural-based approaches (Okpor, 2014).

Nowadays, NLP strategies typically follow rule-based, statistical, or hybrid approaches. Rule-based methods are designed by domain specialists and have the advantage of interpretability. However, as mentioned above, with increasingly complex rule-based systems, interpretability decreases, with rules interacting unpredictably. As such, they become difficult to replicate and update. Because of this, rules handle "ungrammatical" prose very poorly, even though this type of text is comprehensible by humans. Statistical systems, also known as machine learning systems, are designed using training data. In the case of NLP, the training data are large bodies of text (corpora), which have now become widely available and provide the gold standards for evaluation.

As the field of NLP research expanded, more and more corpora have been developed, including specialized data sets for purposes such as sentiment analysis, voice recognition or chatbots, and audio speech data sets, many of which can be found for free online.

2.2. *NLP definitions*

In the following, we explain common sub-problems and associated tasks in NLP.

Low-level NLP tasks:

- *Sentence boundary detection*: Detecting where one sentence ends and another begins.
- *Tokenization*: Separating a piece of text into smaller units called "tokens". Tokens can be broadly classified into words, characters, or subwords.
- *Part-of-speech assignment to individual words ("POS tagging")*: Categorizing words in a text in correspondence with a particular part of speech, depending on the definition of the word and its context.
- *Morphological decomposition*: Comprehending words through decomposition of compound words. Useful sub-tasks include *stemming*, which is a more crude heuristic process of removing the ends of words, and *lemmatization*, which is the conversion of a word to a root, often by removing suffixes.

- *Shallow parsing ("chunking")*: Analyzing a sentence to identify the constituents (noun groups, verbs, verb groups, etc).

Higher-level NLP tasks:

- *Grammatical error correction*: Correcting various errors in text such as spelling, punctuation, grammatical, and word choice errors.
- *Named entity recognition*: Scanning text and pulling out fundamental entities and classifying them into predefined categories. Entities are the most important chunks of a particular sentence, such as noun phrases and verb phrases. Examples of entities include people's names, dates and times, disease names, and geographical locations.
- *Word sense disambiguation*: Determining a homograph's correct meaning, which involves properly identifying words and determining the specific usage of a word in a particular sentence.
- *Negation and uncertainty identification*: Differentiating when a named entity is absent and quantifying the uncertainty of this inference.
- *Relationship extraction*: Extracting semantic relationships from a text, usually occurring between two or more entities of a certain type, and falling into a number of semantic categories.
- *Temporal inferences/relationship extraction*: Making inferences from temporal expressions and relations.
- *Information extraction*: Extracting meaningful information from unstructured text data and presenting it in a structured format. This task often comprises many of the tasks described previously.

2.3. *NLP transformation and representation methods*

Next, we define transformation and representation methods, which are used to convert text into mathematical models that can then be processed. These models typically assign probabilities, frequencies, or weights to words, sequences of words, sections of documents, or whole documents.

- *1-hot encoding*: representing categorical variables as binary vectors. In NLP, the length of the word vector is equal to the length of the vocabulary, and each unique observation (e.g. word) is mapped to an integer value. Then, each integer value is represented as a binary vector that is all zero values except the index of the integer, which is marked with a 1. A list of words creates an array of vectors or a matrix. A list of sentences creates a three-dimensional tensor. This representation does not take into account the relationships between words and does not convey information about their surrounding context.

- *Bag-of-words*: a model that represents the text as an unordered set of words, ignoring their original position in the text and keeping only their frequency. This method of representing text is useful in applications such as sentiment analysis and detecting the language a text is written in.
- *TF–IDF (term frequency–inverse document frequency)*: a statistical measure that evaluates how relevant a word is to a document in a collection of documents. Term frequency is defined as the frequency of the word in the current document. Inverse document frequency is defined as $\log(N/d)$, where N is the total number of documents and d is the number of documents that contain the word. The TF–IDF weight is the product of these two metrics. With TF–IDF, discriminative words with low term frequency in a document but which appear in very few other documents are weighted more highly than terms with have high raw frequency in a document but that appear with high frequency in all documents.
- *N-gram model*: estimates the probability of the next word in a sequence given the previous words. A 2-gram (or bigram) is a two-word sequence of words, and so on. Probabilities for various n-grams can be obtained from large bodies of texts.
- *Word embedding*: techniques that map words or phrases to continuous vector representations that predict the likelihood of those words/phrases occurring in the context of other words/phrases. In general, this involves projecting a word from a dimension equivalent to the vocabulary length to a lower dimensional space. These techniques are primarily used with neural network models.
- *Recurrent neural networks (RNN)*: a variant of neural networks that includes loops and allows information to persist, commonly used in

NLP. The standard input is a word instead of the entire sample (as in the case of a standard neural network). Each word is a separate input occurring at time '*t*' and uses the activation value at '*t*-1' as an input in addition to the input at time '*t*'. The architecture categories are: Many-to-One (many inputs used to give one output, e.g. classification tasks), One-to-Many (generates a series of outputs based on a single input, e.g. music generation), and Many-to-Many (e.g. machine translation). This provides two main advantages: flexibility for the network to work with varying sentence lengths, and sharing features learned across different positions of text. However, RNNs are only capable of capturing the dependencies in one direction of language, and are not very good at capturing long-term dependencies (i.e. the vanishing gradient problem). The following two definitions are the main modified architectures that are used in almost every application of RNNs.

- *Gated recurrent unit (GRU)* (J. Chung *et al.*, 2014): a modification to the basic recurrent unit that consists of an additional memory unit, commonly referred to as an update gate or a reset gate. This unit uses *tanh* as an activation function since its output can be both positive and negative and can be used for scaling up or down. The output from this unit is then combined with the activation input to update the value of the memory cell. Thus, at each step, the value of both the hidden unit and the memory unit are updated. This helps capture long range dependencies and fixes the vanishing gradient problem.
- *Long short-term memory (LSTM)*: instead of having one update gate (as in GRU), there is an update gate and a forget gate. This gives the memory cell an option of keeping or dropping old values, for example, dropping the information regarding an old subject's gender when a new subject is encountered.
- *Transformer Networks*: a simple network architecture based solely on self-attention mechanisms (as opposed to complex RNNs or convolutional neural networks that rely on sequence to sequence models). Attention mechanisms are not reliant on the sequencing and the distance between input or output, but instead gather global dependencies between inputs and outputs. This allows for a deeper understanding of the context and relationship of language. In addition, the model uses multiple attention layers, which are stacked on top of each other.

This maintains information from all prior layers of the network, which avoids the vanishing gradient problem as seen in RNNs.

- *Bidirectional Encoder Representations from Transformers (BERT)* (Devlin *et al.*, 2019): a novel language representation model that applies multi-layer bidirectional training of transformers using Masked Language Model (MLM). Inputs are read in a non-directional fashion by jointly conditioning on both left and right contexts, instead of in a unidirectional (right-to-left or left-to-right) manner. The MLM randomly masks some of the words from unlabeled input with the pre-training objective of predicting the original word based on the context of the other inputs. At the same time, the BERT model is pre-trained for Next Sentence Prediction (NSP) by understanding sentence relationships. These learned, pre-trained parameters are then fine-tuned for specific downstream tasks, which can be done relatively quickly and inexpensively. BERT uses a unified architecture across different tasks; thus, the same model can be applied to a broad variety of NLP tasks and has outperformed many task-specific architectures. A few examples of BERT-based models that apply to the field of medicine include BioBERT (BERT with integration of biomedical corpora for biomedical text mining), UmlsBERT (BERT with integration of clinical domain knowledge using the Unified Medical Language System clinical metathesaurus), and Med-BERT (BERT with integration of structured EMR data set) (Lee *et al.*, 2019; Michalopoulos *et al.*, 2021).

Now that we have defined basic concepts that are fundamental to NLP, we will explore the various ways that NLP is applied within medicine. Then, we will examine the progress in NLP thus far within the field of oncology and then more specifically within radiation oncology throughout the rest of this chapter.

3. NLP in Medicine

In modern medicine, electronic medical records (EMRs) contain most of the clinically important data, most often not encoded within structured data fields but rather in clinician-generated narrative text. These data are often difficult to access, let alone analyze, in a critical, comprehensive, or structured way. Recent changes in health information technology have drastically increased the availability of data for research and quality improvement. The HITECH Act under the 2009 American Recovery and Reinvestment act has encouraged widespread use of EMRs, and their ubiquitous use has led to increasing volume and scope of data collected. However, most of the data cannot be easily extracted in a usable way from EMR. There is, therefore, increasing interest in applying NLP in the clinical setting, and research has been thriving, as evident in the increasing number of articles published about NLP in medicine over the past two decades (Wang *et al.*, 2020).

3.1. *The linguistic string project*

The use of NLP in the clinical setting began in the 1960s. The Linguistic String Project was an early study starting in 1965 that focused on NLP in the medical setting, including a dictionary of medical terms, and addressed issues such as de-identification, parsing, mapping, and normalization of clinical text (Sager *et al.*, 1987). Research in this area increased in the 1970s and 1980s, continuing to demonstrate that it was feasible to structure clinical information occurring in text. The Unified Medical Language System (UMLS) was initiated in 1986 by the National Library of Medicine (NLM), and provided controlled vocabularies of medical concepts with mappings across the vocabularies. Soon, more and more NLP systems were developed that demonstrated the utility of NLP in the clinical domain for data extraction in the late 1980s and 1990s.

3.2. *The realtime outbreak and disease surveillance system*

Another early application of NLP in medicine was the Real-time Outbreak and Disease Surveillance (RODS) System initially deployed in 1999, a public health surveillance system for early detection of disease outbreaks by classifying chief complaints into syndrome categories (Tsui *et al.*, 2003). Detection algorithms monitored complaints from patients in a database of emergency department cases for anomalous patterns of occurrence (Wong *et al.*, 2002). Soon, it was demonstrated that free-text triage chief complaints from emergency department visits could be successfully encoded into diagnostic codes and syndromic categories that could be used for biosurveillance (Chapman *et al.*, 2005). However, due to the varying length and quality of the free-text descriptions within chief complaints and lack of standard nomenclature, use of chief complaint data in decisions and research has been difficult. One possible solution reported has been development of contextual embeddings with the goal of mapping free-text chief complaints to structured labels and deriving a standardized dictionary of chief complaints (Chang *et al.*, 2020).

3.3. *Predicting patient outcomes*

Across various clinical settings, NLP has been incorporated into developing algorithms to predict patient outcomes. Multiple groups have reported on neural network models using NLP to predict disposition including hospital admission from emergency department nursing and physician notes in combination with available clinical data (Zhang *et al.*, 2017). Algorithms have also been developed to predict intensive care unit outcomes, including in-hospital mortality or prolonged ICU stay, with good predictive performance (Marafino *et al.*, 2018). These NLP-augmented models are often developed using clinical trajectory models leveraging predictor variables such as vital signs and laboratory tests and enriching these models with information extracted from clinical notes (Marafino *et al.*, 2018).

3.4. *Monitoring adverse drug events*

NLP has also been applied to monitor adverse drug events (ADEs), in order to quantify the incidence and risk of ADEs, identify patients at risk, and provide earlier and more accurate ADE detection. Several initiatives have emerged to establish and develop a global knowledge base to standardize information regarding drugs and their health outcomes of interest (Boyce *et al.*, 2014). For example, Duke *et al.* developed an NLP application which extracts adverse events from product labels to generate a standardized ADE knowledge base (Duke & Friedlin, 2010). Since then, researchers have been working to identify the optimal sources of information from which to extract ADE data. There has also been research into using clinical narratives to identify ADEs; for example, using existing NLP systems such as MedLEE (Friedman *et al.*, 2004) to process patient records and identify ADEs (Li *et al.*, 2014). Proposed future directions include extraction of information from social media, e.g. online health forums and social networks, as patients increasingly share their experiences with medications online.

3.5. *Processing medical literature for clinician use*

Another area that is of interest is using NLP models to aid in the processing of medical literature, as clinicians who practice evidence-based medicine are required to incorporate the latest scientific research into their practices. In order to develop such models, corpora specific to medical literature are necessary. As discussed in the previous section, modern NLP models are often trained using corpora, many of which are freely available online. However, the data sets available for the medical setting are more limited, and many are recently developed or currently in the works. In the 2000s, studies demonstrated that key elements could be extracted from the abstracts of medical articles, including statistical techniques used and clinically relevant aspects (Demner-Fushman & Lin, 2007). Nye *et al.* at Northeastern University developed *EBM-NLP,* a corpus of about 5,000 abstracts of articles describing clinical randomized controlled trials, annotated using PICO elements (Populations, Interventions, Comparators, and Outcomes) (Huang *et al.*, 2006; Nye *et al.*, 2018; *PICO Extraction*, n.d.). The eventual goal of developing corpora such as *EBM-NLP* would be to provide physicians with a way to easily search and organize the published literature while practicing evidence-based medicine. Examples include improving medical literature search and retrieval systems and extracting structured information to automate knowledge base construction.

3.6. *Design and implementation of clinical trials*

Next, we turn our attention to the design and implementation of clinical trials. Currently, a critical rate-limiting step for clinical trials is defining and identifying the patient cohort for randomized controlled trials.

Poor cohort definition can lead to expensive protocol amendments or failed recruitment. Thus, different avenues to address this using NLP have been explored. First, since eligibility criteria are mostly documented as unstructured free-text, many eligibility criteria representations have been developed (Weng *et al.*, 2010). For example, Tu *et al.* designed the Eligibility Rule Grammar and Ontology for clinical eligibility criteria and demonstrated its effectiveness in transforming free-text eligibility criteria into computable criteria (Tu *et al.*, 2011). Meanwhile, other groups were working on developing information extraction systems to parse and formalize eligibility criteria (Kang *et al.*, 2017). The next step will be transforming the structured eligibility criteria to execute cohort queries on standards-based clinical databases. Yuan *et al.* published their work on Criteria2Query, a hybrid information extraction pipeline using named entity recognition that can be used as a natural language interface to clinical databases, demonstrating usability with a 0.795 and 0.805 F1 score for entity recognition and relation extraction, respectively (Yuan *et al.*, 2019).

3.7. *Future applications/directions*

Research involving NLP in medicine has been developing rapidly over the past few decades, now averaging over 100 publications annually (Wang *et al.*, 2020). As detailed in this section, information extraction and syntax parsing are the most common uses of NLP in the clinical domain. The most common subject area in NLP-assisted medical research is unsurprisingly in oncology, accounting for the highest proportion of studies published about medical NLP. Advances in using NLP to facilitate cancer research will be the focus of the next section in our chapter.

4. NLP in Oncology

As discussed, most of the data archived in EMR is in free text form and cannot be extracted in a readily analyzable form. Free text data allows for personalized documentation for each patient and can capture more nuanced information, especially longitudinally, as oncologic status needs to be monitored over time. However, in a retrospective or research setting, these data then need to be extracted and normalized into useable data, typically in a tabular representation. In addition, there must be inter-operator transferability of information as patients are often cared for in a multidisciplinary fashion and may not stay within the same healthcare network.

4.1. *Radiographic surveillance and diagnosis*

In the realm of oncology, there are many areas in which NLP can have a transformative impact on data extraction (Spasić *et al.*, 2014; Yim *et al.*, 2016). Much of the focus has been on semi-structured texts such as radiology or pathology reports. Hripcsak *et al.* demonstrated the use of NLP in translating clinical prose of radiology findings and impressions reports into structured semantics that could be coded for (Hripcsak *et al.*, 2002). Here, NLP was used to code narratives for 10 years' worth of chest radiographs, which included over 800,000 radiographs, at an urban academic center, and was compared to manual coding, resulting in a sensitivity of 0.81 and specificity of 0.99. This could potentially translate to more accurate hospital diagnosis coding, automated decision, support, and clinical research (Hripcsak *et al.*, 1995). The ability to extract data by a standardized method can pave the way for diagnostic surveillance. Specifically, in regard to potentially malignant lesions where temporal change over time is critically important in addition to new findings on imaging, NLP can be used to alert physicians to critical findings to aid in unmissed surveillance and timely diagnostic work up. Gara *et al.* demonstrated this by developing a system to alert physicians for potentially malignant liver lesions (Garla *et al.*, 2013). Not only is there a role for NLP in detection of malignancy, NLP can also be utilized to characterize a lesion's status over time. For example, Cheng *et al.* utilized NLP to classify tumors in a cohort of brain tumors as stable, progressing, or regressing with 80.8% sensitivity and 91.6% specificity (Cheng *et al.*, 2010).

4.2. *Detailed pathological, molecular, and genomic features*

There has also been work in the use of NLP for extracting information from narrative pathology reports to efficiently gather large volume data and appropriately categorize disease diagnoses (Leyh-Bannurah *et al.*,

2018). Cancer genetics and phenotypes are increasingly being used to tailor therapy (Savova *et al.*, 2017). Extracting specific tumor characteristics, such as histology, staging features, genomics, can allow for selection of appropriate patient cohorts for studies without the tedious human role of parsing out free text forms. In addition, this allows for a wider analysis of biomarkers based on immunohistology reports that may not be specific to a single diagnosis or type of cancer. This, in part, requires an accessible database of known pathological diagnoses with expression of certain biomarkers to aid in diagnosis and prediction of pharmacological response (Lee *et al.*, 2018). Though there exists an online resource from Pathpedia, available data are dependent on journal articles addressing the biomarkers of interest, which is not always the case. Thus, an NLP algorithm to extract these data can be incredibly informative. Given the abundance of information within pathology specimens, institutions are also utilizing NLP to dynamically populate a continuous tumor registry in a comprehensive manner (Oliwa *et al.*, 2019).

4.3. *Identifying patient cohorts from EMR*

Both radiology and pathology in addition to clinical assessment play critical roles in identifying patients within a desired cohort. NLP technology has shown promise in appropriately classifying cancer diagnoses from semi-structured and free-text documentation, identifying terminology related to a cancer diagnosis, and if the relation with the patient is a positive or negative one, often with high F-scores (D'Avolio *et al.*, 2010). Often, billing codes are utilized to identify patient cohorts, though this has been achieved with variable accuracy. Potential areas for error include limited clinical data, diagnostic errors, or miscoded data (Peabody *et al.*, 2004). One should keep in mind that ICD-9 codes were intended for reimbursement purposes, and thus, may not always align with clinical goals; however, this has been an easy method to identify patients. NLP can potentially identify cases that have more complexity than what is captured with a billing code, which may not be as specific. NLP methods have been compared to ICD-9 code methods to identify certain cancers. In evaluating the accuracy of identifying pancreatic cancer in those with IPMN, NLP demonstrated marked greater specificity (94% vs 46%) and PPV

(84% vs 38%), though with a sensitivity of 87% vs 95% when using ICD-9 codes (Friedlin *et al.*, 2010). A combination of ICD-9 and NLP has been suggested to improve case identification (Danforth *et al.*, 2012).

4.4. *Identifying cancer stage from EMR*

In addition to identifying patients with a certain disease, appropriate staging is critical in oncology for both management and predicted outcomes. Often, staging data are missing from large cancer registries, even in those with mandate stage data collection, and can be inaccurate. When data are not entered prospectively, it is even more difficult and labor-intensive to retrospectively stage patients from medical reports (Threlfall *et al.*, 2005). Initially, studies focused on extracting TNM staging from pathology reports as those are more semi-structured data, though this limits M classification (Kim *et al.*, 2014). Soysal *et al.* did, however, show feasibility of developing an NLP system to extract metastasis site and status from pathology reports in a cohort of lung cancer specific patients (Soysal *et al.*, 2017). Clinical staging is often a combination of biopsy, imaging, and clinical assessments, which requires more advanced data extraction methods. Differentiation between pathological and clinical staging is also required. A hybrid system of both pattern matching and machine learning to extract unstructured T, N, M staging in a large cancer registry was developed and achieved an F score of about 0.85 (AAlAbdulsalam *et al.*, 2018). Areas of error included differentiating clinical and pathological staging and confusion of staging vs MRI sequence T2. Ling *et al.* were able to use NLP to extract a metastatic breast cancer cohort, including de novo and recurrent metastatic disease with >85% sensitivity and specificity (Ling *et al.*, 2019).

4.5. *Risk assessment*

The focus on obtaining accurate and detailed oncological characteristics for research and clinical purposes is ultimately with the goal of tailoring therapy and improving outcomes. The ability to predict patient outcomes would aid in discussions for optimal treatment for patients. For example, often surgical candidacy is determined in part by preoperative risk assessments involving structured, discrete features. NLP has the potential to capture a more nuanced clinical assessment for a patient and predict for post-operative complications and readmission with increased accuracy compared to using discrete features alone (Barber *et al.*, 2021).

4.6. *Clinical outcomes*

The ability to assess patients long term is necessary to understand the course of patients' malignancies. These outcomes include oncological status as well as toxicities, complications, quality of life, etc. This is an ongoing area of study as an application of NLP, as it typically involves more free text language. Most research has been centered around detecting cancer recurrence as there is more semi-structured documentation involving radiology or pathology reports (Banerjee *et al.*, 2019). Most cancer registries do not track recurrence status; thus, there is reliance on manual chart review. However, this is often not feasible in large studies. The extraction tools must be able to identify pertinent information in each document, determine the temporal relationship between every event, and determine if the patient meets specified criteria (Ping *et al.*, 2013). Much of the details and nuances in clinical status are retained in clinical documentation such as H&Ps, progress notes, and discharge summaries. In evaluating unstructured texts, Kehl *et al.* recently demonstrated the ability to use assessment and plans from oncology notes to predict clinical outcomes (Kehl *et al.*, 2020). This group developed an algorithm using neural networks to determine retrospectively if the oncology note indicated the presence of cancer and if so, whether there was improvement or progression of disease. They then determined if this translated to differences in outcomes. They found that NLP output of progressive disease was associated with decreased survival, and NLP output of improvement was associated with improved survival. This is exciting as it demonstrates the feasibility and real potential of NLP to identify temporal changes in disease status that may translate to clinical outcomes.

4.7. *Identifying social determinants of care and identifying healthcare gaps*

There is also potential to assess social determinants from the cancer patient population that may affect care such as social isolation, substance use history, and living situation (Hong *et al.*, 2020; Zhu *et al.*, 2019). This may allow for more efficient needs assessment for patients and appropriately allocate resources to support patients. This could also help identify gaps in care and at-risk populations in more detail with more population-based extractions.

4.8. *Summary*

With the burgeoning knowledge in oncology, large volumes of data are continually published. Due to the fast-paced nature of clinical practice as well as the desire to assess patients and start treatment in a timely manner, an efficient method of triaging literature is of value. The generalizability of these tools still needs to be investigated but would greatly enhance the utility of evidence-based medicine in clinical practice.

5. NLP in Radiation Oncology

Radiation oncology is a highly technical field that relies heavily on digital data and computer software and comprises many different healthcare professionals. This combination highlights the number of human–machine interactions that each treatment relies on. Much of the data, including clinical documentation, radiation treatment planning, and dosimetric detail, are stored in various software programs and often require manual extraction. However, research into applications of NLP in radiation oncology has remained limited, despite the advances in the field of oncology. With increasing NLP efforts, there is a large opportunity to analyze data that have previously been difficult and unavailable to access (Bitterman *et al.*, 2021).

5.1. *Big data analysis*

Cancer registries provide databases that allow for epidemiologic studies, surveillance, and outcome measurements. Even large registries, such as SEER or NCDB, lack high-quality radiation therapy data, thereby limiting the ability to conduct population analyses (Jacobs *et al.*, 2019). This has been acknowledged by organizations such as the American Society of

Clinical Oncology (ASCO) and American Society for Radiation Oncology (ASTRO). In response, they launched a collaborative registry in 2018 to improve the quality of data recorded (*New Registry Launched to Track and Improve the Quality of Cancer Care Delivered in the U.S. —American Society for Radiation Oncology (ASTRO)*, 2018). NLP can be used to augment existing registries to obtain more complete information, and moving forward, input additional data. As discussed previously, appropriate patient identification is the first step toward data collection and analysis. In addition, more complete registries can help identify larger cohorts of rare, underreported malignancies, which raises the potential for further research and knowledge of these tumors.

5.2. *Understanding complex radiation histories*

As patients are living longer due to improvements in therapies, more patients are undergoing additional courses of radiation. There is emerging evidence for the use of targeted therapies and immunotherapies in combination with radiation therapy as well as data to support radiation therapy for oligometastatic or oligo-progressive disease. As such, more complex radiation histories will become more common, and our field would benefit from advanced algorithms to analyze these data accurately and efficiently. NLP has already been used to help identify patients who have received radiation and identify the sites treated with good accuracy. The latter is a task that would otherwise be difficult, especially since a single site can often be named differently depending on the treating physician or group (Walker *et al.*, 2019). This is one of the ways that NLP will aid in continued surveillance and updates of cancer registries efficiently.

5.3. *Overcoming non-standardized nomenclature*

A known barrier to aggregating data within radiation oncology is the lack of standardized nomenclature; however, NLP can be used to make these data more accessible. Consistency in nomenclature throughout radiation oncology is necessary for a variety of reasons, including facilitation of large data collection, collaboration among institutions, dosimetric analysis, and transfers of care. As such, this consistency is critical in both the clinical patient care and research settings. Though there does exist a standardized naming system for organs at risk and target structures according to TG-263 developed in 2018, there has not been universal adoption of this system by every institution (Mayo *et al.*, 2017). Some challenges include software limitations in naming, institutional lack of participation or oversight, and difficulties with transitioning from previously used nomenclature. Researchers have, instead, utilized NLP to match unstructured naming from clinical documentation and treatment planning systems to standardized nomenclature (Syed *et al.*, 2020).

5.4. *Improving documentation and communication of radiation histories*

ASTRO is also working to identify a minimum set of data from radiation therapy that needed to be captured within EMR and oncologic databases to facilitate research, quality improvement, interdisciplinary communication, and ease of transfer among hospital systems with the goal of improving patient care (Hayman *et al.*, 2019). This includes data such as treatment site, dose, fractionation, technique, and dates. Often, these data are extracted manually, leaving room for error and can become a documentation burden. A consensus treatment summary has been proposed by the Commission on Cancer to standardize the reporting of radiation treatment, which comprises three sections including a mix of structured and free text (Christodouleas *et al.*, 2020). Thus, implementation of NLP to extract these data in a standardized fashion can help streamline clinical care and ensure data is not lost during transfers of care (Bitterman *et al.*, 2020).

5.5. *Treatment-related toxicity*

A primary source of interest in radiation therapy is the potential toxicities experienced, which can occur during treatment or months to years after treatment. Much of these data are captured in free text forms during on treatment visits, treatment summaries, and follow up notes, which are compared to their baseline, often noted in consultation notes. Though toxicity is graded according to the National Cancer Institute (NCI) Common Terminology Criteria for Adverse Events (CTCAE), there is

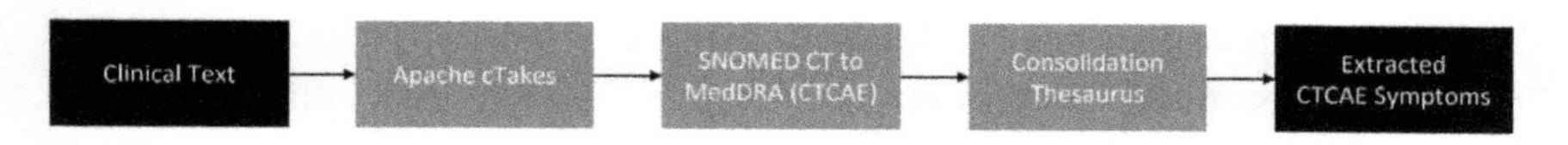

Fig. 1. A natural language processing pipeline, which can be used for extracting CTCAE symptoms from radiation oncology on-treatment visit notes with high accuracy.

often inter-rater variation and retrospective collection is labor-intensive (Fairchild *et al.*, 2020). Thus, the ability of NLP to systematically extract CTCAE symptoms has been of interest (Fig. 1). NLP has shown good precision and recall for common present symptoms, including ones that previously had low human inter-rater reliability; however, negated symptoms have proven to be more difficult (J. C. Hong, Fairchild *et al.*, 2020).

Patient reported outcomes also offer significant insight into adverse events that are symptomatic, and these can be underrepresented based on provider-documented CTCAE (Grewal & Berman, 2019). Thus, the NCI also commissioned the creation of PRO-CTCAE, a patient reported outcome measurement to capture symptomatic toxicity (Basch *et al.*, 2014). Similarly, there are many other questionnaires used by institutions to capture patient reported data, which often contain free text entries (Chung *et al.*, 2019). The details within free text entries stand to benefit from extraction using NLP, as it is often laborious and time consuming to obtain such data manually.

5.6. *Real-time management*

In addition, the use of NLP can potentially play a role in real-time management of patient care. The increasing use of patient portals and messaging platforms made available by EMR systems has translated to change in therapy, such as discontinuation of hormone therapy (Yin *et al.*, 2018). This serves as an additional pool of data that is unstructured and often not utilized, even though it can directly impact management. About 10–20% of patients undergoing radiation treatment or chemoradiation will require acute care, either with an emergency department visit or inpatient admission (Jairam *et al.*, 2019; Waddle *et al.*, 2015). In an effort to reduce the number of preventable visits, machine learning has been used to extract pretreatment and treatment information to predict for emergency department visits during outpatient radiotherapy or chemoradiation (Hong *et al.*,

2018). In a prospective, randomized, single institution study, this NLP pipeline was used to direct intervention. High risk patients were randomized to standard weekly clinical evaluation versus twice weekly evaluation, though both arms were allowed to evaluate patients more frequently based on clinical discretion. Hong *et al.* showed that NLP accurately identified high-risk patients and that additional evaluation of these patients led to a reduction in emergency department admissions (Hong *et al.*, 2020). By accurately identifying these high-risk patients, early supportive care and tailored monitoring can be successfully employed.

6. Conclusion

All in all, applications of NLP in radiation oncology remain in their infancy. Radiation oncology healthcare teams will need to work closely with data scientists to become more well-versed in the field of informatics. Clinically, NLP has the potential to be applied throughout all aspects of patient care. NLP offers a pathway to more efficient individualized care and real-time patient management. It may improve communication of complex radiation histories to other members of the healthcare team and improve transfer of patient information. As standardization of EMR data and radiation oncology nomenclature is still ongoing, NLP offers a way to utilize the vast amounts of EMR data available that would not otherwise be amenable to analysis and reduces the labor-intensive nature of research. The ability of NLP to accurately select patient cohorts for research analysis will be a critical first step to generating reliable real-world data, which will complement prospective clinical trials. Ultimately, NLP has demonstrated enormous potential in multiple applications in the field, but continued research is necessary to optimize its accuracy and reliability.

References

AAlAbdulsalam, A. K., Garvin, J. H., Redd, A., Carter, M. E., Sweeny, C., & Meystre, S. M. (2018). Automated extraction and classification of cancer stage mentions from unstructured text fields in a central cancer registry. *AMIA Summits on Translational Science Proceedings, 2018*, 16–25.

Banerjee, I., Bozkurt, S., Caswell-Jin, J. L., Kurian, A. W., & Rubin, D. L. (2019). Natural language processing approaches to detect the timeline of metastatic recurrence of breast cancer. *JCO Clinical Cancer Informatics*, *3*, 1–12. https://doi.org/10.1200/CCI.19.00034.

Barber, E. L., Garg, R., Persenaire, C., & Simon, M. (2021). Natural language processing with machine learning to predict outcomes after ovarian cancer surgery. *Gynecologic Oncology*, *160*(1), 182–186. https://doi.org/10.1016/j.ygyno.2020.10.004.

Basch, E., Reeve, B. B., Mitchell, S. A., Clauser, S. B., Minasian, L. M., Dueck, A. C., Mendoza, T. R., Hay, J., Atkinson, T. M., Abernethy, A. P., Bruner, D. W., Cleeland, C. S., Sloan, J. A., Chilukuri, R., Baumgartner, P., Denicoff, A., St Germain, D., O'Mara, A. M., Chen, A., … Schrag, D. (2014). Development of the National Cancer Institute's patient-reported outcomes version of the common terminology criteria for adverse events (PRO-CTCAE). *Journal of the National Cancer Institute*, *106*(9), dju244. https://doi.org/10.1093/jnci/dju244.

Bitterman, D. S., Miller, T. A., Harris, D., Lin, C., Finan, S., Warner, J., Mak, R. H., & Savova, G. K. (2020). Extracting radiotherapy treatment details using neural network-based natural language processing. *International Journal of Radiation Oncology, Biology, Physics*, *108*(3), e771–e772. https://doi.org/10.1016/j.ijrobp.2020.07.219.

Bitterman, D. S., Miller, T. A., Mak, R. H., & Savova, G. K. (2021). Clinical natural language processing for radiation oncology: A review and practical primer. *International Journal of Radiation Oncology*Biology*Physics*. *110*(3), 641–655. https://doi.org/10.1016/j.ijrobp.2021.01.044.

Boyce, R. D., Ryan, P. B., Norén, G. N., Schuemie, M. J., Reich, C., Duke, J., Tatonetti, N. P., Trifirò, G., Harpaz, R., Overhage, J. M., Hartzema, A. G., Khayter, M., Voss, E. A., Lambert, C. G., Huser, V., & Dumontier, M. (2014). Bridging islands of information to establish an integrated knowledge base of drugs and health outcomes of interest. *Drug Safety*, *37*(8), 557–567. https://doi.org/10.1007/s40264-014-0189-0.

Chang, D., Hong, W. S., & Taylor, R. A. (2020). Generating contextual embeddings for emergency department chief complaints. *JAMIA Open*, *3*(2), 160–166. https://doi.org/10.1093/jamiaopen/ooaa022.

Chapman, W. W., Christensen, L. M., Wagner, M. M., Haug, P. J., Ivanov, O., Dowling, J. N., & Olszewski, R. T. (2005). Classifying free-text triage chief complaints into syndromic categories with natural language processing. *Artificial Intelligence in Medicine*, *33*(1), 31–40. https://doi.org/10.1016/j.artmed.2004.04.001.

Cheng, L. T. E., Zheng, J., Savova, G. K., & Erickson, B. J. (2010). Discerning tumor status from unstructured MRI reports — completeness of information in existing reports and utility of automated natural language processing. *Journal of Digital Imaging*, *23*(2), 119–132. https://doi.org/10.1007/s10278-009-9215-7.

Christodouleas, J. P., Anderson, N., Gabriel, P., Greene, R., Hahn, C., Kessler, S., Mayo, C. S., McNutt, T., Shulman, L. N., Smith, B. D., West, J., & Williamson, T. (2020). A multidisciplinary consensus recommendation on a synoptic radiation treatment summary: A commission on cancer workgroup report. *Practical Radiation Oncology*, *10*(6), 389–401. https://doi.org/10.1016/j.prro.2020.01.002.

Chung, A. E., Shoenbill, K., Mitchell, S. A., Dueck, A. C., Schrag, D., Bruner, D. W., Minasian, L. M., St. Germain, D., O'Mara, A. M., Baumgartner, P., Rogak, L. J., Abernethy, A. P., Griffin, A. C., & Basch, E. M. (2019). Patient free text reporting of symptomatic adverse events in cancer clinical research using the National Cancer Institute's Patient-Reported Outcomes version of the Common Terminology Criteria for Adverse Events (PRO-CTCAE). *Journal of the American Medical Informatics Association : JAMIA*, *26*(4), 276–285. https://doi.org/10.1093/jamia/ocy169.

Chung, J., Gulcehre, C., Cho, K., & Bengio, Y. (2014). Empirical evaluation of gated recurrent neural networks on sequence modeling. *ArXiv:1412.3555 [Cs]*. http://arxiv.org/abs/1412.3555.

Danforth, K. N., Early, M. I., Ngan, S., Kosco, A. E., Zheng, C., & Gould, M. K. (2012). Automated identification of patients with pulmonary nodules in an integrated health system using administrative health plan data, radiology reports, and natural language processing. *Journal of Thoracic Oncology: Official Publication of the International Association for the Study of Lung Cancer*, *7*(8), 1257–1262. https://doi.org/10.1097/JTO.0b013e31825bd9f5.

D'Avolio, L. W., Nguyen, T. M., Farwell, W. R., Chen, Y., Fitzmeyer, F., Harris, O. M., & Fiore, L. D. (2010). Evaluation of a generalizable approach to clinical information retrieval using the Automated Retrieval Console (ARC). *Journal of the American Medical Informatics Association: JAMIA*, *17*(4), 375–382. https://doi.org/10.1136/jamia.2009.001412.

Demner-Fushman, D. & Lin, J. (2007). Answering clinical questions with knowledge-based and statistical techniques. *Computational Linguistics*, *33*(1), 63–103. https://doi.org/10.1162/coli.2007.33.1.63.

Devlin, J., Chang, M.-W., Lee, K., & Toutanova, K. (2019). BERT: Pre-training of deep bidirectional transformers for language understanding. *ArXiv:1810.04805 [Cs]*. http://arxiv.org/abs/1810.04805.

Duke, J. D. & Friedlin, J. (2010). ADESSA: A real-time decision support service for delivery of semantically coded adverse drug event data. *AMIA ... Annual Symposium Proceedings. AMIA Symposium*, *2010*, 177–181.

Fairchild, A. T., Tanksley, J. P., Tenenbaum, J. D., Palta, M., & Hong, J. C. (2020). Interrater reliability in toxicity identification: Limitations of current standards. *International Journal of Radiation Oncology*Biology*Physics*, *107*(5), 996–1000. https://doi.org/10.1016/j.ijrobp.2020.04.040.

Friedlin, J., Overhage, M., Al-Haddad, M. A., Waters, J. A., Aguilar-Saavedra, J. J. R., Kesterson, J., & Schmidt, M. (2010). Comparing methods for identifying pancreatic cancer patients using electronic data sources. *AMIA Annual Symposium Proceedings*, *2010*, 237–241.

Friedman, C., Shagina, L., Lussier, Y., & Hripcsak, G. (2004). Automated encoding of clinical documents based on natural language processing. *Journal of the American Medical Informatics Association*, *11*(5), 392–402. https://doi.org/10.1197/jamia.M1552.

Garla, V., Taylor, C., & Brandt, C. (2013). Semi-supervised clinical text classification with Laplacian SVMs: An application to cancer case management. *Journal of Biomedical Informatics*, *46*(5), 869–875. https://doi.org/10.1016/j.jbi.2013.06.014.

Grewal, A. S. & Berman, A. T. (2019). Patient-centered outcomes in radiation oncology. *Hematology/Oncology Clinics of North America*, *33*(6), 1105–1116. https://doi.org/10.1016/j.hoc.2019.08.012.

Hayman, J. A., Dekker, A., Feng, M., Keole, S. R., McNutt, T. R., Machtay, M., Martin, N. E., Mayo, C. S., Pawlicki, T., Smith, B. D., Kudner, R., Dawes, S., & Yu, J. B. (2019). Minimum data elements for radiation oncology: An American Society for radiation oncology consensus paper. *Practical Radiation Oncology*, *9*(6), 395–401. https://doi.org/10.1016/j.prro.2019.07.017.

Hong, J. C., Eclov, N. C. W., Dalal, N. H., Thomas, S. M., Stephens, S. J., Malicki, M., Shields, S., Cobb, A., Mowery, Y. M., Niedzwiecki, D., Tenenbaum, J. D., & Palta, M. (2020). System for High-Intensity Evaluation During Radiation Therapy (SHIELD-RT): A prospective randomized study of machine learning–directed clinical evaluations during radiation and chemoradiation. *Journal of Clinical Oncology*, *38*(31), 3652–3661. https://doi.org/10.1200/JCO.20.01688.

Hong, J. C., Fairchild, A. T., Tanksley, J. P., Palta, M., & Tenenbaum, J. D. (2020). Natural language processing for abstraction of cancer treatment toxicities: Accuracy versus human experts. *JAMIA Open*, *3*(4), 513–517. https://doi.org/10.1093/jamiaopen/ooaa064.

Hong, J. C., Niedzwiecki, D., Palta, M., & Tenenbaum, J. D. (2018). Predicting emergency visits and hospital admissions during radiation and chemoradiation: An internally validated pretreatment machine learning algorithm. *JCO Clinical Cancer Informatics*, *2*, 1–11. https://doi.org/10.1200/CCI.18.00037.

Hong, J., Davoudi, A., Yu, S., & Mowery, D. L. (2020). Annotation and extraction of age and temporally-related events from clinical histories. *BMC Medical Informatics and Decision Making*, *20*(suppl 11), 338. https://doi.org/10.1186/s12911-020-01333-5.

Hripcsak, G., Austin, J. H. M., Alderson, P. O., & Friedman, C. (2002). Use of natural language processing to translate clinical information from a database of 889,921 chest radiographic reports. *Radiology*, *224*(1), 157–163. https://doi.org/10.1148/radiol.2241011118.

Hripcsak, G., Friedman, C., Alderson, P. O., DuMouchel, W., Johnson, S. B., & Clayton, P. D. (1995). Unlocking clinical data from narrative reports: A study of natural language processing. *Annals of Internal Medicine*, *122*(9), 681–688. https://doi.org/10.7326/0003-4819-122-9-199505010-00007.

Huang, X., Lin, J., & Demner-Fushman, D. (2006). Evaluation of PICO as a knowledge representation for clinical questions. *AMIA ... Annual Symposium Proceedings. AMIA Symposium*, 359–363.

Jacobs, C. D., Carpenter, D. J., Hong, J. C., Havrilesky, L. J., Sosa, J. A., & Chino, J. P. (2019). Radiation records in the national cancer database: Variations in coding and/or practice can significantly alter survival results. *JCO Clinical Cancer Informatics*, *3*, 1–9. https://doi.org/10.1200/CCI.18.00118.

Jairam, V., Lee, V., Park, H. S., Thomas, C. R., Melnick, E. R., Gross, C. P., Presley, C. J., Adelson, K. B., & Yu, J. B. (2019). Treatment-related complications of systemic therapy and radiotherapy. *JAMA Oncology*, *5*(7), 1028. https://doi.org/10.1001/jamaoncol.2019.0086.

Kang, T., Zhang, S., Tang, Y., Hruby, G. W., Rusanov, A., Elhadad, N., & Weng, C. (2017). EliIE: An open-source information extraction system for clinical trial eligibility criteria. *Journal of the American Medical Informatics Association*, *24*(6), 1062–1071. https://doi.org/10.1093/jamia/ocx019.

Kehl, K. L., Xu, W., Lepisto, E., Elmarakeby, H., Hassett, M. J., Van Allen, E. M., Johnson, B. E., & Schrag, D. (2020). Natural language processing to ascertain cancer outcomes from medical oncologist notes. *JCO Clinical Cancer Informatics*, *4*, 680–690. https://doi.org/10.1200/CCI.20.00020.

Kim, B. J., Merchant, M., Zheng, C., Thomas, A. A., Contreras, R., Jacobsen, S. J., & Chien, G. W. (2014). A natural language processing program effectively extracts key pathologic findings from radical prostatectomy reports. *Journal of Endourology*, *28*(12), 1474–1478. https://doi.org/10.1089/end.2014.0221.

Koehn, P. (2009). *Statistical Machine Translation*. New York: Cambridge University Press.

Lee, J., Song, H.-J., Yoon, E., Park, S.-B., Park, S.-H., Seo, J.-W., Park, P., & Choi, J. (2018). Automated extraction of Biomarker information from pathology reports. *BMC Medical Informatics and Decision Making*, *18*(1), 29. https://doi.org/10.1186/s12911-018-0609-7.

Lee, J., Yoon, W., Kim, S., Kim, D., Kim, S., So, C. H., & Kang, J. (2019). BioBERT: A pre-trained biomedical language representation model for biomedical text mining. *Bioinformatics*, *36*(4), 1234–1240, btz682. https://doi.org/10.1093/bioinformatics/btz682.

Leyh-Bannurah, S.-R., Tian, Z., Karakiewicz, P. I., Wolffgang, U., Sauter, G., Fisch, M., Pehrke, D., Huland, H., Graefen, M., & Budäus, L. (2018). Deep learning for natural language processing in urology: State-of-the-art automated extraction of detailed pathologic prostate cancer data from narratively written electronic health records. *JCO Clinical Cancer Informatics*, *2*, 1–9. https://doi.org/10.1200/CCI.18.00080.

Li, Y., Salmasian, H., Vilar, S., Chase, H., Friedman, C., & Wei, Y. (2014). A method for controlling complex confounding effects in the detection of adverse drug reactions using electronic health records. *Journal of the American Medical Informatics Association: JAMIA*, *21*(2), 308–314. https://doi.org/10.1136/amiajnl-2013-001718.

Ling, A. Y., Kurian, A. W., Caswell-Jin, J. L., Sledge, G. W., Jr, Shah, N. H., & Tamang, S. R. (2019). Using natural language processing to construct a metastatic breast cancer cohort from linked cancer registry and electronic medical records data. *JAMIA Open*, *2*(4), 528–537. https://doi.org/10.1093/jamiaopen/ooz040.

Marafino, B. J., Park, M., Davies, J. M., Thombley, R., Luft, H. S., Sing, D. C., Kazi, D. S., DeJong, C., Boscardin, W. J., Dean, M. L., & Dudley, R. A. (2018). Validation of prediction models for critical care outcomes using natural language processing of electronic health record data. *JAMA Network Open*, *1*(8), e185097. https://doi.org/10.1001/jamanetworkopen.2018.5097.

Mayo, C., Moran, J., Bosch, W., Xiao, Y., McNutt, T., Popple, R., Michalski, J., Feng, M., Marks, L., Fuller, C., Yorke, E., Palta, J., Gabriel, P., Molineu, A., Matuszak, M., Covington, E., Masi, K., Richardson, S., Ritter, T., & Yock, T. (2017). AAPM TG-263: Standardizing nomenclatures in radiation oncology. *International Journal of Radiation Oncology *Biology *Physics*, *100*(4), 1057–1066. https://doi.org/10.1016/j.ijrobp.2017.12.013.

Michalopoulos, G., Wang, Y., Kaka, H., Chen, H., & Wong, A. (2021). UmlsBERT: Clinical domain knowledge augmentation of contextual embeddings using the unified medical language system metathesaurus. *Proceedings of the 2021 Conference of the North American Chapter of the Association for Computational Linguistics: Human Language Technologies*, pp. 1744–1753. https://doi.org/10.18653/v1/2021.naacl-main.139.

New Registry Launched to Track and Improve the Quality of Cancer Care Delivered in the U.S. — American Society for Radiation Oncology (ASTRO) — American Society for Radiation Oncology (ASTRO). (2018). ASTRO. https://www.astro.org/News-and-Publications/News-and-Media-Center/News-Releases/2018/New-registry-launched-to-track-and-improve-the-qua.

Nye, B., Jessy Li, J., Patel, R., Yang, Y., Marshall, I. J., Nenkova, A., & Wallace, B. C. (2018). A corpus with multi-level annotations of patients, interventions and outcomes to support language processing for medical literature. *Proceedings of the Conference. Association for Computational Linguistics. Meeting*, *2018*, 197–207.

Okpor, M. D. (2014). Machine translation approaches: Issues and challenges. *Undefined*. https://www.semanticscholar.org/paper/Machine-Translation-Approaches%3A-Issues-and-Okpor/488bf38420814f742c54f3d1cd2c29a5974698b8.

Oliwa, T., Maron, S. B., Chase, L. M., Lomnicki, S., Catenacci, D. V. T., Furner, B., & Volchenboum, S. L. (2019). Obtaining knowledge in pathology reports through a natural language processing approach with classification, named-entity recognition, and relation-extraction heuristics. *JCO Clinical Cancer Informatics*, *3*, 1–8. https://doi.org/10.1200/CCI.19.00008.

Peabody, J. W., Luck, J., Jain, S., Bertenthal, D., & Glassman, P. (2004). Assessing the accuracy of administrative data in health information systems. *Medical Care*, *42*(11), 1066–1072. https://doi.org/10.1097/00005650-200411000-00005.

PICO Extraction. (n.d.). June 28, 2021. https://ebm-nlp.herokuapp.com/.

Ping, X.-O., Tseng, Y.-J., Chung, Y., Wu, Y.-L., Hsu, C.-W., Yang, P.-M., Huang, G.-T., Lai, F., & Liang, J.-D. (2013). Information extraction for tracking liver cancer patients' statuses: From mixture of clinical narrative report types. *Telemedicine and E-Health*, *19*(9), 704–710. https://doi.org/10.1089/tmj.2012.0241.

Sager, N., Friedman, C., & Lyman, M. S. (1987). *Medical Language Processing: Computer Management of Narrative Data*. Boston: Addison-Wesley Publishing Company.

Savova, G. K., Tseytlin, E., Finan, S., Castine, M., Miller, T., Medvedeva, O., Harris, D., Hochheiser, H., Lin, C., Chavan, G., & Jacobson, R. S. (2017). DeepPhe: A natural language processing system for extracting cancer phenotypes from clinical records. *Cancer Research*, *77*(21), e115–e118. https://doi.org/10.1158/0008-5472.CAN-17-0615.

Soysal, E., Warner, J. L., Denny, J. C., & Xu, H. (2017). Identifying metastases-related information from pathology reports of lung cancer patients. *AMIA Summits on Translational Science Proceedings*, *2017*, 268–277.

Spasić, I., Livsey, J., Keane, J. A., & Nenadić, G. (2014). Text mining of cancer-related information: Review of current status and future directions. *International Journal of Medical Informatics*, *83*(9), 605–623. https://doi.org/10.1016/j.ijmedinf.2014.06.009.

Syed, K., Sleeman IV, W., Ivey, K., Hagan, M., Palta, J., Kapoor, R., & Ghosh, P. (2020). Integrated natural language processing and machine learning models for standardizing radiotherapy structure names. *Healthcare*, *8*(2), 120. https://doi.org/10.3390/healthcare8020120.

Threlfall, T., Wittorff, J., Boutdara, P., Heyworth, J., Katris, P., Sheiner, H., & Fritschi, L. (2005). Collection of population-based cancer staging information in Western Australia — a feasibility study. *Population Health Metrics*, *3*, 9. https://doi.org/10.1186/1478-7954-3-9.

Tsui, F.-C., Espino, J. U., Dato, V. M., Gesteland, P. H., Hutman, J., & Wagner, M. M. (2003). Technical description of RODS: A real-time public health surveillance system. *Journal of the American Medical Informatics Association*, *10*(5), 399–408. https://doi.org/10.1197/jamia.M1345.

Tu, S. W., Peleg, M., Carini, S., Bobak, M., Ross, J., Rubin, D., & Sim, I. (2011). A practical method for transforming free-text eligibility criteria into computable criteria. *Journal of Biomedical Informatics*, *44*(2), 239–250. https://doi.org/10.1016/j.jbi.2010.09.007.

Waddle, M. R., Chen, R. C., Arastu, N. H., Green, R. L., Jackson, M., Qaqish, B. F., Camporeale, J., Collichio, F. A., & Marks, L. B. (2015). Unanticipated hospital admissions during or soon after radiation therapy: Incidence and predictive factors. *Practical Radiation Oncology*, *5*(3), e245–e253. https://doi.org/10.1016/j.prro.2014.08.004.

Walker, G., Soysal, E., & Xu, H. (2019). Development of a natural language processing tool to extract radiation treatment sites. *Cureus*, *11*(10), e6010. https://doi.org/10.7759/cureus.6010.

Wang, J., Deng, H., Liu, B., Hu, A., Liang, J., Fan, L., Zheng, X., Wang, T., & Lei, J. (2020). Systematic evaluation of research progress on natural language processing in medicine over the past 20 years: Bibliometric study on PubMed. *Journal of Medical Internet Research*, *22*(1), e16816. https://doi.org/10.2196/16816.

Weng, C., Tu, S. W., Sim, I., & Richesson, R. (2010). Formal representation of eligibility criteria: A literature review. *Journal of Biomedical Informatics*, *43*(3), 451–467. https://doi.org/10.1016/j.jbi.2009.12.004.

Wong, W.-K., Moore, A., Cooper, G., & Wagner, M. (2002). Rule-based anomaly pattern detection for detecting disease outbreaks. *Eighteenth National Conference on Artificial Intelligence*, 217–223.

Yim, W., Yetisgen, M., Harris, W. P., & Kwan, S. W. (2016). Natural language processing in oncology: A review. *JAMA Oncology*, *2*(6), 797–804. https://doi.org/10.1001/jamaoncol.2016.0213.

Yin, Z., Harrell, M., Warner, J. L., Chen, Q., Fabbri, D., & Malin, B. A. (2018). The therapy is making me sick: How online portal communications between breast cancer patients and physicians indicate medication discontinuation. *Journal of the American Medical Informatics Association : JAMIA*, *25*(11), 1444–1451. https://doi.org/10.1093/jamia/ocy118.

Yuan, C., Ryan, P. B., Ta, C., Guo, Y., Li, Z., Hardin, J., Makadia, R., Jin, P., Shang, N., Kang, T., & Weng, C. (2019). Criteria2Query: A natural language interface to clinical databases for cohort definition. *Journal of the American Medical Informatics Association*, *26*(4), 294–305. https://doi.org/10.1093/jamia/ocy178.

Zhang, X., Kim, J., Patzer, R. E., Pitts, S. R., Patzer, A., & Schrager, J. D. (2017). Prediction of emergency department hospital admission based on natural language processing and neural networks. *Methods of Information in Medicine*, *56*(5), 377–389. https://doi.org/10.3414/ME17-01-0024.

Zhu, V. J., Lenert, L. A., Bunnell, B. E., Obeid, J. S., Jefferson, M., & Halbert, C. H. (2019). Automatically identifying social isolation from clinical narratives for patients with prostate Cancer. *BMC Medical Informatics and Decision Making*, *19*(1), 43. https://doi.org/10.1186/s12911-019-0795-y.

Part 4
AI Applications

Chapter 9

Knowledge-Based Treatment Planning: An Efficient and Reliable Planning Technique towards Treatment Planning Automation

Dalong Pang

Department of Radiation Medicine, Georgetown University Medical Center, Washington, DC 20007, USA

Abstract

Knowledge-based treatment planning (KBP) generates treatment plans by utilizing information and knowledge accumulated from manually generated treatment plans collected in a database. Through categorization of anatomical features, such as target volume and organs at risk (OAR) and the spatial orientation relative to each other, KBP selects DVH parameters achieved in a clinical plan in the database as the DVH objectives for a new patient who has anatomical features similar to the database patient. This methodology therefore eliminates the typical trial-and-error process in treatment planning optimization and reduces the time requirement and plan quality variation in planning. The process of selection, comparison, extraction of data and plan optimization can be automated through scripting to generate a good quality plan in a matter of minutes instead of the typical hours and days. In this chapter, we describe in detail the KBP methodology, present a few representative cases of KBP studies, and discuss its utility and future direction in radiotherapy.

1. Introduction

Radiotherapy is a multiple-step, sequential process that generally follows the following three steps: (1) prescription, (2) treatment planning, and (3) treatment plan delivery (Khan *et al.*, 2021). While each step is important, the ability to produce high-quality treatment plans is arguably the most technically challenging in meeting the treatment requirements specified in the prescription. The skills to generate high-quality treatment plans for various complexities take years of training and practice to develop and are frequently limited to a particular treatment modality only (Bentel, 1996; Xia *et al.*, 2018). As such even within a single radiotherapy institution treatment plan quality varies in a rather wide range due to the various degrees of experience of the treatment planning staff (Kubo *et al.*, 2019; Nelms *et al.*, 2012). Such variations limit operational efficiency, pose challenges to treatment plan quality standardization, and hinder adoption of standardized treatment protocols. Furthermore, from the financial and operational point of view, it takes substantial resources to train staff with no or limited experience to reach a reasonable level of planning competency which has been the case for most radiotherapy facilities in the past decades (Babashov *et al.*, 2017; Das *et al.*, 2009).

Traditionally, treatment planning has been an iterative process that involves many rounds of trial and error. The planner starts from an initial set of optimization parameters to produce a dose distribution, which in most cases will be not clinically satisfactory. The planner will then modify the optimization parameters to start another round of optimization with the intent for improved dose distribution. This process is repeated many times until the dose distribution satisfies the clinical goals. In this process, planner experience plays a very important role in the end outcome of the treatment plans and the amount of time and effort to achieve it. As the treatment technology becomes more sophisticated, the requirement on the planner skills becomes more stringent to achieve desired dose distributions (Gardner *et al.*, 2019). The ability to shorten the learning curve, to generate plans of more consistent and uniform quality and to improve operational efficiency has become ever more desirable.

In the last decade, radiotherapy physicists and other scientists have intensified efforts to achieve the above-mentioned desire to make treatment planning less planner dependent and more automated. The approaches generally can be categorized as the following: (1) knowledge-based planning (Alpuche Aviles *et al.*, 2018; Appenzoller *et al.*, 2012; Babier *et al.*, 2018; Boutilier *et al.*, 2016; Cagni *et al.*, 2017; Chang *et al.*, 2016), (2) protocol-based automatic iterative optimization (Chanyavanich *et al.*, 2011; Chatterjee *et al.*, 2017, 2020; Chin Snyder *et al.*, 2016; Cooper *et al.*, 2016; Cornell *et al.*, 2020), (3) multi-criteria optimization (Buschmann *et al.*, 2016; Craft *et al.*, 2012; Zhang *et al.*, 2019, 2020), (4) artificial-intelligence-based treatment planning (Chen *et al.*, 2019; Ghandour *et al.*, 2015; Kierkels *et al.*, 2015; Liu *et al.*, 2019; Young *et al.*, 2016). In this chapter, we will focus our discussion on knowledge-based treatment planning.

2. Knowledge-Based Treatment Planning (KBP)

KBP may be described as any approach that makes use of knowledge, data, and experience gained in treatment plans collected in a database to predict an achievable dose in a new patient of similar anatomical features to a subset of patients in the database or to derive a better initial set of optimization parameters to reduce the rounds of trial-and-error optimizations. The library-based approach and the model-based approach may be covered under the domain of KBP (Alpuche Aviles *et al.*, 2018; Appenzoller *et al.*, 2012; Babier *et al.*, 2018; Boutilier *et al.*, 2016; Cagni *et al.*, 2017; Chang *et al.*, 2016; Gardner *et al.*, 2019). In the library-based approach, a better initial set of optimization parameters can be derived to reduce the rounds of optimization from the database based on the closest anatomical feature match between a new patient and patients in the database, whereas the model-based KBP utilizes characterization of the anatomical and geometric features for a particular anatomical site to build a DVH model that predicts achievable DVH values for a new patient with anatomical features resembling that in the database (Faught *et al.*, 2018; Fogliata *et al.*, 2014, 2017). In the following sections, we will describe both library-based and model-based approaches to generate treatment plans and discuss their clinical applications.

2.1. *Library-based approach*

Central to the KBP is a library of prior plans for a given anatomic site for a large number of patients. While no studies have specified the number of plans necessary in order to build an adequate database, the smallest database employed 40 patient plans (Hussein *et al.*, 2016). The plans should follow a standardized planning protocol with consistent naming of all anatomic structures of interest. For instance, in the case of H&N, there may be PTV1, PTV2, and PTV3 for a simultaneous integrated boost (SIB) treatment technique to doses of 70, 63, and 58.1 Gy, and a rather large number of OARs that are consistently named (Wang *et al.*, 2019; Wu *et al.*, 2012). Naturally, there will be variation in plan quality amongst the plans, the extent of which depends on the planning skills of the planners. The data should include PTV and OAR sizes, the associated DVH values for each patient, and most importantly, a parameter or a set of parameters that quantify the anatomic configurations between PTVs and OARs that can be used to determine anatomic similarities between patients, in particular, between a new patient whose plan needs to be generated and a patient in the database.

2.2. *Overlap Volume Histogram (OVH)*

While there are several geometric parameters that have been reported in the literature for anatomic similarity evaluation, including OVH, distance to target histograms (DTH), and OAR distance-to-PTV, we will only discuss the most widely used OVH parameter for similarity assessment between database patient and a new patient. The OVH is a geometric parameter that describes the relative orientation and closeness of an OAR to a PTV. It is a one-dimensional, unitless, parameter describing how the percentage of overlap volume between a PTV and an OAR varies as the volume of PTV is made to expand or contract in pre-defined increments. A histogram relating the overlap volume and the expansion/contraction distance is constructed as the process continues until the expanding PTV completely overlaps the OAR or the contracting PTV completely separates from the OAR. Figure 1 shows one example of the OVH curve (Wu *et al.*, 2009).

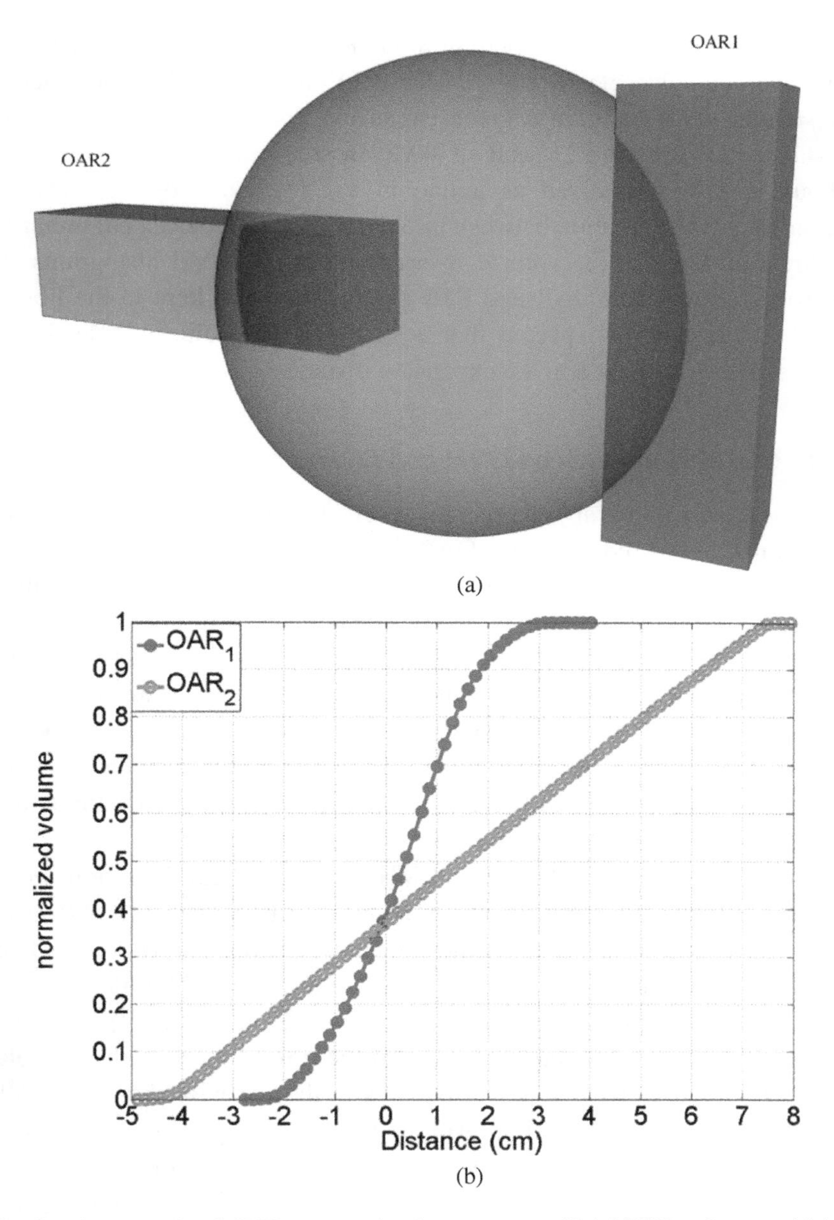

Fig. 1. An example of OVH construction between an artificial PTV and two artificial OARs, where the two OARs have identical volume but oriented differently relative to the PTV. Adapted from Wu *et al.* (2009) with permission, where the distance is the expansion distance (+) or contraction distance (–) from the initial position.

The two curves corresponding to OAR_1 and OAR_2 demonstrate how the overlap volume will vary as the PTV is expanded or contracted. A smaller OVH value at a given expansion distance r implies a closer distance between the PTV and an OAR. Bear in mind that this distance r should not be visualized as a line in a Cartesian coordinate system describing the separation between two points on two objects, but rather an indirect measure of the volume overlapping effect. OVH histograms are constructed for each OAR and PTV permutation and kept in the library database. It can be expected that a smaller OVH value will lead to a greater DVH value at a given expansion distance r.

2.3. *Correlation between OVH and DVH*

The goal of radiotherapy planning is to create treatment plans that maximize tumor dose and minimize OAR dose. The ideal plan is one that only gives dose to the tumor and no dose at all to the OARs. Obviously, this is not possible in realistic situations. In practice, an ideal dose distribution perhaps can be described as such that the isodose surface exactly matches the shape of the target boundary and other isodose surfaces are simply the expansion or contraction of the target boundary with a sharp dose gradient between target and OAR (Wu *et al.*, 2011). The ability to achieve such a result will depend heavily on the target and OAR sizes, locations, and relative orientation. As a descriptor of such configuration, the OVH is predictive of potential achievable DVH for a given configuration. For a given percentage overlap volume v between a PTV and an OAR at an expansion distance r, the larger the r to achieve v, the smaller the DVH of the OAR at v. Therefore, for two OARs relative to a PTV, the one that requires a larger r to yield the same v will have lower DVH at that volume v and therefore easier to control the dose. Based on this correlation, OVH can be used to select patients in the database that have OVH values similar to a new patient. Among the group of patients with similar OVHs, plans with the lowest DVH can be selected as optimization objectives for the new patient (Wu *et al.*, 2012, 2013). In the following section, a description of the selection process will be given.

2.4. *Selection of DVH values as the optimization objectives for a new patient*

Now that a database has been constructed with each patient's PTVs, OARs contoured and the associated DVH values of their plans stored, we can use OVH to select the best plans in the database where the DVH values are used as optimization goals to be achieved or further improved for a new patient's plan.

The process can be outlined in the following steps: (1) compute the new patient's OVH for each PTV/OAR pair; (2) search in the database for a subset of patients with similar OVH values; (3) select the plan with the lowest DVHs in the subset and use its DVH values as the new patient's DVH objectives.

A process like this significantly improves planning efficiency and guarantees a certain level of plan quality. Not only does it eliminate the inefficient trial-and-error process in optimization to generate an acceptable plan, but also it ensures the selection of the highest quality plans in the database. It can be imagined that the application of KBP will significantly reduce the planning time and create plans of better consistency and good quality. In the following section, we will select a few published studies to demonstrate its application and provide a summary of existing literature on this topic.

3. Applications of KBP

Many studies on KBP application have been reported in the literature. KBP has been applied to clinical sites where inverse planning and optimization are required, and treatment protocols have been standardized with consistent structure naming. They include head and neck, prostate, gynecological, breast, and GI cancers.

3.1. *KBP in head and neck cancer*

Due to the high likelihood of lymph nodes involvement of many types of head and neck cancers, the PTVs frequently extend to large areas and bilateral, and require different dose levels for treatment (Orlandi *et al.*, 2010). Furthermore, there are numerous OARs in this region that are in contact with the PTVs. As a result, head and neck planning is frequently the most complex and challenging, requiring high levels of skills to generate quality plans. Therefore, the need for planning automation to minimize reliance on the skills of individual planners is most widely pursued.

Wu *et al.* (2009, 2011, 2012, 2013, 2014, 2017) were one of the earliest in developing a KBP-based methodology in treatment planning for head and neck cancer. They developed the OVH parameter described in the previous sections for similarity quantification of patient anatomy to retrieve DVH parameters in the database as the planning objectives for a new patient plan. In one study, they built a database consisting of 91 HN patient plans and applied the KBP method to generate plans for comparison with the clinical plans. Their comparison showed a non-inferiority of the KBP plans in PTV coverage but with significantly reduced doses to the spinal cord, brainstem and parotid. Furthermore, the KBP plans were generated in substantially shorter times (Wu *et al.*, 2012).

Other investigators have similarly studied KBP application in head and neck cancer. Lian *et al.* (2013) and Yuan *et al.* (2014) took a different approach; instead of directly retrieving plans from a database based on anatomy similarity comparison, they used the database plans to create a DVH prediction model for a new patient. The anatomy feature they used is a distance to target histogram between an OAR and a PTV. The average of model predicted OAR dose indices were found within 2.1% of that of clinical plans.

3.2. *KBP in prostate cancer*

Prostate is another anatomic site where KBP has found many applications. Appenzoller *et al.* (2012) use the minimum distance from a voxel of an OAR to the PTV surface as an OAR–PTV spatial relationship evaluator to predict achievable DVH values for rectum and bladder. Good *et al.* (2013) use a summed BEV projection for PTV, rectum, bladder and the femoral heads from each beam angle as an anatomy similarity quantifier to retrieve DVH values in plans in the database as the predicted new patient DVH values. Their KBP plans have on average more homogeneous doses in the

PTV and statistically lower volumes to receive specified doses to all the three OARs for most of the planning cases although for about 6% of the cases, the KBP plans have yielded worse DVH results than the database plans. Sheng *et al.* (2015) applied another anatomical descriptor, the percent distance to the PTV from each OAR and the concaveness angle formed by seminal vesicle relative to the anterior-posterior axis to retrieve DVH values for a new patient.

3.3. *KBP in lung, breast and GI cancers*

Lung and breast are the other sites where more than a dozen KBP applications have been reported in the literature (Chin Snyder *et al.*, 2016; Cornell *et al.*, 2020; Delaney *et al.*, 2017; Hoffmann *et al.*, 2021; Kavanaugh *et al.*, 2019; Rago *et al.*, 2021; Van't Hof *et al.*, 2019). In all cases, KBP generated plans either outperformed clinical plans or showed non-inferiority to clinical plans.

As mentioned before, the KBP application is not limited to a specific site. Inverse planning and optimization are the only requirements. A few KBP studies have also been reported for other anatomic sites, such as the rectum, pelvis and liver (Celik *et al.*, 2021; Hussein *et al.*, 2016; Sheng *et al.*, 2019; Wu *et al.*, 2016; Zhang *et al.*, 2018).

3.4. *Cross-institutional application of KBP*

In addition to intra-institution evaluation, Wu *et al.* further applied the KBP methodology for cross-institutional application to demonstrate the transferability and quality consistency of the KBP (Wu *et al.*, 2017). They have further extended the methodology to generate VMAT plans from an IMRT plan database (Wu *et al.*, 2013), thus allowing the applicability of KBP to different treatment techniques. Their technique was commercialized in Rapid Plan by Varian.

3.5. *Multi-modality application of KBP*

While most KBP studies are centered on linac-based treatment techniques, Wu *et al.* have extended the KBP methodology to Cyberknife treatment planning (Wu *et al.*, 2014). They constructed a database of 400 patient clinical plans and retrospectively and prospectively generated KBP plans. They found that almost all KBP plans are at least as good as the best-quality plans in the database, demonstrating the applicability of the KBP technique to generate quality plans for other treatment modalities.

4. Summary

From the above discussions, one can see that the traditional treatment planning process based on the individual user's experience using a trial-and-error method is at the stage of being replaced with auto-treatment planning. Knowledge-based treatment planning is just one of the many auto-planning techniques in development and refinement. Gradual and broad implementation of the auto-planning techniques in the radiotherapy community will undoubtedly improve planning efficiency and quality in a significant way.

References

Alpuche Aviles, J. E., Cordero Marcos, M. I., Sasaki, D., Sutherland, K., Kane, B., & Kuusela, E. (2018). Creation of knowledge-based planning models intended for large scale distribution: Minimizing the effect of outlier plans. *Journal of Applied Clinical Medical Physics*, *19*(3), 215–226.

Appenzoller, L. M., Michalski, J. M., Thorstad, W. L., Mutic, S., & Moore, K. L. (2012). Predicting dose-volume histograms for organs-at-risk in IMRT planning. *Medical Physics*, *39*(12), 7446–7461.

Babashov, V., Aivas, I., Begen, M., Cao, J., Rodrigues, G., D'Souza, D., Lock, M., & Zaric, G. (2017). Reducing patient waiting times for radiation therapy and improving the treatment planning process: A discrete-event simulation model (radiation treatment planning). *Clinical Oncology*, *29*(6), 385–391.

Babier, A., Boutilier, J. J., McNiven, A. L., & Chan, T. C. (2018). Knowledge-based automated planning for oropharyngeal cancer. *Medical Physics*, *45*(7), 2875–2883.

Bentel, G. C. (1996). *Radiation Therapy Planning* (Vol. 162). New York: McGraw-Hill.

Boutilier, J. J., Craig, T., Sharpe, M. B., & Chan, T. C. (2016). Sample size requirements for knowledge-based treatment planning. *Medical Physics*, *43*(3), 1212–1221.

Buschmann, M., Seppenwoolde, Y., Wiezorek, T., Weibert, K., & Georg, D. (2016). Advanced optimization methods for whole pelvic and local prostate external beam therapy. *Physica Medica*, *32*(3), 465–473.

Cagni, E., Botti, A., Micera, R., Galeandro, M., Sghedoni, R., Orlandi, M., Iotti, C., Cozzi, L., & Iori, M. (2017). Knowledge-based treatment planning: An inter-technique and inter-system feasibility study for prostate cancer. *Physica Medica, 36*, 38–45.

Celik, E., Baues, C., Claus, K., Fogliata, A., Scorsetti, M., Marnitz, S., & Cozzi, L. (2021). Knowledge-based intensity-modulated proton planning for gastroesophageal carcinoma. *Acta Oncologica, 60*(3), 285–292.

Chang, A. T., Hung, A. W., Cheung, F. W., Lee, M. C., Chan, O. S., Philips, H., Cheng, Y.-T., & Ng, W.-T. (2016). Comparison of planning quality and efficiency between conventional and knowledge-based algorithms in nasopharyngeal cancer patients using intensity modulated radiation therapy. *International Journal of Radiation Oncology* Biology* Physics, 95*(3), 981–990.

Chanyavanich, V., Das, S. K., Lee, W. R., & Lo, J. Y. (2011). Knowledge-based IMRT treatment planning for prostate cancer. *Medical Physics, 38*(5), 2515–2522.

Chatterjee, A., Serban, M., Abdulkarim, B., Panet-Raymond, V., Souhami, L., Shenouda, G., Sabri, S., Jean-Claude, B., & Seuntjens, J. (2017). Performance of knowledge-based radiation therapy planning for the glioblastoma disease site. *International Journal of Radiation Oncology* Biology* Physics, 99*(4), 1021–1028.

Chatterjee, A., Serban, M., Faria, S., Souhami, L., Cury, F., & Seuntjens, J. (2020). Novel knowledge-based treatment planning model for hypofractionated radiotherapy of prostate cancer patients. *Physica Medica, 69*, 36–43.

Chen, X., Men, K., Li, Y., Yi, J., & Dai, J. (2019). A feasibility study on an automated method to generate patient-specific dose distributions for radiotherapy using deep learning. *Medical Physics, 46*(1), 56–64.

Chin Snyder, K., Kim, J., Reding, A., Fraser, C., Gordon, J., Ajlouni, M., Movsas, B., & Chetty, I. J. (2016). Development and evaluation of a clinical model for lung cancer patients using stereotactic body radiotherapy (SBRT) within a knowledge-based algorithm for treatment planning. *Journal of Applied Clinical Medical Physics, 17*(6), 263–275.

Cooper, B. T., Li, X., Shin, S. M., Modrek, A. S., Hsu, H. C., DeWyngaert, J., Jozsef, G., Lymberis, S. C., Goldberg, J. D., & Formenti, S. C. (2016). Preplanning prediction of the left anterior descending artery maximum dose based on patient, dosimetric, and treatment planning parameters. *Advances in Radiation Oncology, 1*(4), 373–381.

Cornell, M., Kaderka, R., Hild, S. J., Ray, X. J., Murphy, J. D., Atwood, T. F., & Moore, K. L. (2020). Noninferiority study of automated knowledge-based planning versus human-driven optimization across multiple disease sites. *International Journal of Radiation Oncology* Biology* Physics, 106*(2), 430–439.

Craft, D. L., Hong, T. S., Shih, H. A., & Bortfeld, T. R. (2012). Improved planning time and plan quality through multicriteria optimization for intensity-modulated radiotherapy. *International Journal of Radiation Oncology* Biology* Physics, 82*(1), e83–e90.

Das, I. J., Moskvin, V., & Johnstone, P. A. (2009). Analysis of treatment planning time among systems and planners for intensity-modulated radiation therapy. *Journal of the American College of Radiology, 6*(7), 514–517.

Delaney, A. R., Dahele, M., Tol, J. P., Slotman, B. J., & Verbakel, W. F. (2017). Knowledge-based planning for stereotactic radiotherapy of peripheral early-stage lung cancer. *Acta Oncologica*, *56*(3), 490–495.

Faught, A. M., Olsen, L., Schubert, L., Rusthoven, C., Castillo, E., Castillo, R., Zhang, J., Guerrero, T., Miften, M., & Vinogradskiy, Y. (2018). Functional-guided radiotherapy using knowledge-based planning. *Radiotherapy and Oncology*, *129*(3), 494–498.

Fogliata, A., Belosi, F., Clivio, A., Navarria, P., Nicolini, G., Scorsetti, M., Vanetti, E., & Cozzi, L. (2014). On the pre-clinical validation of a commercial model-based optimisation engine: Application to volumetric modulated arc therapy for patients with lung or prostate cancer. *Radiotherapy and Oncology*, *113*(3), 385–391.

Fogliata, A., Reggiori, G., Stravato, A., Lobefalo, F., Franzese, C., Franceschini, D., Tomatis, S., Mancosu, P., Scorsetti, M., & Cozzi, L. (2017). RapidPlan head and neck model: The objectives and possible clinical benefit. *Radiation Oncology*, *12*(1), 1–12.

Gardner, S. J., Kim, J., & Chetty, I. J. (2019). Modern radiation therapy planning and delivery. *Hematology/Oncology Clinics*, *33*(6), 947–962.

Ghandour, S., Matzinger, O., & Pachoud, M. (2015). Volumetric-modulated arc therapy planning using multicriteria optimization for localized prostate cancer. *Journal of Applied Clinical Medical Physics*, *16*(3), 258–269.

Good, D., Lo, J., Lee, W. R., Wu, Q. J., Yin, F.-F., & Das, S. K. (2013). A knowledge-based approach to improving and homogenizing intensity modulated radiation therapy planning quality among treatment centers: An example application to prostate cancer planning. *International Journal of Radiation Oncology* Biology* Physics*, *87*(1), 176–181.

Hoffmann, L., Knap, M., Alber, M., & Møller, D. (2021). Optimal beam angle selection and knowledge-based planning significantly reduces radiotherapy dose to organs at risk for lung cancer patients. *Acta Oncologica*, *60*(3), 293–299.

Hussein, M., South, C. P., Barry, M. A., Adams, E. J., Jordan, T. J., Stewart, A. J., & Nisbet, A. (2016). Clinical validation and benchmarking of knowledge-based IMRT and VMAT treatment planning in pelvic anatomy. *Radiotherapy and Oncology*, *120*(3), 473–479.

Kavanaugh, J. A., Holler, S., DeWees, T. A., Robinson, C. G., Bradley, J. D., Iyengar, P., Higgins, K. A., Mutic, S., & Olsen, L. A. (2019). Multi-institutional validation of a knowledge-based planning model for patients enrolled in RTOG 0617: Implications for plan quality controls in cooperative group trials. *Practical Radiation Oncology*, *9*(2), e218–e227.

Khan, F. M., Sperduto, P. W., & Gibbons, J. P. (2021). *Khan's Treatment Planning in Radiation Oncology*. Philadelphia: Lippincott Williams & Wilkins.

Kierkels, R. G., Visser, R., Bijl, H. P., Langendijk, J. A., van't Veld, A. A., Steenbakkers, R. J., & Korevaar, E. W. (2015). Multicriteria optimization enables less experienced planners to efficiently produce high quality treatment plans in head and neck cancer radiotherapy. *Radiation Oncology*, *10*(1), 1–9.

Kubo, K., Monzen, H., Ishii, K., Tamura, M., Nakasaka, Y., Kusawake, M., Kishimoto, S., Nakahara, R., Matsuda, S., & Nakajima, T. (2019). Inter-planner variation in treatment-plan quality of plans created with a knowledge-based treatment planning system. *Physica Medica*, *67*, 132–140.

Lian, J., Yuan, L., Ge, Y., Chera, B. S., Yoo, D. P., Chang, S., Yin, F., & Wu, Q. J. (2013). Modeling the dosimetry of organ-at-risk in head and neck IMRT planning: An intertechnique and interinstitutional study. *Medical Physics*, *40*(12), 121704.

Liu, Z., Fan, J., Li, M., Yan, H., Hu, Z., Huang, P., Tian, Y., Miao, J., & Dai, J. (2019). A deep learning method for prediction of three-dimensional dose distribution of helical tomotherapy. *Medical Physics*, *46*(5), 1972–1983.

Nelms, B. E., Robinson, G., Markham, J., Velasco, K., Boyd, S., Narayan, S., Wheeler, J., & Sobczak, M. L. (2012). Variation in external beam treatment plan quality: An inter-institutional study of planners and planning systems. *Practical Radiation Oncology*, *2*(4), 296–305.

Orlandi, E., Palazzi, M., Pignoli, E., Fallai, C., Giostra, A., & Olmi, P. (2010). Radiobiological basis and clinical results of the Simultaneous Integrated Boost (SIB) in Intensity Modulated Radiotherapy (IMRT) for head and neck cancer: A review. *Critical Reviews in Oncology/Hematology*, *73*(2), 111–125.

Rago, M., Placidi, L., Polsoni, M., Rambaldi, G., Cusumano, D., Greco, F., Indovina, L., Menna, S., Placidi, E., & Stimato, G. (2021). Evaluation of a generalized knowledge-based planning performance for VMAT irradiation of breast and locoregional lymph nodes — Internal mammary and/or supraclavicular regions. *PLoS One*, *16*(1), e0245305.

Sheng, Y., Li, T., Zhang, Y., Lee, W. R., Yin, F.-F., Ge, Y., & Wu, Q. J. (2015). Atlas-guided prostate intensity modulated radiation therapy (IMRT) planning. *Physics in Medicine & Biology*, *60*(18), 7277.

Sheng, Y., Zhang, J., Wang, C., Yin, F.-F., Wu, Q. J., & Ge, Y. (2019). Incorporating case-based reasoning for radiation therapy knowledge modeling: A pelvic case study. *Technology in Cancer Research & Treatment*, *18*, 1533033819874788.

Van't Hof, S., Delaney, A. R., Tekatli, H., Twisk, J., Slotman, B. J., Senan, S., Dahele, M., & Verbakel, W. F. (2019). Knowledge-based planning for identifying high-risk stereotactic ablative radiation therapy treatment plans for lung tumors larger than 5 cm. *International Journal of Radiation Oncology* Biology* Physics*, *103*(1), 259–267.

Wang, Y., Heijmen, B. J., & Petit, S. F. (2019). Knowledge-based dose prediction models for head and neck cancer are strongly affected by interorgan dependency and dataset inconsistency. *Medical Physics*, *46*(2), 934–943.

Wu, B., Kusters, M., Kunze-Busch, M., Dijkema, T., McNutt, T., Sanguineti, G., Bzdusek, K., Dritschilo, A., & Pang, D. (2017). Cross-institutional Knowledge-Based Planning (KBP) implementation and its performance comparison to Auto-Planning Engine (APE). *Radiotherapy and Oncology*, *123*(1), 57–62.

Wu, B., McNutt, T., Zahurak, M., Simari, P., Pang, D., Taylor, R., & Sanguineti, G. (2012). Fully automated simultaneous integrated boosted–intensity modulated radiation therapy treatment planning is feasible for head-and-neck cancer: A prospective clinical study. *International Journal of Radiation Oncology* Biology* Physics*, *84*(5), e647–e653.

Wu, B., Pang, D., Lei, S., Gatti, J., Tong, M., McNutt, T., Kole, T., Dritschilo, A., & Collins, S. (2014). Improved robotic stereotactic body radiation therapy plan quality and planning efficacy for organ-confined prostate cancer utilizing overlap-volume histogram-driven planning methodology. *Radiotherapy and Oncology*, *112*(2), 221–226.

Wu, B., Pang, D., Simari, P., Taylor, R., Sanguineti, G., & McNutt, T. (2013). Using overlap volume histogram and IMRT plan data to guide and automate VMAT planning: A head-and-neck case study. *Medical Physics*, *40*(2), 021714.

Wu, B., Ricchetti, F., Sanguineti, G., Kazhdan, M., Simari, P., Chuang, M., Taylor, R., Jacques, R., & McNutt, T. (2009). Patient geometry-driven information retrieval for IMRT treatment plan quality control. *Medical Physics*, *36*(12), 5497–5505.

Wu, B., Ricchetti, F., Sanguineti, G., Kazhdan, M., Simari, P., Jacques, R., Taylor, R., & McNutt, T. (2011). Data-driven approach to generating achievable dose–volume histogram objectives in intensity-modulated radiotherapy planning. *International Journal of Radiation Oncology* Biology* Physics*, *79*(4), 1241–1247.

Wu, H., Jiang, F., Yue, H., Li, S., & Zhang, Y. (2016). A dosimetric evaluation of knowledge-based VMAT planning with simultaneous integrated boosting for rectal cancer patients. *Journal of Applied Clinical Medical Physics*, *17*(6), 78–85.

Xia, P., Godley, A., Shah, C., Videtic, G. M., & Suh, J. (2018). *Strategies for Radiation Therapy Treatment Planning*. New York: Springer Publishing Company.

Young, M. R., Craft, D. L., Colbert, C. M., Remillard, K., Vanbenthuysen, L., & Wang, Y. (2016). Volumetric-modulated arc therapy using multicriteria optimization for body and extremity sarcoma. *Journal of Applied Clinical Medical Physics*, *17*(6), 283–291.

Yuan, L., Wu, Q. J., Yin, F. F., Jiang, Y., Yoo, D., & Ge, Y. (2014). Incorporating single-side sparing in models for predicting parotid dose sparing in head and neck IMRT. *Medical Physics*, *41*(2), 021728.

Zhang, J., Ge, Y., Sheng, Y., Wang, C., Zhang, J., Wu, Y., Wu, Q., Yin, F.-F., & Wu, Q. J. (2020). Knowledge-based tradeoff hyperplanes for head and neck treatment planning. *International Journal of Radiation Oncology* Biology* Physics*, *106*(5), 1095–1103.

Zhang, J., Ge, Y., Sheng, Y., Yin, F. F., & Wu, Q. J. (2019). Modeling of multiple planning target volumes for head and neck treatments in knowledge-based treatment planning. *Medical Physics*, *46*(9), 3812–3822.

Zhang, Y., Li, T., Xiao, H., Ji, W., Guo, M., Zeng, Z., & Zhang, J. (2018). A knowledge-based approach to automated planning for hepatocellular carcinoma. *Journal of Applied Clinical Medical Physics*, *19*(1), 50–59.

Chapter 10

Artificial Intelligence in Radiation Therapy Treatment Planning

Xiaofeng Zhu*, Jiajin Fan*, Ashish Chawla* and Dandan Zheng[†]

**Inova Schar Cancer Institute, Falls Church VA, USA*
[†]University of Rochester Medical Center, Rochester NY, USA

Abstract

Treatment planning is arguably the most critical step in the radiation oncology workflow, and has traditionally involved intense manual work, highly trained expertise, and interactions between experts. Over the past decade, there have been fruitful strides and intense research efforts on automating treatment planning with algorithms powered by Artificial Intelligence (AI). These algorithms can be divided into soft-AI, including knowledge-based algorithms, rule-based algorithms, and algorithms exploring multi-criteria optimization, and hard-AI algorithms.

This chapter will provide an overview of these four categories of algorithms, and introduce the mathematical foundation and technical basis from the soft-AI methods to the hard-AI algorithms. Popular methods such as principal component analysis, convolutional neural network, generative adversarial network, and reinforcement learning will be discussed. Further, in this chapter we will also review the current success of these methods in improving the efficiency, consistency, and quality of treatment planning.

1. Introduction

Radiation therapy is a main treatment modality for cancer and is used for over half of cancer patients. Treatment planning is an essential and effort-consuming step of the radiation therapy workflow. It has become more sophisticated over the past couple of decades with the help of operation research and computer science, enabling planners to design highly complex radiation therapy plans to minimize normal tissue damage and maximize tumor control. Like how it is applied to automate and improve many other medical fields, artificial intelligence (AI) has also been employed to automate and improve radiation therapy treatment planning. In addition to the cost-saving provided by automating the labor-intensive plan optimization process, AI-powered radiation therapy treatment planning offers several other main advantages. The improved plan-generating speed compared with manual planning is highly desirable for scenarios where a quick turnaround time is needed, such as online adaptive radiation therapy and emergent treatments. The consistent quality of AI plans reduces healthcare disparities by making advanced treatment planning expertise broadly available. Potentially, advanced AI could also offer better plan quality than manual planners could achieve en masse. In this chapter, we will describe the technical basis as well as current clinical implementations of AI in radiation therapy treatment planning.

Radiation therapy treatment plans can be created through a forward or an inverse fashion. Forward planning is usually employed for simple planning tasks, in which the planner designs beam apertures to create plans with dose desired by the physician. Inverse planning typically involves more complex dose designs, in which structures are outlined based on the patient anatomy, the physician desired dose distribution is specified as dose prescription and dose volume constraints, and the plan is generated inversely via optimizing a cost function based on the constraints. These machine planning algorithms can be loosely categorized into two main categories, the soft-AI approaches that have been implemented in current clinical software and the hard-AI approaches that are currently under active research, some in-house deployment, and recently released commercial software. Both categories contain various algorithmic approaches. Although radiation therapy treatment planning automation is rapidly progressing into a hard-AI era, in this chapter we also include the soft-AI methods as they lay the foundation for the hard-AI methods and still dominate current clinical applications. It is our hope that the knowledge of the mathematics of the simpler methods will help readers better understand the more complex, newer methods.

2. Radiation Therapy Treatment Planning Workflow and Automation

An inverse planning workflow is depicted in Fig. 1 for the manual planning process (A), three soft-AI processes including Automated Rule Implementation and Reasoning (ARIR, B), knowledge-based planning with dose volume histogram-based predictions (KBP, C), and multicriteria optimization (MCO, D), as well as a generic hard-AI process (E).

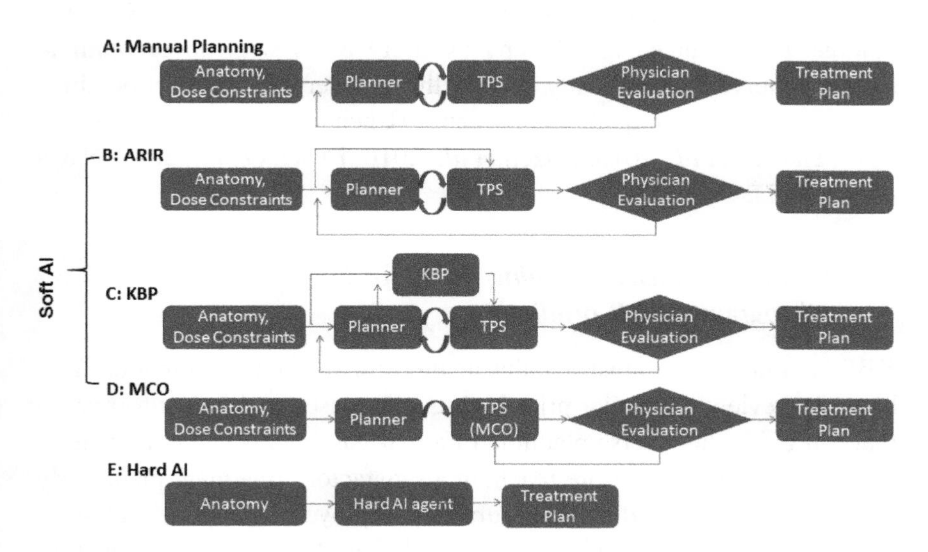

Fig. 1. Workflow of (A) manual, (B) ARIR, (C) KBP, (D) MCO, and (E) hard-AI in treatment planning. AI indicates artificial intelligence; ARIR, automated rule implementation and reasoning; KBP, knowledge-based planning; MCO, multicriteria optimization. Reprinted from Wang *et al.* (2019) with permission.

2.1. *Automated Rule Implementation and Reasoning (ARIR)*

A typical manual planning process involves the planner setting up beams and optimization dose objectives and iteratively fine-tuning them to yield a satisfactory plan. Physicians' inputs are integrated into the process via one or more rounds of plan evaluation, depending on if changes are suggested from the evaluation. An ARIR algorithm mimics the manual process via hard-coded rules and "if-then" actions. The most popular ARIR algorithm is Auto-Planning^{TM} implemented in Pinnacle treatment planning system (TPS) (Philips Radiation Oncology Systems, Fitchburg, Wisconsin). With Auto-Planning^{TM}, the planner specifies a planning technique that includes the basic target prescription and organ at risk (OAR) sparing goals, for a type of treatment instead of individual patients' treatment. For individual patients, the Auto-Planning^{TM} algorithms automatically generate auxiliary planning structures and fine-tune the optimization objectives in several cycles of iterations based on the technique, emulating a human planner. Since its advent about a decade ago, Auto-Planning^{TM} has been documented in many clinical studies to yield clinically acceptable intensity modulated radiation therapy (IMRT) and volumetric modulated arc therapy (VMAT) plans with no or minimal manual interventions, greatly reduce the planner-TPS interaction time, and improve the plan quality consistency (Chen *et al.*, 2018; Gintz *et al.*, 2016; Hansen *et al.*, 2016; Hazell *et al.*, 2016; Kusters *et al.*, 2017; Nawa *et al.*, 2017).

2.2. *Knowledge-based Planning (KBP) for Dose Volume Histogram (DVH) prediction*

KBP is arguably the most popular method for planning automation. It is based on reviewing similar prior high-quality cases to derive information that can guide the inverse planning of a new case and hence reduce iterative plan adjustments before reaching a satisfactory treatment plan. Early developments in this direction, currently deployed in commercial solutions, use dose volume histogram (DVH)-based prediction and inverse optimization. DVH is one important metric that physicians use to evaluate a treatment plan. Such evaluations are usually discrete, by checking only certain points on each DVH to assess whether they satisfy the target or

OAR dose tolerances derived from evidence and previous clinical experience on tumor control or normal tissue toxicity. Therefore, a typical manual plan optimization is also based on these point objectives, as the toxicity evidence and human experience are often only quantified at these discrete points. The advent of DVH-based KBP methods not only automated the treatment planning process, but also changed point objectives into line objectives in the optimization although point objectives can still be similarly applied. This is because unlike human experts who are limited to using only discrete points, the KBP AIs predict and quantify the entire DVH.

The most popular KBP algorithm currently in clinical use is RapidPlan™ implemented in Eclipse TPS (Varian Medical System, Palo Alto, California). Because statistical or simple machine learning methods are used in KBP algorithms with DVH-based prediction goals, the required training case numbers is moderate, typically as few as a couple dozen. From these training cases, characteristic relationships between the DVHs and anatomical/geometrical features of target(s)/OARs are established during the modeling process. The geometry of an OAR relative to the target is represented by the distance-to-target histogram (DTH). To reduce the number of model variables, the features of DTH and DVH are learned and extracted via methods such as principal component analysis (PCA). Numerous studies have been published on development and clinical applications of RapidPlan™ and similar in-house algorithms (Fogliata *et al.*, 2014 2015; Wu *et al.*, 2011; Zhu *et al.*, 2011a). Like Auto-Planning™, RapidPlan™ was also found to greatly improve the treatment planning efficiency and consistency (Berry *et al.*, 2016b; Kubo *et al.*, 2017; Rice *et al.*, 2019; Scaggion *et al.*, 2018; Schubert *et al.*, 2017). Because no iterative optimization objective fine-tuning is involved, the plan generation speed is even faster for RapidPlan™, while the plan quality was found to be comparable between the two algorithms (Smith *et al.*, 2019).

2.3. *Multicriteria Optimization (MCO)*

In inverse planning, the task is mathematically the minimization of a cost function, defined with a weighted sum of the penalty for deviations from target and normal tissue dosimetric constraints. In the iterative process of manual plan generation, the planner fine-tunes both the dosimetric criteria and their weights. Yet, the optimal tradeoff between the conflicting criteria identified by the planner may not be acceptable to the physician due to clinical factors, and the communication and understanding between the planner and the physician. In the manual process when a plan is rejected by the physician and new priorities communicated, the planner re-initiates a new set of constraints for a more suitable solution. In contrast, MCO generates multiple anchoring Pareto plans simultaneously instead of a single plan in the initial inverse planning process. Based on these Pareto-optimal plans where the dose constraints of a single OAR are optimized without compromising the target constraints, the physician can navigate through the pre-generated series of Pareto-optimal plans along different Pareto surfaces and interactively select the desired tradeoff (Breedveld *et al.*, 2009; Chen *et al.*, 2012; Romeijn *et al.*, 2004; van de Water *et al.*, 2013).

MCO can be implemented in an *a posteriori* approach, where the Pareto database of feasible plans are browsed and the users select the optimal plan by adjusting the combination of dosimetric criteria through interactive sliding bars, or an *a priori* approach, where an explicit set of dosimetric preferences are defined before the inverse optimization to sequentially minimize the criteria based on the ascribed priorities to reach a single optimal plan on the Pareto surface (Biston *et al.*, 2021; Breedveld *et al.*, 2007, 2012). Currently, two commercial TPSs have implemented MCO, both using the *a posteriori* approach: the pioneer MCO system RayStation (RaySearch, Stockholm, Sweden) and, more recently, Eclipse (Varian Medical System, Palo Alto, California).

2.4. *Voxel dose prediction and hard-AI*

A major drawback of the DVH-based KBP, ARIR, and MCO soft-AI approaches is the lack of spatial dose information. Some important spatially relevant dosimetric endpoints are hence missed by such methods. Therefore, current AI RT planning research has focused on spatial dose distribution or voxel dose-based approaches. Voxel dose prediction is not only able to provide accurate spatial dose information to guide the machine decision-making, but also enable fully automated treatment planning workflow without the need for DVH-based inverse optimization. There has been intense voxel-dose-based AI planning research. Many of them used KBP, but other approaches such as MCO were also developed (Babier *et al.*, 2018, 2020b; Fan *et al.*, 2019a; Kearney *et al.*, 2018a; Li *et al.*, 2021b; Ma *et al.*, 2021b; Mashayekhi *et al.*, 2022; McIntosh & Purdie, 2017; McIntosh *et al.*, 2017). Because of the increased complexity in the prediction compared with DVH-based prediction, deep learning-based approaches are usually used in these hard-AI agents. In the following sections, some most relevant deep learning algorithms will be introduced, along with current clinical developments using such algorithms. The algorithms and process for the simpler case of KBP with DVH prediction will first be described to lay some foundation for and to contrast with the more complex algorithms.

3. AI Approaches in Radiation Therapy Treatment Planning

Visual feature extraction and pattern recognition is at the foundation of various AI RT planning approaches. Feature extraction reduces dimensionalities, where smaller data sets are easier to explore and visualize. It makes analyzing data much easier and faster without extraneous variables to process. Here we will introduce a few of the most popular AI approaches/algorithms used in radiation therapy treatment planning: (1) manual feature extraction to characterize dose distribution, applied in DVH-based KBP; (2) auto feature extraction using deep learning for dose prediction; (3) generative adversarial network; and (4) reinforcement learning using state-action pairs to explore machine parameter prediction.

3.1. *Manual Feature Extraction in Dose Volume Histogram (DVH)-based Knowledge-based Planning (KBP)*

In radiation therapy, each plan's dose distribution is determined by the individual patient's anatomy. AI algorithms thus use key characteristics called features to deduce the relationship between anatomy and dose for prediction and automation. Both ARIR and KBP employ manual feature extraction, such as using dose volume histogram (DVH) and distance to target histogram (DTH). Classic machine learning tools such as principal component analysis (PCA) are often used in these implementations to reduce number of dimensionalities. In the following paragraphs, we will use DVH-based KBP as an example to introduce the basic process and important concepts of manual feature extraction.

A common goal of both the DVH-based KBP algorithms and the hard-AI algorithms with deep architecture and compositionality is to develop good models that can fit dose outputs from anatomy or imaging inputs. As both images and dose maps are high dimensional data with very large numbers of voxels, dimension reduction is needed for a model to be fitted by computer. In DVH-based KBP, substantial dimension reduction is achieved via manual feature extraction on both ends, i.e. using DTH as the input and using DVH as the output. By doing so, the 3D data from both the input end (image) and the output end (dose) are reduced to 1D data. The histogram data are further dimension reduced using classic machine learning tools such as PCA, through which the 1D curve is often reduced to two or three parameters.

Figure 2 shows example key plots for the DVH-based KBP process. Figure 2(a) shows the voxel dose of a given OAR as a function of the minimal 3D distance from the voxel to the tumor target. Intuitively, since the tumor target is where high radiation dose is delivered, dose in the normal tissue voxels decreases as its distance to the tumor target increases. In this plot, each symbol represents a voxel of the OAR, and different colors denote the voxels on different axial CT slices. This explains that different doses at the same distances are related to those distances to the radiation beam.

By projecting all points to the dose axis, we obtain a cumulative DVH, where the 3D dose cloud of the OAR is reduced to a 1D DVH curve, shown in Fig. 2(b). The number of variables is reduced from thousands (the 3D dose cloud) to about a hundred, depending on the resolution. Similarly, by projecting the 3D distance cloud to the distance axis, the geometric information of the distance map is also compressed to the 1D DTH curve as shown in Fig. 2(c).

The 1D DTH is then taken as the input data for model training to predict the 1D DVH output. During the modeling, the 1D data usually

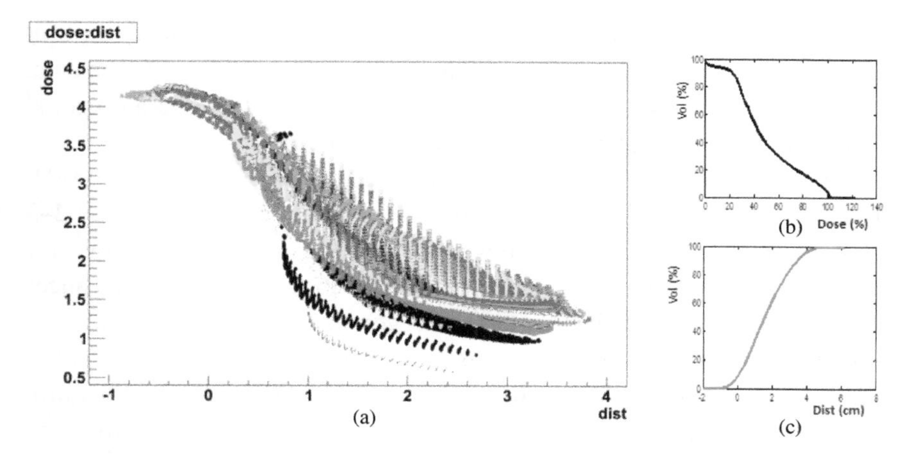

Fig. 2. Manual feature extraction in KBP. (a) Aggregated dose-to-distance histograms. Voxels of the same CT slice are plotted with same color and symbol, showing that dose to normal tissue decreases as the distance from tumor increases. Manual feature extraction is performed in this approach by reducing the 3D data to 1D: (b) yielding DVH via projecting to the dose axis (output of the prediction), and (c) yielding DTH via projecting to the distance axis (input of the prediction).

further go through dimension reduction by application of methods such as PCA.

PCA uses covariance calculation to find relationships within high-dimensional data sets (*X*, *Y*, *Z*, etc.). It can be thought of as fitting a multi-dimensional ellipsoid to the data, where each axis of the ellipsoid represents a principal component. If some axis of the ellipsoid is small, then the variance along that axis is also small, so it can be removed for dimensionality reduction. To find the axes of the ellipsoid, we must first subtract the mean of each variable from the data set to center the data on the origin. Then, we compute the covariance matrix of the data and calculate the eigenvalues and corresponding eigenvectors of this covariance matrix. Equation (1) shows the calculation of the covariance between *X* and *Y*,

$$Cov\left(X,Y\right)=\frac{\sum_{i=1}^{n}(X_i-\overline{X})(Y_i-\overline{Y})}{(n-1)} \tag{1}$$

where n is the number of data points, and $\overline{X}$ and $\overline{Y}$ are the averages, respectively. Each orthogonal eigenvector is then normalized to turn it into a unit vector. Once this is done, each of the mutually orthogonal, unit eigenvectors can be interpreted as an axis of the ellipsoid fitted to the data. This choice of basis will transform the covariance matrix into a diagonal form with the diagonal elements representing the variance of each axis.

In simple KBP, PCA is usually applied on the DTH and the DVH. Through PCA, each curve is often characterized and reconstructed by 2–3 PCA components. Therefore, the whole input data are reduced to a vector of about 10 variables. An example is shown in Fig. 3 for a prostate cancer radiation therapy case. In this case, the geometry input was reduced to 9 variables, 3 DTH principal components each for bladder and rectum, and the volumes of the PTV, and of the two OARs (bladder and rectum). As shown in Fig. 3, a parallel coordinates plot is used to visualize the

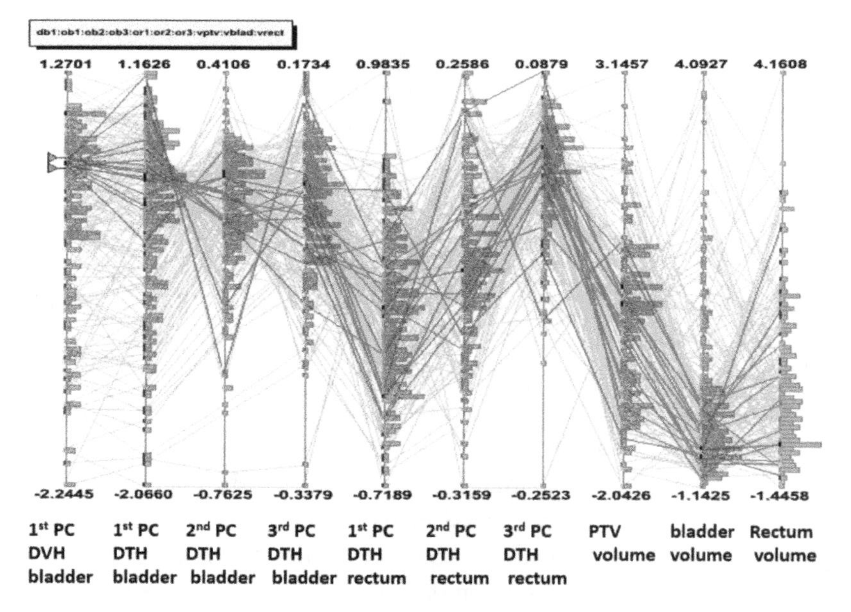

Fig. 3. An example DVH-based KBP modeling case for prostate cancer showing a parallel coordinates plot to assist feature visualization and modeling. The plot shows how one output parameter (First principal component of the bladder DVH) is connected with the 9 input parameters (3 DTH principal components each for bladder and rectum, the volumes of the PTV, and the two OARs). Variables from the same patient plan are linked by the green lines. The blue lines highlight the patients with output parameters within the narrow brackets denoted with the two arrows on the left.

non-linear correlation between the input data and to assist modeling based on a database of ~200 patient cases.

With the dimension reduction by 1D histogram projection and further PCA decomposition, the modeling problem of the DVH-based KBP approach then involves modeling from ~10 input variables to a few output variables, as shown in the complete workflow plotted in Fig. 4. Using PCA, the input DTH data are compressed to a vector X of ~10 variables. Those variables are mapped to the output vector Y, which is also the PC variables reduced from the training DVH. The mapping process is called modeling, which could use either simple statistical methods or classical machine learning methods such as support vector regression or artificial neural network.

As a forerunner of radiation therapy treatment planning AI, the simple KBP approach has been actively studied and broadly applied. Different manual feature extraction and modeling methods were explored (Berry *et al.*, 2016a; Yuan *et al.*, 2012; Zhang *et al.*, 2018; Zhu *et al.*, 2011b). Sometimes when the mapping (modeling) task is simple and the training data set size is limited, a simple statistical model may perform

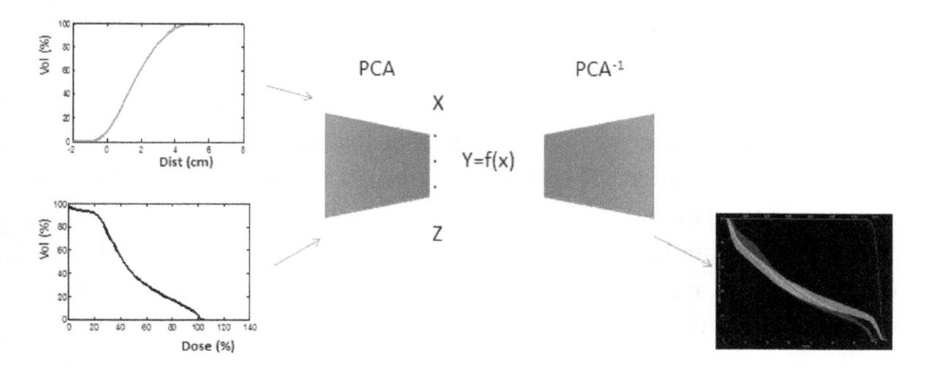

Fig. 4. Workflow for DVH-based KBP showing the downsample and upsample processes: PCA is used for dimensionality reduction, inverse PCA for DVH curve reconstruction. Both input (DTH) and output (DVH) are compressed using PCA to reduce them to a simple input vector X and output vector Y, each containing ~10 variables. Mapping from X to Y can be achieved using statistical or simple machine learning methods. For new patients, the predicted Y is then converted back to predicted DVHs through an inverse PCA. In this example, the predicted DVHs of the two OARs are shown in the bottom right plot, with the semi-transparent bands showing the uncertainty or confidence intervals.

non-inferiorly or even superiorly to machine learning methods (Landers *et al.*, 2018). Besides DVH prediction, it has also been used to predict beam angle arrangement prediction, etc. for facilitating automated treatment planning (Yuan *et al.*, 2015; Zhang, *et al.*, 2011). As the approach was commercialized in clinical treatment planning systems, it has been widely applied in treatment planning for all kinds of cancer sites and showed improved treatment efficiency and consistency, with clinically acceptable treatment plan quality that sometimes outperforms average human planners (Amaloo *et al.*, 2019; Chang *et al.*, 2016; Fogliata *et al.*, 2017, 2019; Kubo *et al.*, 2017; Scaggion *et al.*, 2018; Smith *et al.*, 2019; Tinoco *et al.*, 2020; Tol *et al.*, 2015; Wu *et al.*, 2016a, 2016b).

3.2. *Automatic feature extraction: Convolutional Neural Network (CNN)*

Compared with soft-AI methods with manual feature extraction, the more recent hard-AI methods apply automatic feature extraction using deep learning and other AI methods. These deep learning methods further remove human interactions using algorithms inspired by the structure and function of human brains.

One popular deep learning method is convolutional neural network (CNN). This method mimics human visual neurons and is widely used to reduce data dimension by extracting spatial features in applications such as image segmentation. This method is based on convolution filters, a common feature extraction tool in imaging processing. Figure 5(a) shows a simplified example: a 3 × 3 2D matrix represents CT voxels labeled as tumor or organs at risks (OARs); a matrix of its distance to target; a matrix of dose where tumor is expecting 100% dose with fast dose fall off at OARs. Figure 5(b) shows a dose fall off feature extraction and dimension reduction using convolution/deconvolution filters, also termed encoder/decoder filters. In this example, using a 2 × 2 encoder filter, a 3 × 3 input image/dose matrix is reduced to a 2 × 2 compressed matrix. This encoder filter is chosen to highlight the dose difference along the diagonal direction. The compressed matrix can then be reconstructed back using a decoder filter to restore the resolution and feature of the original input. Clearly, the convolution step is down sampling, and the transpose

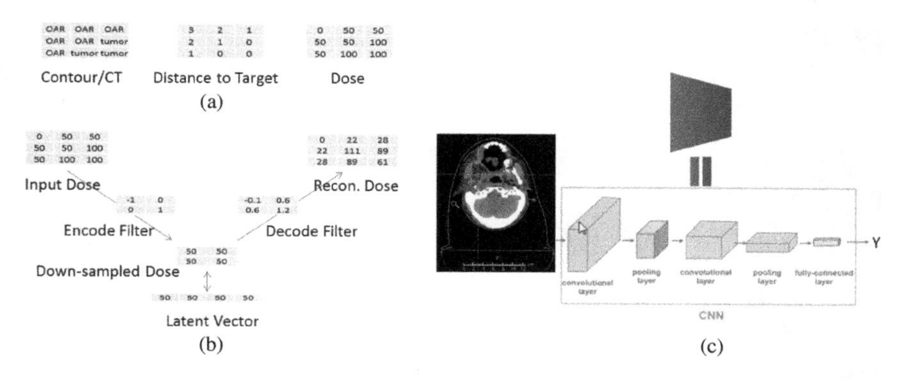

Fig. 5. A simple convolution/deconvolution process example demonstrating auto feature extraction in CNN-based automated treatment planning: (a) inputs of 3 × 3 matrices consisting of CT/Contour, distance to target, and ideal dose. (b) downsampling from a 3 × 3 input image matrix to a 2 × 2 compressed matrix with an encoder filter, then reconstructed back to a 3 × 3 output matrix with a decoder filter; (c) showcasing the building blocks of a feature extraction CNN for automated treatment planning: A 3D CT/contour/dose feature extraction is compressed to a 1D array *Y*, the latent vector.

convolution is the reverse. In transpose convolution, the transpose kernel is placed over each pixel. The pixel values are multiplied by the kernel weights to produce the upsampled matrix/images. Ideally, the reconstructed output would be identical to the input. The decoder filter is then least-square fitted by minimizing the difference between the input and the reconstructed output.

Unlike the 1D conversion used in the manual feature extraction case presented in the last section, a CNN applies convolution filters directly onto the input image. Figure 5(c) shows the building blocks of a feature extraction CNN, including convolution, activation, and pooling layers. The convolution layer reduces the image data size by using a bank of small filters, which characterizes limited spatial feature only seen by one neuron. To mimic the activation of a neuron, the output of convolution is fed to an activation function. For instance, Rectified Linear Unit (ReLU): $g(x) = \max(0, x)$, with fast computation and non-linearity, is a widely used activation function in CNN. The output of activation could be further reduced using a pooling layer such as a maximum pool local filter, which simply calculates the maximum value for patches of the feature map. Small variation of translation, rotation, and scaling of the input will not

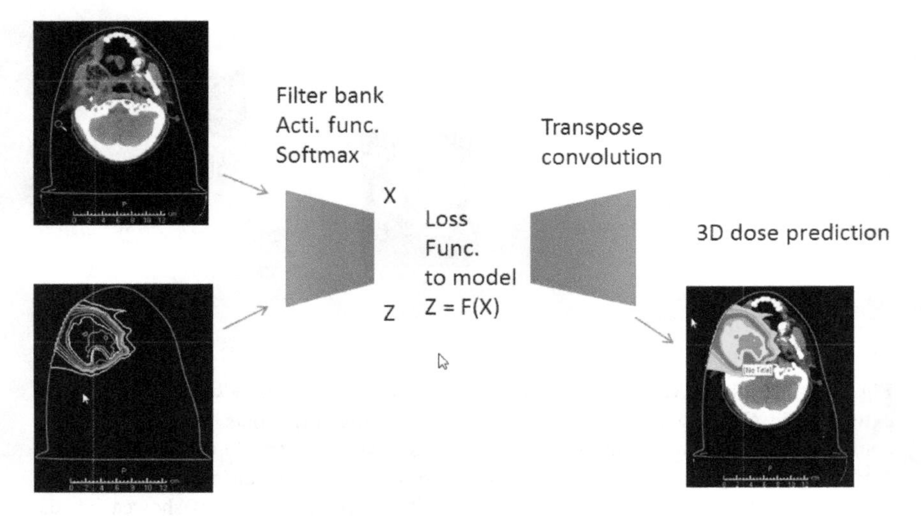

Fig. 6. 3D dose prediction achieved using downsampling and upsampling CNN architecture. The latent vector, *Y*, is the input for the transpose convolution.

affect the convolution-pooling results. The spatial invariance is maintained within the multiple layers of convolution and pooling network for feature extraction and dimension reduction. The last layer is always made of a fully connected neural network, with an output of a 1D data array, *Y*, the latent vector, which is the final extracted feature.

Therefore, the latent vector is a low-dimensional representation of the higher-dimensional input data that can be applied for dose prediction as shown in Fig. 6, and can similarly be applied to other applications such as classification and segmentation (contouring) through the upsampling of the latent vector.

At the time of this writing, CNN has been arguably the most popular deep learning method used for hard-AI treatment planning. Various network architectures have been studied such as U-net originally developed for biomedical image segmentation, DenseNet, and ResNet. In these applications, dose is predicted from patient images, target and OAR contours, and manual dosimetric or distance features are also sometimes added to the input to improve the prediction efficiency and accuracy (Barragan-Montero *et al.*, 2019; Kajikawa *et al.*, 2019; Kandalan *et al.*,

2020; Kearney *et al.*, 2018a, 2018b; Liu *et al.*, 2019; Ma *et al.*, 2021a; Ma *et al.*, 2019a, 2019b; Nguyen *et al.*, 2019a 2019b).

Auto feature extraction could be achieved with or without data labeling. When the upsampling network is reconstructing the original input, data labeling can be omitted. In this case, the later vectors X and Y make up a bottleneck hidden layer forcing the network to learn compressed representation and find its hidden structure. Model training is hence through minimizing the loss function shown in Eq. (2), as follows:

$$L = (\text{Reconstruction loss}) + (\text{Regularization term}) \tag{2}$$

The reconstruction loss is the difference between the prediction and training. The regularization term is used to tune the network to avoid overfitting due to limited training data set. Through training of the neural network, the weight would be increased for convolution filters that emphasize dose fall off outside the tumor. Finally, the one feature that must be automatically modeled by a successful neural network is that dose decreases when its distance to the tumor increases.

3.3. *Generative Adversarial Neural network (GAN)*

Huge data are essential for the success of CNN, which relies on training millions of parameters. While the sampling size in radiation therapy is very limited, usually it results in biased sample distribution. To overcome overfitting and data biasing, Generative Adversarial Network (GAN) is another deep learning approach that was introduced to address the complex sample distribution. Using upsampling to build a generator network, it creates fake samples from learning the representation of data distribution. Figure 7(a) presents the GAN architecture. The generator and discriminator will be trained iteratively by competing with each other. Its loss function is defined as

$$L = minmax\ E\ [log\ D(G(img)) + log(1 - D(img))] \tag{3}$$

where D is the probability that the discriminator estimates the image to be a true image; G is the generator's fake image output from noise; E is the

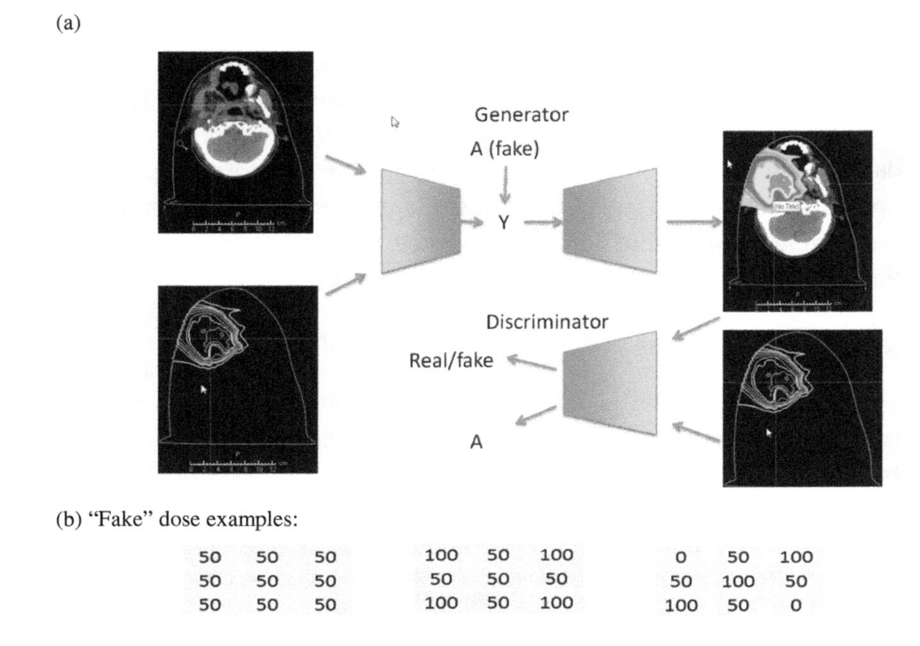

Fig. 7. (a) Outline of a GAN: Generator tries to synthesize fake images that fool the best discriminator; the discriminator tries to identify the synthesized images; (b) Following the example in Fig. 5(a), a three sample dose matrix where dose doesn't fall off outside tumor will be identified by the discriminator as "fake", while the dose sample in 5(a) will be "real".

expected value over all data instances; L is the loss function that G tries to minimize while D tries to maximize. Following the example in Fig. 5(a), three fake dose samples were created by the generator in Fig. 5(a). Those doses in the three samples do not decrease as their distances to target increase, so $D(G(img))$ is close to 0, and the loss function will approach ∞.

GAN is gaining popularity as a treatment planning AI with reported recent successes, trained by radiation therapy data of small sample sizes (Babier *et al.*, 2020a; Fan *et al.*, 2019b; Kearney *et al.*, 2020; Li *et al.*, 2020, 2021a; Murakami *et al.*, 2020). Some of these applications directly predict radiation fluence maps instead of the dose distribution. Due to the degenerative nature that varying fluence maps can yield similar 3D dose distribution, GAN is suitable for identifying the non-unique fluence map solutions.

3.4. *Reinforcement Learning (RL): Optimize machine parameters*

Reinforcement Learning (RL) develops from dynamic system theory, as the optimal control of incompletely-known Markov decision process, where exact mathematical models and methods are infeasible. The planning of Volume-Modulated Arc Therapy (VMAT) represents such a challenge. For instance, the MLC aperture has almost infinite number of shapes for selection in the optimization process.

RL uses short-term reward, r_t, at a step t, to evaluate an agent's action, a_t, at a certain state S_t. The total reward including its long-term impact is defined as $R_t = \Sigma_{k=t}^{\infty} \gamma^k r_k$ discounted by the factor γ ($0 < \gamma < 1$). The Q-function captures the estimated total future reward. To achieve optimality, the Q-function is updated by the Bellman equation described in Eq. (4),

$$Q(s,a) = Q(s,a) + \alpha\{r + \gamma\, max_{a'} Q(s',a') - Q(s,a)\}. \quad (4)$$

The training of the Q network is through minimizing the loss function between the target and the predicted in Eq. (5):

$$L = E\{\| r + \gamma\, max_{a'} Q(s',a') - Q(s,a) \|\}^2 \quad (5)$$

For an application in VMAT planning, the term 'step' is naturally defined as the Linac gantry angle gap or control point in VMAT; the action includes the Linac dose rate and MLC leaf positions; dose difference between the prescribed and the current setup is defined as the rewards to compute the discounted cumulative cost in the Q-value. RL was performed to determine a policy to minimize the Q-value, and the policy will guide the MLC position and dose rate selection at each control point.

An example is shown in Fig. 8: a single deep Q learning (DQN) agent is implemented to control the dose rate and MLC leaves. The DQN

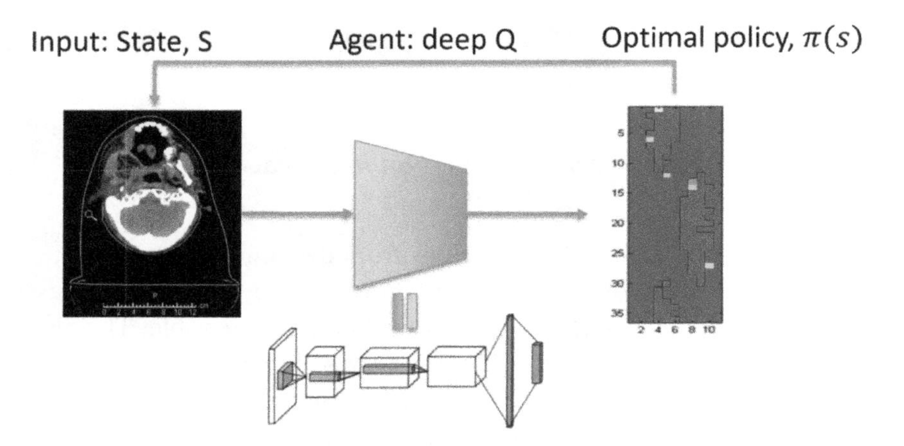

Fig. 8. Training of the deep-Q-network: optimizing the MLC aperture and dose rate at each step to achieve final high-quality treatment plan.

consists of three convolutional layers followed by a fully connected layer and a final output layer (with ReLU activation). The DQN training follows the ε–greedy algorithms to balance the exploration–exploitation tradeoff. By assigning an ε between 0 and 1. With a probability of ε at each step, the dose rate and leaf position will change randomly, as does the Q-value. The Q-value is maximized with a probability of 1-ε. At the initial training, ε is chosen close to 1 to allow more searching freedom. During training, ε will be decreased to speed up convergence, similar to the simulated annealing process.

Due to the complexity in radiation therapy treatment planning and the strength of RL to solve very complex problems, RL began to be studied for this application. While this line of efforts is relatively new, some preliminary success has been demonstrated. RL application has also been expanded from external beam radiation therapy to high dose rate brachytherapy (Hrinivich & Lee, 2020; Shen *et al.*, 2020).

4. Other AI Methods and Considerations

In addition to the methods introduced above, there are also other approaches being researched for AI-based radiation therapy treatment planning. For example, there are atlas-based approaches by selecting the atlas closest to the new image from the training atlas pool for dose mimicking (Conroy *et al.*, 2021; McIntosh *et al.*, 2017, 2021; McIntosh & Purdie, 2016, 2017).

As with other AI applications, AI treatment planning shares many common challenges and considerations. For example, the data set size limitation is usually present because unlike millions of natural images available for other semantic segmentation problems, the number of radiation therapy treatment plans available for AI training is usually only a few hundreds or less. In addition, despite the fact that radiation oncology is one of the most evidence-based medical field using standard care, dosimetric constraint and prescription differences still exist among individual practitioners and institutions. Generalizability is therefore an important consideration for treatment planning AIs. Furthermore, as the AI methods become increasingly automated and complicated, they function more and more like a black box. Efforts are also devoted to improve the interpretability of treatment planning AI agents. Lastly, as with other medical AIs, there exist various biases both within the data set used to train the AI and in steps of the AI workflow itself. The developers and users need to discover and understand these biases to mitigate and correct their effects in the treatment planning AIs.

Acknowledgment

The authors thank Leigh Conroy, PhD, and Tom Purdie, PhD, for internal critical review of the manuscript.

References

Amaloo, C., Hayes, L., Manning, M., Liu, H., & Wiant, D. (2019). Can automated treatment plans gain traction in the clinic? *Journal of Applied Clinical Medical Physics, 20*(8), 29–35. https://doi.org/10.1002/acm2.12674.

Babier, A., Boutilier, J. J., McNiven, A. L., & Chan, T. C. Y. (2018). Knowledge-based automated planning for oropharyngeal cancer. *Medical Physics, 45*(7), 2875–2883. https://doi.org/10.1002/mp.12930.

Babier, A., Mahmood, R., McNiven, A. L., Diamant, A., & Chan, T. C. Y. (2020a). Knowledge-based automated planning with three-dimensional generative adversarial networks. *Medical Physics, 47*(2), 297–306. https://doi.org/10.1002/mp.13896.

Babier, A., Mahmood, R., McNiven, A. L., Diamant, A., & Chan, T. C. Y. (2020b). Knowledge-based automated planning with three-dimensional generative adversarial networks. *Medical Physics, 47*(2), 297–306. https://doi.org/10.1002/mp.13896.

Barragan-Montero, A. M., Nguyen, D., Lu, W., Lin, M. H., Norouzi-Kandalan, R., Geets, X., ... Jiang, S. (2019). Three-dimensional dose prediction for lung IMRT patients with deep neural networks: Robust learning from heterogeneous beam configurations. *Medical Physics, 46*(8), 3679–3691. https://doi.org/10.1002/mp.13597.

Berry, S. L., Ma, R., Boczkowski, A., Jackson, A., Zhang, P., & Hunt, M. (2016a). Evaluating inter-campus plan consistency using a knowledge based planning model. *Radiotherapy and Oncology: Journal of the European Society for Therapeutic Radiology and Oncology, 120*(2), 349–355. https://doi.org/10.1016/j.radonc.2016.06.010.

Berry, S. L., Ma, R., Boczkowski, A., Jackson, A., Zhang, P., & Hunt, M. (2016b). Evaluating inter-campus plan consistency using a knowledge based planning model. *Radiotherapy & Oncology, 120*(2), 349–355. https://doi.org/10.1016/j.radonc.2016.06.010.

Biston, M. C., Costea, M., Gassa, F., Serre, A. A., Voet, P., Larson, R., & Gregoire, V. (2021). Evaluation of fully automated a priori MCO treatment planning in VMAT for head-and-neck cancer. *Physica Medica: PM: An International Journal Devoted to the Applications of Physics to Medicine and Biology: Official Journal of the Italian Association of Biomedical Physics, 87*, 31–38. https://doi.org/10.1016/j.ejmp.2021.05.037.

Breedveld, S., Storchi, P. R., & Heijmen, B. J. (2009). The equivalence of multi-criteria methods for radiotherapy plan optimization. *Physics in Medicine and Biology, 54*(23), 7199–7209. https://doi.org/10.1088/0031-9155/54/23/011.

Breedveld, S., Storchi, P. R., Keijzer, M., Heemink, A. W., & Heijmen, B. J. (2007). A novel approach to multi-criteria inverse planning for IMRT. *Physics in Medicine and Biology, 52*(20), 6339–6353. https://doi.org/10.1088/0031-9155/52/20/016.

Breedveld, S., Storchi, P. R., Voet, P. W., & Heijmen, B. J. (2012). iCycle: Integrated, multicriterial beam angle, and profile optimization for generation of coplanar and noncoplanar IMRT plans. *Medical Physics, 39*(2), 951–963. https://doi.org/10.1118/1.3676689.

Chang, A. T. Y., Hung, A. W. M., Cheung, F. W. K., Lee, M. C. H., Chan, O. S. H., Philips, H., ... Ng, W. T. (2016). Comparison of planning quality and efficiency between conventional and knowledge-based algorithms in nasopharyngeal cancer patients using intensity modulated radiation therapy. [Comparative Study Evaluation Study]. *International Journal of Radiation Oncology, Biology, Physics, 95*(3), 981–990. https://doi.org/10.1016/j.ijrobp.2016.02.017.

Chen, H., Wang, H., Gu, H., Shao, Y., Cai, X., Fu, X., & Xu, Z. (2018). Study for reducing lung dose of upper thoracic esophageal cancer radiotherapy by auto-planning: Vvolumetric-modulated arc therapy vs intensity-modulated radiation therapy. [Comparative Study]. *Medical Dosimetry: Official Iournal of the American Association of Medical Dosimetrists, 43*(3), 243–250. https://doi.org/10.1016/j.meddos.2017.09.001.

Chen, W., Unkelbach, J., Trofimov, A., Madden, T., Kooy, H., Bortfeld, T., & Craft, D. (2012). Including robustness in multi-criteria optimization for intensity-modulated proton therapy. *Physics in Medicine and Biology, 57*(3), 591–608. https://doi.org/10.1088/0031-9155/57/3/591.

Conroy, L., Khalifa, A., Berlin, A., McIntosh, C., & Purdie, T. G. (2021). Performance stability evaluation of atlas-based machine learning radiation therapy treatment planning in prostate cancer. *Physics in Medicine and Biology, 66*(13), 134001. https://doi.org/10.1088/1361-6560/abfff0.

Fan, J., Wang, J., Chen, Z., Hu, C., Zhang, Z., & Hu, W. (2019a). Automatic treatment planning based on three-dimensional dose distribution predicted from deep learning technique. *Medical Physics, 46*(1), 370–381. https://doi.org/10.1002/mp.13271.

Fan, J., Wang, J., Chen, Z., Hu, C., Zhang, Z., & Hu, W. (2019b). Automatic treatment planning based on three-dimensional dose distribution predicted from deep learning technique. *Medical Physics, 46*(1), 370–381. https://doi.org/10.1002/mp.13271.

Fogliata, A., Belosi, F., Clivio, A., Navarria, P., Nicolini, G., Scorsetti, M., ... Cozzi, L. (2014). On the pre-clinical validation of a commercial model-based optimisation engine: Application to volumetric modulated arc therapy for patients with lung or prostate cancer. [Research Support, Non-U.S. Gov't Validation Study]. *Radiotherapy & Oncology, 113*(3), 385–391. https://doi.org/10.1016/j.radonc.2014.11.009.

Fogliata, A., Cozzi, L., Reggiori, G., Stravato, A., Lobefalo, F., Franzese, C., ... Scorsetti, M. (2019). RapidPlan knowledge based planning: Iterative learning process and model ability to steer planning strategies. *Radiation Oncology, 14*(1), 187. https://doi.org/10.1186/s13014-019-1403-0.

Fogliata, A., Nicolini, G., Bourgier, C., Clivio, A., De Rose, F., Fenoglietto, P., ... Cozzi, L. (2015). Performance of a knowledge-based model for optimization of volumetric modulated arc therapy plans for single and bilateral breast irradiation. [Research Support, Non-U.S. Gov't]. *PloS one, 10*(12), e0145137. https://doi.org/10.1371/journal.pone.0145137.

Fogliata, A., Reggiori, G., Stravato, A., Lobefalo, F., Franzese, C., Franceschini, D., ... Cozzi, L. (2017). RapidPlan head and neck model: The objectives and possible clinical benefit. *Radiation Oncology, 12*(1), 73. https://doi.org/10.1186/s13014-017-0808-x.

Gintz, D., Latifi, K., Caudell, J., Nelms, B., Zhang, G., Moros, E., & Feygelman, V. (2016). Initial evaluation of automated treatment planning software. [Evaluation Study]. *Journal of Applied Clinical Medical Physics, 17*(3), 331–346. https://doi.org/10.1120/jacmp.v17i3.6167.

Hansen, C. R., Bertelsen, A., Hazell, I., Zukauskaite, R., Gyldenkerne, N., Johansen, J., ... Brink, C. (2016). Automatic treatment planning improves the clinical quality of head and neck cancer treatment plans. *Clinical and Translational Radiation Oncology, 1*, 2–8. https://doi.org/10.1016/j.ctro.2016.08.001.

Hazell, I., Bzdusek, K., Kumar, P., Hansen, C. R., Bertelsen, A., Eriksen, J. G., ... Brink, C. (2016). Automatic planning of head and neck treatment plans. [Research Support, Non-U.S. Gov't]. *Journal of Applied Clinical Medical Physics, 17*(1), 272–282. https://doi.org/10.1120/jacmp.v17i1.5901.

Hrinivich, W. T. & Lee, J. (2020). Artificial intelligence-based radiotherapy machine parameter optimization using reinforcement learning. *Medical Physics, 47*(12), 6140–6150. https://doi.org/10.1002/mp.14544.

Kajikawa, T., Kadoya, N., Ito, K., Takayama, Y., Chiba, T., Tomori, S., ... Jingu, K. (2019). A convolutional neural network approach for IMRT dose distribution prediction in prostate cancer patients. *Journal of Radiation Research, 60*(5), 685–693. https://doi.org/10.1093/jrr/rrz051.

Kandalan, R. N., Nguyen, D., Rezaeian, N. H., Barragan-Montero, A. M., Breedveld, S., Namuduri, K., ... Lin, M. H. (2020). Dose prediction with deep learning for prostate cancer radiation therapy: Model adaptation to different treatment planning practices. [Research Support, N.I.H., Extramural]. *Radiotherapy and Oncology: Journal of the European Society for Therapeutic Radiology and Oncology, 153*, 228–235. https://doi.org/10.1016/j.radonc.2020.10.027.

Kearney, V., Chan, J. W., Haaf, S., Descovich, M., & Solberg, T. D. (2018a). DoseNet: A volumetric dose prediction algorithm using 3D fully-convolutional neural networks. *Physics in Medicine and Biology, 63*(23), 235022. https://doi.org/10.1088/1361-6560/aaef74.

Kearney, V., Chan, J. W., Valdes, G., Solberg, T. D., & Yom, S. S. (2018b). The application of artificial intelligence in the IMRT planning process for head and neck cancer. [Review]. *Oral Oncology, 87*, 111–116. https://doi.org/10.1016/j.oraloncology.2018.10.026.

Kearney, V., Chan, J. W., Wang, T., Perry, A., Descovich, M., Morin, O., ... Solberg, T. D. (2020). DoseGAN: A generative adversarial network for synthetic dose prediction using attention-gated discrimination and generation. *Scientific Reports, 10*(1), 11073. https://doi.org/10.1038/s41598-020-68062-7.

Kubo, K., Monzen, H., Ishii, K., Tamura, M., Kawamorita, R., Sumida, I., ... Nishimura, Y. (2017). Dosimetric comparison of RapidPlan and manually optimized plans in volumetric modulated arc therapy for prostate cancer. [Comparative Study]. *Physica Medica: PM: An International Journal Devoted to the Applications of Physics to Medicine and Biology: Official Journal of the Italian Association of Biomedical Physics, 44*, 199–204. https://doi.org/10.1016/j.ejmp.2017.06.026.

Kusters, J., Bzdusek, K., Kumar, P., van Kollenburg, P. G. M., Kunze-Busch, M. C., Wendling, M., ... Kaanders, J. (2017). Automated IMRT planning in Pinnacle: A study in head-and-neck cancer. [Comparative Study Evaluation Study].

Strahlentherapie und Onkologie: Organ der Deutschen Rontgengesellschaft ... [et al.], 193(12), 1031–1038. https://doi.org/10.1007/s00066-017-1187-9.

Landers, A., Neph, R., Scalzo, F., Ruan, D., & Sheng, K. (2018). Performance comparison of knowledge-based dose prediction techniques based on limited patient data. *Technology in Cancer Research & Treatment, 17*, 1533033818811150. https://doi.org/10.1177/1533033818811150.

Li, X., Wang, C., Sheng, Y., Zhang, J., Wang, W., Yin, F. F., ... Ge, Y. (2021a). An artificial intelligence-driven agent for real-time head-and-neck IMRT plan generation using conditional Generative Adversarial Network (cGAN). *Medical Physics, 48*(6), 2714–2723. https://doi.org/10.1002/mp.14770.

Li, X., Wang, C., Sheng, Y., Zhang, J., Wang, W., Yin, F. F., ... Ge, Y. (2021b). An artificial intelligence-driven agent for real-time head-and-neck IMRT plan generation using conditional Generative Adversarial Network (cGAN). *Medical Physics, 48*(6), 2714–2723. https://doi.org/10.1002/mp.14770.

Li, X., Zhang, J., Sheng, Y., Chang, Y., Yin, F. F., Ge, Y., ... Wang, C. (2020). Automatic IMRT Planning via Static Field Fluence Prediction (AIP-SFFP): A deep learning algorithm for real-time prostate treatment planning. *Physics in Medicine and Biology, 65*(17), 175014. https://doi.org/10.1088/1361-6560/aba5eb.

Liu, Z., Fan, J., Li, M., Yan, H., Hu, Z., Huang, P., ... Dai, J. (2019). A deep learning method for prediction of three-dimensional dose distribution of helical tomotherapy. *Medical Physics, 46*(5), 1972–1983. https://doi.org/10.1002/mp.13490.

Ma, J., Nguyen, D., Bai, T., Folkerts, M., Jia, X., Lu, W., ... Jiang, S. (2021a). A feasibility study on deep learning-based individualized 3D dose distribution prediction. *Medical Physics, 48*(8), 4438–4447. https://doi.org/10.1002/mp.15025.

Ma, J., Nguyen, D., Bai, T., Folkerts, M., Jia, X., Lu, W., ... Jiang, S. (2021b). A feasibility study on deep learning-based individualized 3D dose distribution prediction. *Medical Physics, 48*(8), 4438–4447. https://doi.org/10.1002/mp.15025.

Ma, M., Kovalchuk, N., Buyyounouski, M. K., Xing, L., & Yang, Y. (2019a). Incorporating dosimetric features into the prediction of 3D VMAT dose distributions using deep convolutional neural network. [Research Support, N.I.H., Extramural Research Support, Non-U.S. Gov't]. *Physics in Medicine and Biology, 64*(12), 125017. https://doi.org/10.1088/1361-6560/ab2146.

Ma, M., M, K. B., Vasudevan, V., Xing, L., & Yang, Y. (2019b). Dose distribution prediction in isodose feature-preserving voxelization domain using deep convolutional neural network. *Medical Physics, 46*(7), 2978–2987. https://doi.org/10.1002/mp.13618.

Mashayekhi, M., Tapia, I. R., Balagopal, A., Zhong, X., Barkousaraie, A. S., McBeth, R., ... Nguyen, D. (2022). Site-Agnostic 3D dose distribution prediction with deep learning neural networks. *Medical Physics, 49*(3), 1391–1406. https://doi.org/10.1002/mp.15461.

McIntosh, C., Conroy, L., Tjong, M. C., Craig, T., Bayley, A., Catton, C., ... Purdie, T. G. (2021). Clinical integration of machine learning for curative-intent radiation treatment of patients with prostate cancer. [Research Support, Non-U.S. Gov't]. *Nature Medicine, 27*(6), 999–1005. https://doi.org/10.1038/s41591-021-01359-w.

McIntosh, C. & Purdie, T. G. (2016). Contextual atlas regression forests: Multiple-atlas-based automated dose prediction in radiation therapy. [Research Support, Non-U.S. Gov't]. *IEEE Transactions on Medical Imaging, 35*(4), 1000–1012. https://doi.org/10.1109/TMI.2015.2505188.

McIntosh, C. & Purdie, T. G. (2017). Voxel-based dose prediction with multi-patient atlas selection for automated radiotherapy treatment planning. *Physics in Medicine and Biology, 62*(2), 415–431. https://doi.org/10.1088/1361-6560/62/2/415.

McIntosh, C., Welch, M., McNiven, A., Jaffray, D. A., & Purdie, T. G. (2017). Fully automated treatment planning for head and neck radiotherapy using a voxel-based dose prediction and dose mimicking method. *Physics in Medicine and Biology, 62*(15), 5926–5944. https://doi.org/10.1088/1361-6560/aa71f8.

Murakami, Y., Magome, T., Matsumoto, K., Sato, T., Yoshioka, Y., & Oguchi, M. (2020). Fully automated dose prediction using generative adversarial networks in prostate cancer patients. [Research Support, Non-U.S. Gov't]. *PloS one, 15*(5), e0232697. https://doi.org/10.1371/journal.pone.0232697.

Nawa, K., Haga, A., Nomoto, A., Sarmiento, R. A., Shiraishi, K., Yamashita, H., & Nakagawa, K. (2017). Evaluation of a commercial automatic treatment planning system for prostate cancers. [Evaluation Study]. *Medical Dosimetry: Official Journal of the American Association of Medical Dosimetrists, 42*(3), 203–209. https://doi.org/10.1016/j.meddos.2017.03.004.

Nguyen, D., Jia, X., Sher, D., Lin, M. H., Iqbal, Z., Liu, H., & Jiang, S. (2019a). 3D radiotherapy dose prediction on head and neck cancer patients with a hierarchically densely connected U-net deep learning architecture. [Research Support, Non-U.S. Gov't]. *Physics in Medicine and Biology, 64*(6), 065020. https://doi.org/10.1088/1361-6560/ab039b.

Nguyen, D., Long, T., Jia, X., Lu, W., Gu, X., Iqbal, Z., & Jiang, S. (2019b). A feasibility study for predicting optimal radiation therapy dose distributions of prostate cancer patients from patient anatomy using deep learning. [Research Support, Non-U.S. Gov't]. *Scientific Reports, 9*(1), 1076. https://doi.org/10.1038/s41598-018-37741-x.

Rice, A., Zoller, I., Kocos, K., Weller, D., DiCostanzo, D., Hunzeker, A., & Lenards, N. (2019). The implementation of RapidPlan in predicting deep inspiration breath-hold candidates with left-sided breast cancer. *Medical Dosimetry: Official Journal of the American Association of Medical Dosimetrists, 44*(3), 210–218. https://doi.org/10.1016/j.meddos.2018.06.007.

Romeijn, H. E., Dempsey, J. F., & Li, J. G. (2004). A unifying framework for multi-criteria fluence map optimization models. *Physics in Medicine and Biology, 49*(10), 1991–2013. https://doi.org/10.1088/0031-9155/49/10/011.

Scaggion, A., Fusella, M., Roggio, A., Bacco, S., Pivato, N., Rossato, M. A., ... Paiusco, M. (2018). Reducing inter- and intra-planner variability in radiotherapy plan output with a commercial knowledge-based planning solution. *Physica Medica: PM: An International Journal Devoted to the Applications of Physics to Medicine and*

Biology: Official Journal of the Italian Association of Biomedical Physics, 53, 86–93. https://doi.org/10.1016/j.ejmp.2018.08.016.

Schubert, C., Waletzko, O., Weiss, C., Voelzke, D., Toperim, S., Roeser, A., ... Cozzi, L. (2017). Intercenter validation of a knowledge based model for automated planning of volumetric modulated arc therapy for prostate cancer. The experience of the German RapidPlan Consortium. [Multicenter Study]. *PloS one, 12*(5), e0178034. https://doi.org/10.1371/journal.pone.0178034.

Shen, C., Nguyen, D., Chen, L., Gonzalez, Y., McBeth, R., Qin, N., ... Jia, X. (2020). Operating a treatment planning system using a deep-reinforcement learning-based virtual treatment planner for prostate cancer intensity-modulated radiation therapy treatment planning. *Medical Physics, 47*(6), 2329–2336. https://doi.org/10.1002/mp.14114.

Smith, A., Granatowicz, A., Stoltenberg, C., Wang, S., Liang, X., Enke, C. A., ... Zheng, D. (2019). Can the student outperform the master? A plan comparison between pinnacle auto-planning and eclipse knowledge-based rapidplan following a prostate-bed plan competition. *Technology in Cancer Research & Treatment, 18*, 1533033819851763. https://doi.org/10.1177/1533033819851763.

Tinoco, M., Waga, E., Tran, K., Vo, H., Baker, J., Hunter, R., ... Court, L. (2020). RapidPlan development of VMAT plans for cervical cancer patients in low- and middle-income countries. [Validation Study]. *Medical Dosimetry: Official Journal of the American Association of Medical Dosimetrists, 45*(2), 172–178. https://doi.org/10.1016/j.meddos.2019.10.002.

Tol, J. P., Dahele, M., Delaney, A. R., Slotman, B. J., & Verbakel, W. F. (2015). Can knowledge-based DVH predictions be used for automated, individualized quality assurance of radiotherapy treatment plans? [Research Support, Non-U.S. Gov't]. *Radiation Oncology, 10*, 234. https://doi.org/10.1186/s13014-015-0542-1.

van de Water, S., Kraan, A. C., Breedveld, S., Schillemans, W., Teguh, D. N., Kooy, H. M., ... Hoogeman, M. S. (2013). Improved efficiency of multi-criteria IMPT treatment planning using iterative resampling of randomly placed pencil beams. *Physics in Medicine and Biology, 58*(19), 6969–6983. https://doi.org/10.1088/0031-9155/58/19/6969.

Wang, C., Zhu, X., Hong, J. C., & Zheng, D. (2019). Artificial Intelligence in radiotherapy treatment planning: Present and future. [Review]. *Technology in Cancer Research & Treatment, 18*, 1533033819873922. https://doi.org/10.1177/1533033819873922.

Wu, B., Ricchetti, F., Sanguineti, G., Kazhdan, M., Simari, P., Jacques, R., ... McNutt, T. (2011). Data-driven approach to generating achievable dose-volume histogram objectives in intensity-modulated radiotherapy planning. [Research Support, Non-U.S. Gov't]. *International Journal of Radiation Oncology, Biology, Physics, 79*(4), 1241–1247. https://doi.org/10.1016/j.ijrobp.2010.05.026.

Wu, H., Jiang, F., Yue, H., Li, S., & Zhang, Y. (2016a). A dosimetric evaluation of knowledge-based VMAT planning with simultaneous integrated boosting for rectal cancer patients. [Evaluation Study]. *Journal of Applied Clinical Medical Physics, 17*(6), 78–85. https://doi.org/10.1120/jacmp.v17i6.6410.

Wu, H., Jiang, F., Yue, H., Zhang, H., Wang, K., & Zhang, Y. (2016b). Applying a RapidPlan model trained on a technique and orientation to another: A feasibility and dosimetric evaluation. *Radiation Oncology, 11*(1), 108. https://doi.org/10.1186/s13014-016-0684-9.

Yuan, L., Ge, Y., Lee, W. R., Yin, F. F., Kirkpatrick, J. P., & Wu, Q. J. (2012). Quantitative analysis of the factors which affect the interpatient organ-at-risk dose sparing variation in IMRT plans. *Medical Physics, 39*(11), 6868–6878. https://doi.org/10.1118/1.4757927.

Yuan, L., Wu, Q. J., Yin, F., Li, Y., Sheng, Y., Kelsey, C. R., & Ge, Y. (2015). Standardized beam bouquets for lung IMRT planning. [Randomized Controlled Trial Research Support, N.I.H., Extramural Research Support, Non-U.S. Gov't]. *Physics in Medicine and Biology, 60*(5), 1831–1843. https://doi.org/10.1088/0031-9155/60/5/1831.

Zhang, J., Wu, Q. J., Xie, T., Sheng, Y., Yin, F. F., & Ge, Y. (2018). An ensemble approach to knowledge-based intensity-modulated radiation therapy planning. *Frontiers in Oncology, 8*, 57. https://doi.org/10.3389/fonc.2018.00057.

Zhang, X., Li, X., Quan, E. M., Pan, X., & Li, Y. (2011). A methodology for automatic intensity-modulated radiation treatment planning for lung cancer. [Research Support, N.I.H., Extramural]. *Physics in Medicine and Biology, 56*(13), 3873–3893. https://doi.org/10.1088/0031-9155/56/13/009.

Zhu, X., Ge, Y., Li, T., Thongphiew, D., Yin, F. F., & Wu, Q. J. (2011a). A planning quality evaluation tool for prostate adaptive IMRT based on machine learning. [Research Support, Non-U.S. Gov't]. *Medical Physics, 38*(2), 719–726. https://doi.org/10.1118/1.3539749.

Chapter 11

Clinical Application of AI for Radiation Therapy Treatment Planning

Leigh Conroy* and Thomas G. Purdie†

**Department of Radiation Oncology, University of Toronto, Princess Margaret Cancer Centre, 700 University Ave, Toronto, ON M5G 1X7, Canada*
†Departments of Radiation Oncology and Medical Biophysics, University of Toronto, Princess Margaret Cancer Centre, 700 University Ave, Toronto, ON M5G 1X7, Canada

Abstract

There are numerous high-performing technical solutions for Artificial Intelligence (AI)-based treatment planning; however, clinical use of these algorithms as standard-of-care in the clinic remains low. Challenges in real-world clinical use of AI treatment planning include the ongoing applicability in the dynamic clinical setting, gaining clinician trust, workflow integration, and a lack of guidance on Quality Assurance (QA), re-training, and algorithm maintenance. This chapter provides an overview of considerations and strategies for safe implementation and routine clinical use of AI for radiation treatment planning.

1. Introduction

Artificial Intelligence (AI) has the potential to revolutionize healthcare by increasing efficiency and improving patient outcomes (Hong *et al.*, 2020); however, most medical AI technologies do not ultimately reach clinical patient care. Many algorithms, despite their technical performance, are not clinically relevant or are not designed to integrate with the clinical setting (Hollon *et al.*, 2020; McCarroll *et al.*, 2018; Nimri *et al.*, 2020; Wijnberge *et al.*, 2020). Even AI with validation results that approach or surpass human performance are not adopted into routine clinical practice due to logistical challenges in translation from the ideal, simulated research environment into clinical workflows (Gaube *et al.*, 2021; Wiens *et al.*, 2019). Radiation therapy treatment planning is an ideal testbed for prospective AI deployment as dose prediction for automated radiation treatment planning represents a classic computer vision problem for which there is tremendous active research interest (McIntosh *et al.*, 2021).

However, even with AI algorithms demonstrating high performance in the research setting, real-world clinical use of these algorithms remains low (Topol, 2019). In radiation treatment planning, the transition from research to clinical implementation of AI is challenged by (i) the ongoing applicability of AI in the dynamic clinical setting (e.g., clinical practice changes over time based on clinical and technical considerations), (ii) clinical end user familiarity with AI outputs in order for clinicians to gain trust and confidence in AI, (iii) integration of AI into well-established clinical workflows with minimal disruption, and (iv) lack of guidance on quality assurance (QA), re-training AI models, AI algorithm maintenance, and systematic processes for data curation (Challen *et al.*, 2019; Parikh *et al.*, 2019; Tonekaboni *et al.*, 2019). This chapter provides an overview of considerations and strategies for safe implementation and routine clinical use of AI for radiation treatment planning.

A framework for stepwise implementation of AI into the Radiation Oncology clinic for AI radiation treatment planning requires evaluation of the AI by specific stakeholders and should assess AI performance using the appropriate methods and metrics (Fig. 1). Machine Learning (ML) algorithm development for AI deployment should be executed by a multi-disciplinary team formed at the outset of algorithm design and data curation. This core team should include computer scientists, medical physicists, and radiation oncologists, with expertise from other members of the clinical team including dosimetrists/planners. The framework steps for successful clinical deployment are highlighted throughout the chapter.

2. Problem Definition, Scope, and Data Curation

The first stage of development for an AI algorithm intended to be deployed in the clinic is to define the scope of the problem to be solved. For treatment planning this may include factors such as treatment site(s), patient population(s), who will use the algorithm, and at what point in the clinical workflow the algorithm will be implemented. It is imperative that both clinical and technical stakeholders are involved in defining the problem and scope. Clinical expertise is needed to ensure that the problem is not only clinically relevant, but also desired by the clinical care team to avoid development of an algorithm for which the clinical team will not see sufficient value to support future implementation (Saria & Subbaswamy, 2019). The clinicians involved in the early development stages can later become champions during clinical validation and implementation (Shah *et al.*, 2019). Conversely, the technical experts that will be developing the algorithm, including computer scientists and ML developers, should be involved in early problem definition discussions to provide expert advice about the possibilities, limitations, and potential pitfalls for various design and training considerations. Ethical implications should be considered by all team members at this earliest design stage, including privacy, safety, and fair treatment of patients (He *et al.*, 2019).

Both clinical and technical expertise is required for data curation. Radiation treatment planning is often viewed as an ideal AI application due to the abundance of labeled image data (e.g., delineated regions of interests and spatial radiation dose); however, historical treatment plans were not labeled nor created for the purpose of training an AI. A clinical

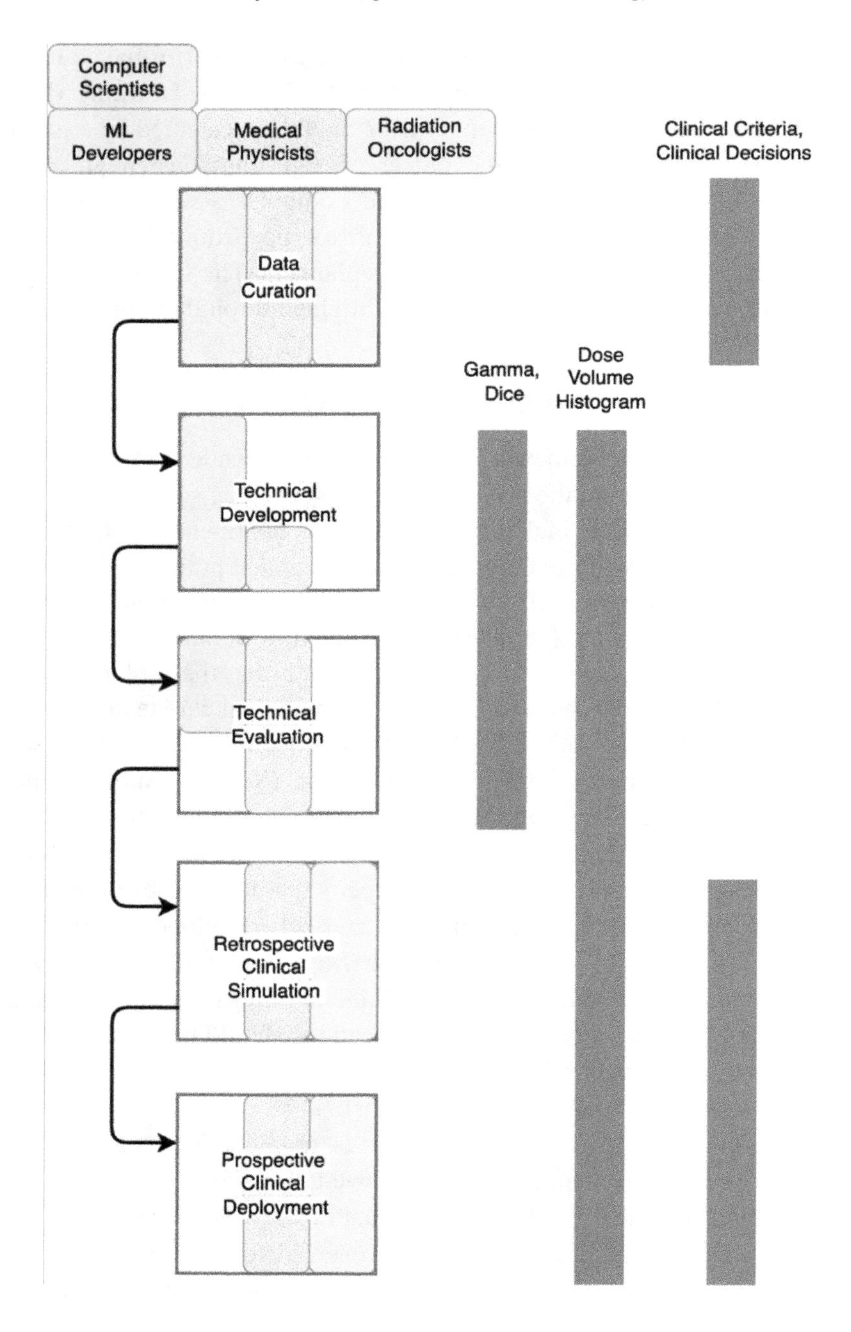
Computer Scientists
ML Developers
Medical Physicists
Radiation Oncologists
Clinical Criteria, Clinical Decisions
Data Curation
Gamma, Dice
Dose Volume Histogram
Technical Development
Technical Evaluation
Retrospective Clinical Simulation
Prospective Clinical Deployment

radiation treatment plan that may be clinically acceptable for an individual patient's treatment may not be appropriate for model training. While clinical treatment plan data is likely to be more applicable than simulated treatment plan data (i.e., planned retrospectively, often without consideration of clinical factors), blind, non-curated collation of historical clinically approved treatment plans for training may negatively impact the real-world performance of the AI. Furthermore, the rapid pace of change in radiation oncology practice warrants caution in using even recent historical data. Clinicians must be engaged at the start of data training to help identify cases that are most relevant to current treatments, and to provide input on future directions to avoid training a model that is out-of-date before it reaches the clinic.

From a prospective data curation perspective, the concept of ontologies and harmonization of data elements in radiation oncology are well understood and establishing standardized nomenclatures (Mayo *et al.*, 2018) for components of treatment plans (e.g., dose specification, treatment site definition, clinical intent, imaging specifications, etc.) are important to improve the quality of data for AI treatment planning. The implementation and clinical integration of data harmonization concepts will require top-down data policies and clinical department buy-in (including across departments or across an entire hospital) providing another important set of stakeholders to engage for AI deployments.

The potential for bias in the training data should be considered at the data curation stage (Obermeyer *et al.*, 2019). Algorithmic bias occurs when data for certain populations are underrepresented. An example of a potential bias in treatment planning is when there is a small sample of patients with a clinically relevant organ-at-risk volume for a given

Fig. 1. (*Continued on Facing Page*) A framework for the stepwise implementation of ML into the Radiation Oncology clinic for AI radiation treatment planning. Each step of successful clinical deployment requires evaluation of the AI by specific stakeholders and should assess AI performance using the appropriate methods and metrics. The outcome of each step is two-fold: validation of the technical or clinical utility of the AI and understanding of the limitations (technical, clinical, or social) of the algorithm. At the conclusion of each step, the team must decide whether to modify the algorithm or how it is used within the workflow or accept the limitations of the algorithm and ensure end users are educated to understand and expect the known limitations.

treatment protocol that is not routinely delineated in a treatment plan (e.g., for conventional locally advanced lung treatment planning, the right brachial plexus is only delineated for superior right lung targets and is otherwise not included in the treatment plan). Without intentional consideration of patient selection in historical data sets, bias in training data may extend to other patient factors not explicitly considered during treatment planning such as body mass index (BMI) or ethnicity. These biases in training data may be easy to predict and detect, similar to cases with less common organ-at-risk volumes, or may be hidden without careful thought. Bias may also present as patterns for a department, clinic, individual physician, or dosimetrist/planner. It is the responsibility of the development team to ensure that adequate data are used for training for all populations and subpopulations for which the algorithm will be used. Methods to interrogate algorithmic bias and stability are discussed in Section 6 of this chapter.

3. Technical Validation

The first validation step toward clinical deployment is to ensure the AI algorithm meets the specified performance based on technical parameters. This validation is performed by the technical development team, including computer scientists and medical physicists. Technical validation metrics will depend on the nature of the AI treatment planning algorithm. Common technical validation metrics (McIntosh *et al.*, 2021; McIntosh & Purdie, 2016) and their relevance to treatment planning are described as follows:

Dice Similarity Coefficient (DSC): The DSC is traditionally used to compare segmented anatomy on images i.e., from different contouring sources such as between physicians or between physician ground truth and an automated method. The DSC is

$$\mathrm{DSC} = 2|\mathrm{Union}\{\mathrm{A},\mathrm{B}\}|/(|\mathrm{A}|+|\mathrm{B}|)$$

The DSC compares the overlap between segmented volumes in which a score of 0% indicates no overlap and 100% indicates identical volumes.

The DSC is useful for evaluating treatment planning dose distribution comparing the binary mask of individual isodose line values between the ground truth dose distribution and the dose distribution generated using AI. DSC provides a simple metric that is straightforward to implement and evaluate but is limited in that it practically provides an independent evaluation of only discrete dose levels.

Gamma Index: The Gamma Index was developed and is traditionally used to evaluate the delivery of a radiation treatment plan to a dosimeter compared with the dose calculated by the treatment planning system, for example, in patient specific QA. The Gamma Index provides a composite quantity for the number of points measured passing or failing a defined criteria based on the percent dose deviation at each point and the distance from each point to achieve the same dose. Therefore, the index can be a useful metric to evaluate entire dose distributions generated in dose prediction and automated planning by replacing the discrete measurement points in the traditional implementation with the dose at each voxel in the dose distribution. The thresholds for evaluation of the Gamma Index in the case of voxel-based assessment are not well established and will vary depending on the use case. In addition, an appropriate cutoff dose below which the dose distribution is not used for analysis should be established to avoid biasing results to lower dose areas for which dose prediction algorithms will typically have learned large variations in low doses relative to the prescription dose.

Receiver Operating Characteristic (ROC) curve: The ROC curve is a graph that shows the performance of a classification model at all classification thresholds. This curve plots two parameters:

True Positive Rate (TPR), on the *y*-axis, which is a synonym for recall and is defined as

$$TPR = TP/(TP + FN)$$

False Positive Rate (FPR), on the *x*-axis, defined as

$$FPR = FP/(FP + TN)$$

where TP is True Positive, FP is False Positive, TN is True Negative, and FN is False Negative.

Area Under the ROC Curve (AUC): AUC is a measure of the two-dimensional area underneath the ROC curve. AUC provides an aggregate measure of performance across all possible classification thresholds. One way of interpreting AUC is as the probability that the model ranks a random positive example more highly than a random negative example. A perfect classifier has an AUC of 1.0, and a model with no discrimination capacity has an AUC of 0.5. AUC is scale-invariant; it measures how well predictions are ranked, rather than their absolute values. AUC is classification-threshold-invariant. It measures the quality of the model's predictions irrespective of what classification threshold is chosen. In radiation treatment planning, AUC is most helpful to investigate the clinical decisions and preferences for AI treatment planning methods.

In addition to the technical metrics above, to estimate model performance different validation strategies can be deployed depending on the size of the available data set and considerations about computational intensity (Fig. 2). The following approaches can be used as tools for performance estimation, model tuning, and parameter optimization:

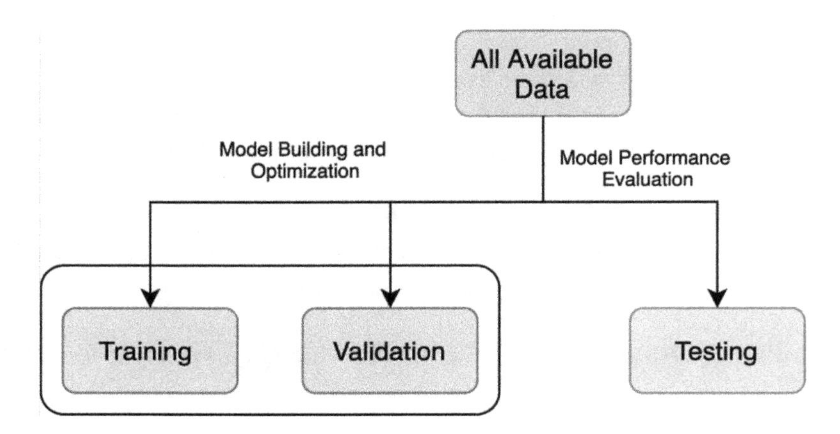

Fig. 2. Generalized data organization for model validation and testing. For holdout validation, the data set is split once, and the data do not change between training, validation, and testing. For cross-validation, data is randomly split in each group multiple times. In leave-one-out cross-validation, the number of splits is equal to the number of instances of data with each sample used for validation in each split.

Holdout set: The data set is split once; and data do not change between training, validation, and testing. This is the preferred method when computational resources are a consideration and a truly independent testing set that has never been used for training is desired. This approach can only be employed with large data sets and is useful when the testing set is intended to be fixed.

N-fold cross-validation: The data set is split multiple times to create multiple instances of training and testing data. This approach requires fewer overall data because there is no holdout data. Data are used for both training and testing, but not within the same instance. Cross-validation can provide confidence intervals and provides a more generalized understanding of model performance and evaluation.

Leave-one-out validation: The data set is split multiple times but is a special case of cross-validation, where the number of splits equals the number of instances in the data set. Thus, the learning algorithm is applied once for each instance, using all other instances as a training set and using the selected instance as a single-item test set.

Holdout is often used synonymously with validation with independent test sets, although there are crucial differences between splitting the data set randomly and designing a validation experiment for independent testing. Independent test sets can be used to measure performance that cannot be measured by resampling or holdout validation, for example performance for unknown future cases (cases that are acquired after the training is finished). This approach can provide information about the current performance of an existing model for new data. More generally, this may be described as measuring the extrapolation performance to define the limits of applicability.

A practical matter for implementing a holdout approach is that it is more straightforward to ensure that training and testing data are properly separated, compared with resampling validation in which data splitting and random assignment of cases is required. In addition, a common data set for testing has benefits for QA and re-training as discussed in Section 6 of this chapter.

4. Clinical Validation

The results of AI technology developed and tested in retrospective environments may not be realized in real-world clinical environments. The translation of AI to the clinic is often confounded by the separation between technical development and clinical implementation creating a disconnect between computer algorithms and clinical care. Retrospective or 'simulated' settings can overestimate impact and fail to account for real-world clinical factors and biases (McIntosh *et al.*, 2021). Employing an iterative, multidisciplinary feedback approach for clinical integration of AI technology is essential to ensure that the AI technology successfully reaches patient care. Direct integration and monitoring of human interaction with the AI technology provides quantitative clinical feedback metrics and may help with identification of barriers to clinical adoption (Elish, 2019).

Following rigorous technical validation, clinical validation is the next step toward clinical use. The purpose of the clinical validation step is to determine the fitness of the algorithm for clinical deployment and to monitor the impact of the AI on the clinical environment.

Quantitative metrics for clinical adoption should be based on those used in clinical treatment plan evaluation by dosimetrists/planners, radiation oncologists, and medical physicists (e.g., dose-volume constraints, treatment plan complexity metrics, quantitative measurements). However, clinical validation also must include qualitative evaluation by clinical experts based on their human experience and judgement (e.g., visual isodose inspection, appropriateness of the treatment plan given the patient's clinical history, evaluation of dose-volume features that may not be reflected in dose-volume histograms such as hotspot location). Evaluation of these judgement-based metrics is critical prior to clinical deployment to avoid surprises in AI treatment plan rejection rates and potential loss of trust in the approach by clinicians and the clinical team.

Retrospective or 'simulated' treatment plan review is the first step in clinical validation and is necessary to evaluate clinical expert judgement and fitness of the AI for clinical deployment (Fig. 3). The retrospective evaluation should be based on metrics directly used for clinical evaluation and measuring expert human judgement to provide a preliminary

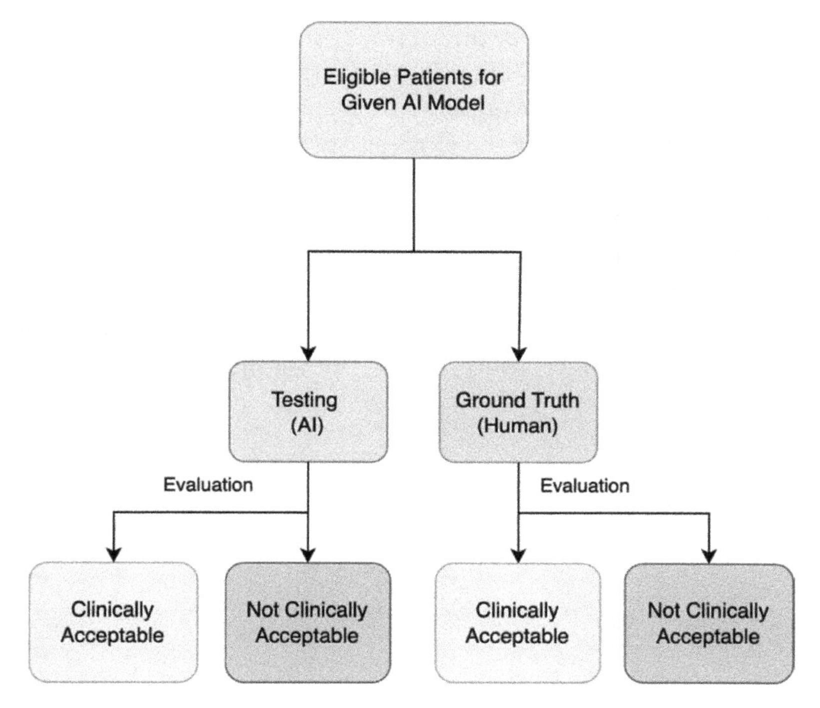

Fig. 3. Simplified framework for understanding baseline AI clinical acceptability against current clinical ground truth process, i.e., human-generated radiation therapy treatment plans.

understanding of the impact AI will have on the clinical environment. The results from retrospective evaluation should also be tempered by the fact that when deployed, clinical decision-making may be altered from the purely retrospective setting. Therefore, the retrospective evaluation provides the ceiling of clinical applicability for AI as the simulated environment has more control over the evaluation process and represents a more idealized evaluation setting that does not contend with clinical timelines, variation in clinical staff, peer-consultation, among other factors that are part of the normal course of clinical care that can influence the evaluation process and results.

There is evidence to suggest that there could be a disconnect between clinical utilization of AI between the retrospective and prospective settings (McIntosh *et al.*, 2021), highlighting that clinical validation must include a prospective component before clinical deployment. AI technology cannot be provided to clinical end users in a silo and needs to be integrated with the clinical workflow also requiring validation. Prospective clinical evaluation is a crucial and necessary step for clinical acceptance and safe deployment of AI in the clinic with various clinical evaluations based on the level of AI automation of the clinical AI deployment (Fig. 4).

Furthermore, just as a single clinician curating data to build an AI treatment planning model may not capture the clinical practice of the entire clinician group, the inclusion of many end users provides a more reliable mechanism for ensuring wide clinical applicability. A natural

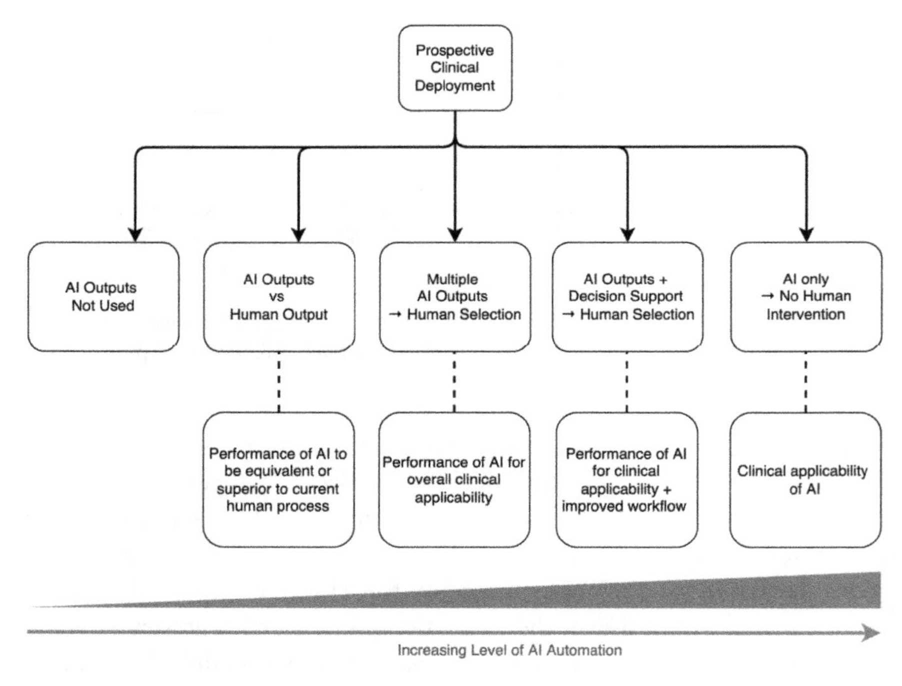

Fig. 4. Progressive automation of treatment planning process through prospective clinical AI deployment. There are various approaches to quantify the clinical applicability of AI for treatment planning depending on the level of rigor and goal of implementing AI for use. Although the ultimate goal may be a fully automated process, it should be recognized that fail-safe methods must exist when AI does not perform to a clinically acceptable level. Clearly, having human experts in the loop enables greater adoption, promotes a collaborative environment, and will provide a framework for getting buy-in and gaining trust at least initially.

extension of multiple end user evaluation is multi-institutional evaluation, although this requires considering higher levels of the implementation framework (Fig. 1) to ensure there is clear alignment with clinical practice guidelines regarding contouring, clinical objective of treatment, as well as harmony between data used for model building and the input data required to generate treatment plans.

5. Clinician Trust, AI Explainability, and Bias

In addition to technical and clinical testing, the successful integration of AI treatment planning requires refined understanding of end user perception, including dosimetrists/planners. physicians, medical physicists, and even patients. AI outputs are often difficult to interpret by clinicians and fail to provide sufficient information to the end user. It is difficult for end users to feel confident in AI predictions as AI algorithms often do not provide sufficient evidence for their outputs, resulting in end users lacking trust in AI and ultimately failing to adopt AI in routine clinical practice. Healthcare providers not only expect high accuracy from AI, but also expect AI to agree with their own views (including biases), even when, in practice, large inter-clinician variation exists (Challen *et al.*, 2019; Parikh *et al.*, 2019). With a well-defined problem, significant patient volumes, and tasks highly amenable to AI, radiation therapy treatment planning is an ideal space for prospective AI deployment to not only improve patient care, but to establish processes for clinical integration of AI around clinician adoption, bias, and real-world impact.

As in any healthcare application of AI, lack of explainability (e.g., "black-box" algorithms) of AI outputs are a major barrier to clinical adoption (Holzinger, 2018; Holzinger *et al.*, 2019). Although we rely on various technology and algorithms for the entire treatment planning process including image acquisition, segmentation, dose calculation, image visualization, dose statistics, etc., the outputs from AI algorithms are fundamentally different from these other algorithms as AI predictions are learned from historical data and end users are usually at arm's length from the data curation process on which the outputs are based. Furthermore, it may not be clear to end users how the training data are being used specifically for an individual patient.

In order to increase trust in the deployment and clinical implementation of AI, it is paramount that there is focus on training all relevant end users including dosimetrists/planners, radiation oncologists, and medical physics. While all end users need not understand all the technical details of an AI algorithm, trust increases when there is shared understanding of the clinical applicability of the algorithm, including scenarios in which it is expected or likely to fail (Cutillo *et al.*, 2020). Upfront design of interpretable AI, such as confidence in prediction scores, outlier flags, or heat maps, will improve transparency and end user trust in algorithms (Haibe-Kains *et al.*, 2020). Interpretable AI interfaces should be deployed using the same framework as the AI, and require significant end user (i.e. physician) input throughout the deployment process (Luo *et al.*, 2019).

One of the final considerations in the clinical deployment of AI for treatment planning to understand the clinical applicability of AI is to measure physician bias toward or against AI (Fig. 5). By including physician bias, a more fundamental evaluation of AI beyond more objective metrics can capture the perceptions of physician end-users and their clinical decisions impacting AI evaluation results and separate any algorithmic, data, or technical deficiencies of AI. Clearly, physician bias analysis is not a requirement for clinical deployment; however, in cases where a preliminary evaluation of AI is being undertaken, the ability to capture the entire decision-making process will enable differentiation between treatment plan quality based on objective measurements vs quality considering how treatment plans were generated (AI vs human).

The physician bias analysis captures variation in physicians' acceptability criteria and provides insight into clinical practice versus the established clinical protocols that are to be followed. This will ultimately provide data to support the requirement for further standardization, changes in clinical protocols, and potentially exposes true or perceived deficiencies in the AI treatment plans that have not been captured previously.

With the ultimate goal of improving treatment plan quality with AI, as with all facets of medicine, if there is a disconnect between AI treatment plans being technically or objectively superior to treatment plans used for patient treatment, in practice AI has failed. And the physician bias analysis can readily quantify this disconnect.

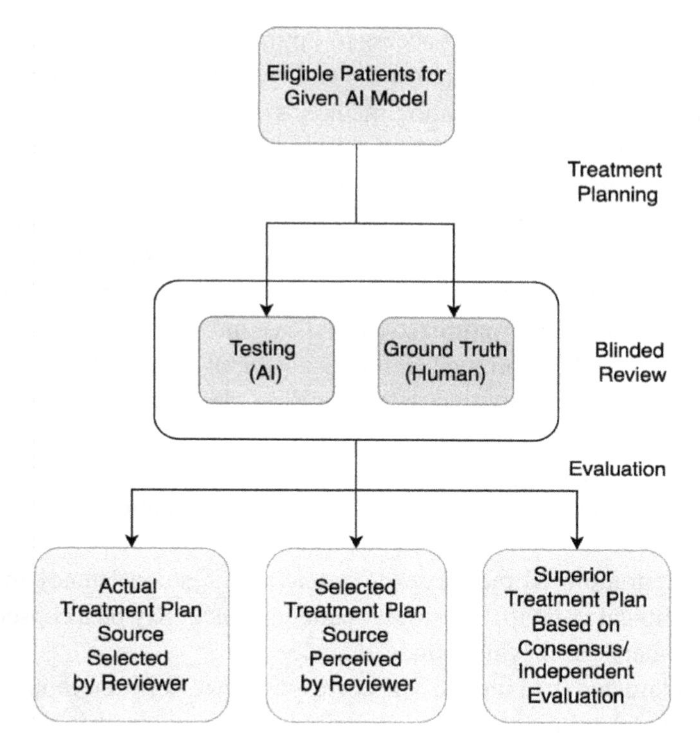

Fig. 5. Requirement in study design for understanding and evaluating bias toward or against AI. (1) providing a framework where the physician has access to simultaneously review both AI-generated and human-generated treatment plans in a blinded fashion. (2) The physicians' perception of the source of the treatment plan (AI vs human). (3) An independent evaluation of the actual superior treatment plan (including one or more of the following: quantitative metrics, group consensus review, independent review, etc.). This framework would enable quantification using AUC as described above.

6. Special Considerations for AI Treatment Planning Implementation

It is clear that AI introduces new challenges for workflow integration and clinical implementation from previous technology that has been deployed for radiation treatment planning. Radiation treatment planning and the technology to generate higher quality treatment plans is constantly becoming more automated and at the same time becoming more complex. There are parallels between AI and the introduction of optimization in treatment planning, however, even with access to optimization methods, the process is still highly manual and requires the end user to understand fundamental concepts of how the optimization method works even if they don't understand how their decisions are being used by the underlying mathematics of the optimization algorithm. With AI, the analogous manual work is done well before the end user is generating a treatment plan including algorithm development, data curation, and algorithm testing. The shift in the upstream manual effort for AI also highlights a fundamental difference between the clinical integration of optimization and AI into the clinical workflow. Optimization methods provide end users a general-purpose tool that can be applied to practically any treatment requiring planning. By contrast, AI is more rigid to end users, as the AI model is directly linked to specific treatment plan requirements. These clinical workflow factors introduce different considerations for downstream clinical implementation:

(1) Data curation: AI model development requires consistency in deciding clinical tradeoffs for similar patients which may be a consequence of human bias driving clinical decisions.
(2) Standardized data inputs: The correspondence between input data for AI model training and novel patients to be planned is paramount. Inconsistency in contouring practice, the inclusion/exclusion of delineated targets and organs, and including an essential organ that has not been used for training may render the model not appropriate for use (as described in Section 2)
(3) Stability Bias: For a given AI model, the training data is static but clinical practice is constantly changing over time, including different clinical teams with different acceptability preferences, major and minor updates to clinical protocols, and changes in equipment affecting the dose distributions presented to clinicians.
(4) AI model applicability: AI models are often specific for a particular clinical use case and therefore it is imperative to understand the limitation of the models (e.g., using an AI model trained on one dose-fractionation applied to treatment plan for a different dose-fractionation) may produce potentially deleterious outputs (as described in Section 7 that follows).

(5) Automation Bias: Physician preference for or against AI (as described in Section 4) enables a better understanding when AI failures are a result of model and algorithm limitations that can potentially be improved through data or better methodologies.

7. Quality Assurance, Re-Training, and Maintenance

Clinical best practice and workflows are constantly changing, which presents significant barriers to the deployment and long-term use of ML models in clinical medicine. Clinical treatment planning practice varies widely between institutions and can evolve rapidly, driven by advances in technology and clinical management.

As a result, the initial technical and clinical validation of an ML model prior to deployment must be continuously verified. Despite the historical importance of robust QA programs in Radiation Oncology, systematic methods for training, validation, and testing of ML treatment planning methods are not well established (Kalet *et al.*, 2020).

There should also be periodic testing of models against the original model to ensure the introduction of new data is not adversely affecting the results. This represents yet another fundamental difference between optimization methods and AI (as discussed in Section 5). The QA process for optimization algorithms is typically limited without formal analysis. The onus is placed on the end users to navigate the optimization space and build the necessary regions of interests needed for optimization, setting objectives and weights, and evaluating treatment plans between optimization iterations. In the case of AI, as models are built or re-trained a formal process is required to ensure models are emulating the intended clinical practice.

One of the fundamental steps in the QA process is to understand for cases which failed or provided inadequate clinical results the source of the failure. In cases that in fact conform to the protocol, the failure may indicate a limitation of the training data and the failed sample provides a useful source of new data for training. In other cases, the issue may be that the model does not actually apply or there is insufficient/missing data that is resulting in the failure. In this case, the sample may not apply to any current or future model.

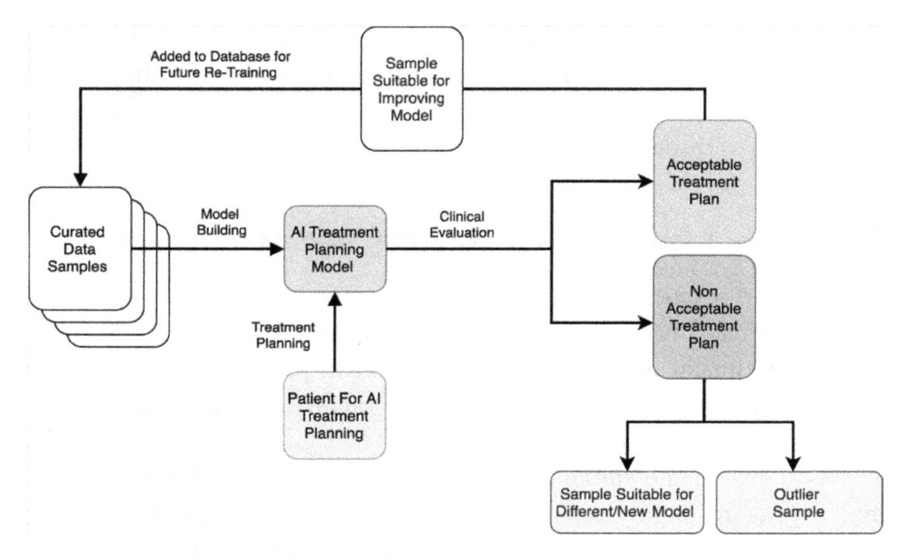

Fig. 6. General simplified framework for quality assurance (QA), model re-training, and maintenance. The above structure establishes treatment plans that will be useful for future model re-training and will enhance model performance. For treatment plans that are deemed to be clinically unacceptable or inferior to a treatment plan that was available for decision making, the sample may be used to build an entirely new model or may be an appropriate sample that is consistent with data used to supplement an existing model. In all cases, QA processes must be built to ensure data curation. There should also be interim analysis of samples as a function of time to understand if there are deviations in practice as changes in practice occur. The concept of removing older data is a solution (moving average).

There are several approaches to ensure maintenance of a given AI model for treatment planning. At the most fundamental level, adding data (Fig. 6) or removing data from a model should not decrease previous performance that has been accepted by the clinical team. Therefore, a common set of patients that represents the normal variation in clinical presentation should be retained for testing purposes over the lifetime of a model and which can be readily reviewed (preferably in head-to-head comparison) by multiple end users. Re-training has the potential to change the output for certain use cases while other use cases will be unchanged even from a quantitative point of view (e.g., evaluating dose-volume clinical criteria) and limits for changes must be established initially as a first evaluation. For example, it may be acceptable to have changes in treatment plans between models based on (1) dose-volume criteria limits that are less than a predefined percentage of the criteria value and (2) dose-volume limits that are still passing the clinical acceptability criteria. Furthermore, image-based metrics such the Gamma Index, Dice Similarity Coefficient of relevant isodose lines, or evaluation of entire dose-volume histogram curves can be compared and quantified. These will provide further technical metrics to understand differences between treatment plans pre and post model update. In cases where the re-trained model is different from the previous model based on the established criteria, further training would be required or reverting to the previous model.

The second level of model maintenance and QA evaluation should include clinical review to understand quality of treatment plans generated with an updated model that is not captured with quantitative metrics. Similar to the above evaluation, the same test set of patients can be used to ensure clinical treatment plan acceptability generated with the updated model.

One potential consideration for QA, maintenance, and re-training are changes in clinical practice that may occur over time and can be incorporated into the data used for model training. Changes to contouring practice, including changes to expansion margins for targets or differences in organ contouring practice could introduce undesirable variation in data that will generate an inferior model for re-training (Conroy *et al.*, 2021). Furthermore, including or excluding organs and/or targets can also have adverse effects on the quality of treatment plans for the new model. This is particularly a challenge for evaluation as the test set of treatment plans may not have these additional organs and/or targets even available for analysis.

8. Summary

There are numerous high-performing technical solutions for AI-based treatment planning; however, clinical use of these algorithms as standard-of-care in the clinic remains low. Challenges in real-world clinical use of AI-based treatment planning include applicability in the clinical setting, gaining clinician trust, workflow integration, and a lack of guidance on algorithm maintenance, testing, and re-training. Strategies must be developed and implemented into the routine clinical process to ensure the safe and effective use of AI for radiation treatment planning.

References

Challen, R., Denny, J., Pitt, M., Gompels, L., Edwards, T., & Tsaneva-Atanasova, K. (2019). Artificial intelligence, bias and clinical safety. *BMJ Quality & Safety*, *28*(3), 231–237. https://doi.org/10.1136/bmjqs-2018-008370.

Conroy, L., Khalifa, A., Berlin, A., McIntosh, C., & Purdie, T. G. (2021). Performance stability evaluation of atlas-based machine learning radiation therapy treatment planning in prostate cancer. *Physics in Medicine & Biology*, *66*(13), 134001. https://doi.org/10.1088/1361-6560/abfff0.

Cutillo, C. M., Sharma, K. R., Foschini, L., Kundu, S., Mackintosh, M., & Mandl, K. D. (2020). Machine intelligence in healthcare — perspectives on trustworthiness, explainability, usability, and transparency. *Npj Digital Medicine*, *3*(1), 47. https://doi.org/10.1038/s41746-020-0254-2.

Elish, M. C. (2019). Moral crumple zones: Cautionary tales in human-robot interaction. *Engaging Science, Technology, and Society*, *5*, 40. https://doi.org/10.17351/ests2019.260.

Gaube, S., Suresh, H., Raue, M., Merritt, A., Berkowitz, S. J., Lermer, E., Coughlin, J. F., Guttag, J. V., Colak, E., & Ghassemi, M. (2021). Do as AI say: Susceptibility in deployment of clinical decision-aids. *Npj Digital Medicine*, *4*(1), 31. https://doi.org/10.1038/s41746-021-00385-9.

Haibe-Kains, B., Adam, G. A., Hosny, A., Khodakarami, F., Waldron, L., Wang, B., McIntosh, C., Goldenberg, A., Kundaje, A., Greene, C. S., Broderick, T., Hoffman, M. M., Leek, J. T., Korthauer, K., Huber, W., Brazma, A., Pineau, J., Tibshirani, R., Hastie, T., … Aerts, H. J. W. L. (2020). Transparency and reproducibility in artificial intelligence. *Nature*, *586*(7829), E14–E16. https://doi.org/10.1038/s41586-020-2766-y.

He, J., Baxter, S. L., Xu, J., Xu, J., Zhou, X., & Zhang, K. (2019). The practical implementation of artificial intelligence technologies in medicine. *Nature Medicine*, *25*(1), 30–36. https://doi.org/10.1038/s41591-018-0307-0.

Hollon, T. C., Pandian, B., Adapa, A. R., Urias, E., Save, A. V., Khalsa, S. S. S., Eichberg, D. G., D'Amico, R. S., Farooq, Z. U., Lewis, S., Petridis, P. D., Marie, T., Shah, A. H., Garton, H. J. L., Maher, C. O., Heth, J. A., McKean, E. L., Sullivan, S. E., Hervey-Jumper, S. L., … Orringer, D. A. (2020). Near real-time intraoperative brain tumor diagnosis using stimulated Raman histology and deep neural networks. *Nature Medicine*, *26*(1), 52–58. https://doi.org/10.1038/s41591-019-0715-9.

Holzinger, A. (2018). From machine learning to explainable AI. *DISA 2018 — IEEE World Symposium on Digital Intelligence for Systems and Machines, Proceedings*, 55–66. https://doi.org/10.1109/DISA.2018.8490530.

Holzinger, A., Langs, G., Denk, H., Zatloukal, K., & Müller, H. (2019). Causability and explainability of artificial intelligence in medicine. *WIREs Data Mining and Knowledge Discovery*, *9*(4), 1–13. https://doi.org/10.1002/widm.1312.

Hong, J. C., Eclov, N. C. W., Dalal, N. H., Thomas, S. M., Stephens, S. J., Malicki, M., Shields, S., Cobb, A., Mowery, Y. M., Niedzwiecki, D., Tenenbaum, J. D., & Palta,

M. (2020). System for High-Intensity Evaluation During Radiation Therapy (SHIELD-RT): A prospective randomized study of machine learning–directed clinical evaluations during radiation and chemoradiation. *Journal of Clinical Oncology*, *38*(31), 3652–3661. https://doi.org/10.1200/JCO.20.01688.

Kalet, A. M., Luk, S. M. H., & Phillips, M. H. (2020). Radiation therapy quality assurance tasks and tools: The many roles of machine learning. *Medical Physics*, *47*(5), 1–10. https://doi.org/10.1002/mp.13445.

Luo, Y., Tseng, H.-H., Cui, S., Wei, L., Ten Haken, R. K., & El Naqa, I. (2019). Balancing accuracy and interpretability of machine learning approaches for radiation treatment outcomes modeling. *BJR|Open*, *1*(1), 20190021. https://doi.org/10.1259/bjro.20190021.

Mayo, C. S., Moran, J. M., Bosch, W., Xiao, Y., McNutt, T., Popple, R., Michalski, J., Feng, M., Marks, L. B., Fuller, C. D., Yorke, E., Palta, J., Gabriel, P. E., Molineu, A., Matuszak, M. M., Covington, E., Masi, K., Richardson, S. L., Ritter, T., ... Yock, T. I. (2018). American Association of Physicists in Medicine Task Group 263: Standardizing nomenclatures in radiation oncology. *International Journal of Radiation Oncology *Biology *Physics*, *100*(4), 1057–1066. https://doi.org/10.1016/j.ijrobp.2017.12.013.

McCarroll, R. E., Beadle, B. M., Balter, P. A., Burger, H., Cardenas, C. E., Dalvie, S., Followill, D. S., Kisling, K. D., Mejia, M., Naidoo, K., Nelson, C. L., Peterson, C. B., Vorster, K., Wetter, J., Zhang, L., Court, L. E., & Yang, J. (2018). Retrospective validation and clinical implementation of automated contouring of organs at risk in the head and neck: A step toward automated radiation treatment planning for low- and middle-income countries. *Journal of Global Oncology*, *4*, 1–11. https://doi.org/10.1200/jgo.18.00055.

McIntosh, C., Conroy, L., Tjong, M. C., Craig, T., Bayley, A., Catton, C., Gospodarowicz, M., Helou, J., Isfahanian, N., Kong, V., Lam, T., Raman, S., Warde, P., Chung, P., Berlin, A., & Purdie, T. G. (2021). Clinical integration of machine learning for curative-intent radiation treatment of patients with prostate cancer. *Nature Medicine*, *27*(6), 999–1005. https://doi.org/10.1038/s41591-021-01359-w.

McIntosh, C. & Purdie, T. G. (2016). Contextual atlas regression forests: Multiple-atlas-based automated dose prediction in radiation therapy. *IEEE Transactions on Medical Imaging*, *35*(4), 1000–1012. https://doi.org/10.1109/TMI.2015.2505188.

Nimri, R., Battelino, T., Laffel, L. M., Slover, R. H., Schatz, D., Weinzimer, S. A., Dovc, K., Danne, T., & Phillip, M. (2020). Insulin dose optimization using an automated artificial intelligence-based decision support system in youths with type 1 diabetes. *Nature Medicine*, *26*(9), 1380–1384. https://doi.org/10.1038/s41591-020-1045-7.

Obermeyer, Z., Powers, B., Vogeli, C., & Mullainathan, S. (2019). Dissecting racial bias in an algorithm used to manage the health of populations. *Science*, *366*(6464), 447–453. https://doi.org/10.1126/science.aax2342.

Parikh, R. B., Teeple, S., & Navathe, A. S. (2019). Addressing bias in artificial intelligence in health care. *JAMA*, *322*(24), 2377. https://doi.org/10.1001/jama.2019.18058.

Saria, S. & Subbaswamy, A. (2019). *Tutorial: Safe and Reliable Machine Learning*. arXiv, abs/1904.07204.

Shah, N. H., Milstein, A., & Bagley, PhD, S. C. (2019). Making machine learning models clinically useful. *JAMA*, *322*(14), 1351. https://doi.org/10.1001/jama.2019.10306.

Tonekaboni, S., Joshi, S., McCradden, M. D., Goldenberg, A., & Ai, A. G. (2019). What clinicians want: Contextualizing explainable machine learning for clinical end use. In F. Doshi-Velez, J. Fackler, K. Jung, D. Kale, R. Ranganath, B. Wallace, & J. Wiens (Eds.), *Proceedings of the 4th Machine Learning for Healthcare Conference* (Vol. 106, pp. 359–380). PMLR.

Topol, E. J. (2019). High-performance medicine: The convergence of human and artificial intelligence. *Nature Medicine*, *25*(1), 44–56. https://doi.org/10.1038/s41591-018-0300-7.

Wiens, J., Saria, S., Sendak, M., Ghassemi, M., Liu, V. X., Doshi-Velez, F., Jung, K., Heller, K., Kale, D., Saeed, M., Ossorio, P. N., Thadaney-Israni, S., & Goldenberg, A. (2019). Do no harm: A roadmap for responsible machine learning for health care. *Nature Medicine*, *25*(9), 1337–1340. https://doi.org/10.1038/s41591-019-0548-6.

Wijnberge, M., Geerts, B. F., Hol, L., Lemmers, N., Mulder, M. P., Berge, P., Schenk, J., Terwindt, L. E., Hollmann, M. W., Vlaar, A. P., & Veelo, D. P. (2020). Effect of a machine learning-derived early warning system for intraoperative hypotension vs standard care on depth and duration of intraoperative hypotension during elective noncardiac surgery: The HYPE randomized clinical trial. *JAMA — Journal of the American Medical Association*, *323*(11), 1052–1060. https://doi.org/10.1001/jama.2020.0592.

Chapter 12

Using AI to Predict Radiotherapy Toxicity Risk Based on Patient Germline Genotyping

Jung Hun Oh, Sangkyu Lee, Maria Thor and Joseph O. Deasy

Department of Medical Physics, Memorial Sloan Kettering Cancer Center, New York NY, USA

Abstract

The collateral irradiation of normal tissues can result in damage that reduces the quality of life for cancer survivors. The variability of toxicity risk has been increasingly recognized as multifactorial, involving patient-specific genetics, dose-volume levels, and other risk factors. The association between genetics and radiotherapy (RT)-induced toxicity, referred to as radiogenomics, has received increasing attention. Traditional statistical analyses have mainly focused on testing the effect of individual genetic variants without considering non-linear interactions of variants. We have shown that artificial intelligence (AI) methods, including machine learning approaches, can efficiently leverage large-scale genetic variants (e.g., single nucleotide polymorphisms [SNPs]), taking into account the complex interactions among genetic markers. In addition, novel post-modeling analyses, employing bioinformatics network techniques, can identify key genes associated with tissue-specific toxicity. The next challenge of genetic prediction models will be to integrate genetic and RT dose-volume factors. Such models have the potential to identify patients at high risk for the development of toxicity and thus offer individualized risk-specific treatment planning. In this chapter, we review results for multiple endpoints yielding usable stratifications of odds ratios for a significant fraction of patients treated with RT. Progress in radiogenomics has been slow primarily due to a lack of data sets and other analytical obstacles. We discuss these issues that need to be addressed when handling genome-wide variants. We conclude by looking to a future when germline genomics is combined with RT dose-volume factors to personalize RT-induced toxicity risk.

1. Introduction

Many normal tissue complication probability (NTCP) models have been developed to predict symptomatic radiotherapy (RT)-induced complications with the ultimate goal to guide individualized risk-specific RT treatment planning (Marks *et al.*, 2010). Risk factors for RT-induced toxicity are multifactorial including RT dose, co-morbidities, as well as genetic factors (Kerns *et al.*, 2015). Researchers have explored associations between the risk of RT-induced toxicity and germline genetic variants at a genome-wide level to identify plausible biomarkers and better understand patient-specific radiosensitivity (West *et al.*, 2014). The establishment of the Radiogenomics Consortium (RGC) in 2009 accelerated the field of research (West & Rosenstein, 2010; West *et al.*, 2010). The radiogenomics study is grounded in the fact that differences in phenotypes or traits are in part attributed to individual genetic variations. The term radiogenomics is here used to refer to studies of genetic variation vs. RT toxicity. (Note: a different use of the term 'radiogenomics' refers to the relationship between tumor image characteristics and genomic characteristics.)

The healing process following radiation damage to normal tissues is complicated, involving coordinated processes at different scales of molecular processing and inter-cellular processing, and is dependent on the tissue type and other characteristics of the host (Denham & Hauer-Jensen,

2002). Like other complex phenotypes or traits, the radiation response is expected to be dependent on many genetic variants with mostly small effects (Sun *et al.*, 2021; Yang *et al.*, 2010). It is not surprising that methods searching for single genetic variants with large effects have mostly been unproductive. Even though some causal variants have been identified, they apply only to a modest fraction of the population with the given alleles (Kerns *et al.*, 2020). Our hypothesis, confirmed in multiple studies, is that robust predictive models can be constructed by layering on small effects from many (dozens or even hundreds) of genetic variants in different genomic regions. In particular, we focus on common genetic variants (single nucleotide polymorphisms [SNPs]) carried in the germline as opposed to infrequent, rare variants (Pitter *et al.*, 2021). A successful model need not be restricted to causal genetic factors only; success can be achieved if the overall predictions are validated and accurate, leading to clinically usable odds ratios (>2 between the safest 1/3 of patients and the riskiest 1/3 of patients treated in a conventional manner). Machine learning/artificial intelligence (AI) is well-suited to this task. Moreover, the resulting models can be interpreted using bioinformatics network approaches, as we will discuss, identifying key biomarkers.

In this chapter, we review the application of AI to predictive modeling on large-scale genetic variants and further propose to employ such modeling methods in radiogenomics studies, investigating incorporated genetic variants and dose-volume factors to stratify patients for the development of RT-induced toxicity, potentially aiming to guide treatment planning.

2. Machine Learning Approaches to GWAS

A typical genome-wide association studies (GWAS) analysis investigates common variants across the whole genome collected from a number of individuals and the statistical relationship with a target trait or phenotype. There are two main approaches used in GWAS analysis: statistical analysis and machine learning. In this section, we first sketch the statistical analysis approach followed by machine learning-based modeling methods that have been used in GWAS.

2.1. *Statistical analysis approaches*

Traditional statistical analysis is often carried out to identify genetic susceptibility loci strongly associated with a trait or phenotype. The statistical power of a given SNP association depends on the frequency of occurrence in the population, the effect size, and the number of endpoint events. To compute the individual significance of each SNP, univariate single SNP-trait association analysis is performed using chi-square test or regression analysis. Clinical variables known as high-risk predictors can be added in the univariate regression analysis to adjust the *p*-values of individual SNPs. The degree of association is represented by a so-called Manhattan or QQ (quantile–quantile) plot. In general, most putative risk loci have small effect sizes (odds ratio <1.5) (Hindorff *et al.*, 2009). In statistical analysis approaches, a power calculation can be made before GWAS to compute the effect sample size to achieve sufficient statistical power while minimizing false negative and false positive findings (Hong & Park, 2012). In the following, the considerations in GWAS analysis are described.

2.1.1. *Multiple hypothesis correction*

Multiple hypothesis testing is a major issue in GWAS due to the large number of SNPs tested simultaneously. The Bonferroni correction method and permutation testing are common approaches for dealing with this issue (Hendricks *et al.*, 2014). A permutation test, wherein endpoint values are randomly re-assigned among samples to judge the likelihood of a random correlation, is a general technique to control a type-I error (false positive significance). However, permutation testing is computationally expensive for high-throughput data. The Bonferroni correction, in contrast, simply adjusts the standard *p*-value threshold under the assumption that multiple tests are statistically independent. The Bonferroni correction is widely used in GWAS, but it is overly conservative. Bonferroni analysis may result in the overcorrection of single SNP associations due to non-independent SNPs that are partially correlated due to linkage disequilibrium (LD) across the genome (Kang *et al.*, 2018). This situation is further exacerbated when genotyping data are imputed, which increases the number of SNPs within LD blocks (Bohmanova *et al.*, 2010).

2.1.2. *Population structure correction*

Population stratification is a key concern in GWAS, which arises when systematic genetic differences in allele frequencies exist in a study population, leading to inflated false positive and false negative error rates (Hellwege *et al.*, 2017; Naret *et al.*, 2018). Therefore, correction for population stratification is important prior to association tests. Typically, a few principal components that describe the genetic structure of the cohort are used in regression modeling as covariates, which results in corrected univariate association *p*-values (Price *et al.*, 2006).

2.1.3. *Genotype imputation*

Current GWAS arrays typically produce a million genotypes per blood sample. Yet, the number of SNPs in the full genome is much larger. To improve genome coverage and increase the power of potential higher associations, genotype imputation is widely used, which results in more than 10 million additional un-genotyped SNPs utilizing common population references (Malhotra *et al.*, 2014; Marchini & Howie, 2010; Pei *et al.*, 2010). Although genotype imputation is a powerful tool to boost statistical power in an association analysis, it further increases the challenge of *p*-value corrections as described above (Schurz *et al.*, 2019). Imputation also facilitates meta-analysis across multiple studies where different GWAS arrays are used. After imputation, quality control for imputed variants is important. This includes the removal of SNPs with low imputation accuracy (e.g., $R2 < 0.3$), as well as the removal of SNPs that do not appear often in the population, referred to as a low minor allele frequency (MAF). A cutoff of ignoring SNPs with an MAF of less than 5% is common. The PLINK software tool is useful for the processing of GWAS data, including quality filtering and computationally efficient significance tests (Purcell *et al.*, 2007). Two imputation servers are publicly available: the TOPMed Imputation Server (https://imputation.biodatacatalyst.nhlbi.nih.

gov) and the Michigan Imputation Server (https://imputationserver.sph.umich.edu); both provide a user-friendly interface for genotype imputation, and both use the Minimac4 algorithm for genotype imputation (Das *et al.*, 2016).

2.1.4. *Fine mapping*

The group of SNPs that capture the local genomic allelic variations are called 'tag SNPs'. Hence, tag SNPs can be used to reconstruct the rest of non-tag SNPs (Hyten *et al.*, 2007; Ilhan & Tezel, 2013). It is important to note that significant SNPs identified from GWAS are not necessarily causal to the phenotype of interest, but are rather correlated to true causal SNPs due to the genomic LD structure (Stram, 2004). Thus, GWAS is typically followed by the post-GWAS processing to search for causal SNPs, referred to as 'fine mapping' (Spain & Barrett, 2015), based on the tag SNPs and genomic structure that surrounds the tag SNPs. This can be heuristically conducted by examining the GWAS signals from the SNPs within the same region of statistically correlated SNPs with the tag SNP in LD, using a software tool such as Haploview (Barrett, 2009). The two main quantitative approaches for fine mapping are penalized regression and Bayesian methods, both of which can be used to jointly analyze the SNPs in the vicinity of the tag SNPs and either result in a smaller set of putative causal SNPs (penalized regression) or posterior probability of causal SNPs (Bayesian method). More details on these approaches can be found in a review paper by Schaid *et al.* (Schaid *et al.*, 2018).

2.2. *Machine learning approaches*

2.2.1. *Selecting genomic features as inputs to model building*

While statistical approaches seek a high degree of confidence that identified SNPs are at least statistically related to the endpoint in the patient population, machine learning modeling can take an unbiased and integrative approach to build predictive models. The use of machine learning methods allows for a de-emphasis on SNP identification with a gain in ability to build more robust predictive models. However, the large number of SNPs requires feature reduction. Fortunately, a univariate approach that identifies a large, but not too large, number of SNPs as inputs to model building is a practical approach.

2.2.2. *Validating machine learning models*

Universal agreement on the best approach to model validation is elusive. Most studies set aside data for a final test of a model. This can either be a second data set, not mixed with data for the model building, or a fraction of the original data set that is randomly sampled to form a separate data set. Due to the decreased need for data when the model is fixed, less data are used for validation in general. A split of 70/30 is a common method. Within the 70% of data for model building, it is common to repeatedly split the data into similar training/testing cohorts. Most machine learning algorithms have parameters that need to be fixed for the model to be applied; these are called 'hyper-parameters'. The model building process then consists of multiple shuffles of the data to create training/testing splits. The hyper-parameters are gradually modified or locked in based on the testing cohort results. Drilling further into the use of the training/testing strategy, common practice is to use cross-validation to estimate performance. In the so-called k-fold cross-validation, data are split into k sub-groups with equal size (Koul *et al.*, 2018). In each iteration, the samples in the k–1 folds are used for model fitting, and the remaining samples are used to estimate model performance, repeating the process for each fold. In particular, when the number of samples in the data is small, leave-one-out cross-validation can be used with $k = n$ (number of samples) (Cheng *et al.*, 2017). Bootstrapping is another resampling method such that the training samples are randomly selected from the whole data with replacement, and the samples that do not belong to the training data are used for testing.

2.2.3. *Methods for developing prediction signatures from GWAS*

Several machine learning methods have been proposed for GWAS to develop predictive multi-SNP models, which we review.

2.2.3.1. Support vector machines

Wei *et al.* (2009) employed a support vector machine (SVM) method for predicting disease risk for type 1 diabetes, using a GWAS data set and validating the model on an independent data set, wherein both resulted in an area under the curve (AUC) of about 0.84 (Wei *et al.*, 2009). Kim *et al.* (2013) proposed a prediction method for GWAS, consisting of two steps: (a) a MAX test, based on the maximum of three trend test statistics derived for recessive, additive, and dominant models, was employed to identify genetic models of each SNP and (b) a final predictive model was built employing penalized SVMs on the SNPs (Kim *et al.*, 2013). Mittag *et al.* (2012) conducted GWAS analyses for seven diseases from the Wellcome Trust Case-Control Consortium (WTCCC), employing several machine learning methods, and found that predictive power of machine learning methods was similar, therefore suggesting simple models for GWAS such as linear SVMs for better model interpretation (Mittag *et al.*, 2015).

2.2.3.2. Penalized logistic regression

In another study, Wei *et al.* (2013) adopted penalized logistic regression with an L1 penalty to build a predictive model of inflammatory bowel disease. Due to the desirable nature of L1 regularized models, redundant SNPs with high correlations, in particular within LD, are likely to be filtered out while fitting a predictive model (Wei *et al.*, 2013). Thus, this approach has the advantage of performing feature selection and predictive modeling, simultaneously. For this reason, penalized logistic regression is an attractive approach as a filtering step prior to applying other machine learning methods. In addition, the estimation of effect sizes for SNPs as assessed from L1 coefficient values quantifies individual SNP contributions. Yang *et al.* (2020) introduced a permutation-assisted tuning procedure for the selection of the L1 LASSO (least absolute shrinkage and selection operator) tuning parameter in a joint multiple-SNP regression model to identify phenotype-associated SNPs (Yang *et al.*, 2020). More recently, Nouira and Azencott (2022) developed a multitask group LASSO method, MuGLasso, for the multivariate analysis of multi-population

GWAS data (Nouira & Azencott, 2022). In this method, feature selection was conducted at the level of LD-groups with each task corresponding to a subpopulation.

2.2.3.3. Random forest models

Random forest is the most extensively used machine learning method in GWAS (Botta *et al.*, 2014; Cosgun *et al.*, 2011; Nguyen *et al.*, 2015; Oh *et al.*, 2017), being well-suited to unbiased model building with many possible predictors and non-linear interactions. The random forest algorithm is an ensemble method that builds a group of decision trees for each application (Denisko & Hoffman, 2018). There are two random selection processes at work in random forest construction. Each tree, consisting of decision nodes based on single variables, is constructed using bootstrapped data randomly sampled with replacement, having the same number of samples as the original data. For the random process in feature selection, a random subset of features is selected at each node split, and the SNP feature that yields the lowest mean squared error is chosen. By building up a 'forest' of such decision trees, the model yields unbiased estimate despite the fact that any individual tree overfits to the randomly sampled data. Correspondingly, individual SNPs and decision trees do not dominate the prediction result. Nguyen *et al.* (2015) proposed a two-stage random forest approach for GWAS (Nguyen *et al.*, 2015). In the first step, the importance scores of SNPs were computed and p-values were assessed against the maximum important score of injected SNPs, resulting in the identification of informative vs. irrelevant SNPs. Only informative SNPs were then used during random forest modeling. Botta *et al.* (2014) proposed a tree-based ensemble method, called T-Trees, designed to consider the correlation structure observed in LD across genome-wide variants, which replaced the univariate linear split functions by multivariate non-linear split functions on several SNPs located in the same block (Botta *et al.*, 2014). Cosgun *et al.* (2011) tested several machine learning methods, including random forest regression, boosted regression tree, and support vector regression, to build a predictive model of warfarin maintenance dose for African Americans, using GWAS data (Cosgun *et al.*, 2011).

In various warfarin dose-response tests, random forest regression with 200 SNPs achieved the best accuracy.

2.2.3.4. Deep learning

Multiple deep learning approaches have recently been developed for GWAS analysis and prediction. Mieth *et al.* (2021) introduced a deep learning-based approach, called DeepCOMBI, to identify SNP-phenotype associations in GWAS (Mieth *et al.*, 2021). In this modeling approach, a layer-wise relevance propagation (LRP) method was adopted to compute SNP relevance scores and only a set of SNPs that were selected based on the relevance scores were tested for statistical associations (Bach *et al.*, 2015). Sun *et al.* (2020) proposed a multi-hidden-layer Cox-based survival model employing a feedforward deep neural network (DNN) where the last output layer produces a prognostic index (Sun *et al.*, 2020). Arloth *et al.* (2020) presented a deep learning model, called DeepWAS, which can identify potential disease/trait-associated SNPs (Arloth *et al.*, 2020).

2.2.3.5. Network analysis

The basic premise of using networks to represent biological networks is that the genes or loci that are functionally correlated (via gene–gene interaction, pathways, or expression quantitative trait loci [eQTL]) are more likely to have joint causal effects (Oti & Brunner, 2007). Azencott *et al.* (2013) proposed a network-based approach, called SConES, to identify sets of genetic loci that are likely associated with a phenotype based on an underlying network, employing a minimum cut reformulation (Azencott *et al.*, 2013). In their study, three network types were proposed: (a) a genomic sequence network wherein SNPs adjacent on the genome sequence are connected, (b) a gene membership network wherein SNPs near the same gene are connected, and (c) a gene interaction network wherein SNPs belonging to two genes connected in a gene–gene interaction network are linked together. Table 1 summarizes the various machine learning methods applied to GWAS.

Table 1. Machine learning methods used in GWAS.

Method	Algorithm	Disease/Trait	Reference
SVM		Type 1 diabetes	(Wei *et al.*, 2009)
SVM		Chronic myelogenous leukemia	(Kim *et al.*, 2013)
SVM		WTCCC	(Mittag *et al.*, 2015)
LASSO		Inflammatory bowel disease	(Wei *et al.*, 2013)
LASSO		Cardiovascular disease	(S. Yang *et al.*, 2020)
LASSO	MuGLasso	Breast cancer	(Nouira & Azencott, 2022)
RF		Warfarin dose	(Cosgun *et al.*, 2011)
RF	T-Trees	WTCCC	(Botta *et al.*, 2014)
RF	ts-RF	Parkinson and Alzheimer diseases	(Nguyen *et al.*, 2015)
RF	PRFR	Radiotherapy toxicity in prostate cancer	(Oh *et al.*, 2017)
DL		Age-related macular degeneration	(T. Sun *et al.*, 2020)
DL	DeepWAS	Multiple sclerosis, major depressive disorder, height	(Arloth *et al.*, 2020)
DL	DeepCOMBI	WTCCC	(Mieth *et al.*, 2021)
Network	SConES	Arabidopsis flowering time phenotypes	(Azencott *et al.*, 2013)

Note: WTCCC: Wellcome Trust Case Control Consortium; SVM: support vector machine; LASSO: least absolute shrinkage and selection operator; RF: random forest; DL: deep learning.

2.3. *A hybrid method of machine learning and statistical analysis*

Oh *et al.* (2017) proposed a hybrid method that integrates statistical analysis with machine learning (Oh *et al.*, 2017) in GWAS, referred to as pre-conditioned random forest regression (PRFR). First, before the modeling, SNPs with univariate p-values >0.001 for a target endpoint are omitted, making the problem tractable. This p-value threshold is modest in comparison with the genome-wide significance level (often, 5×10^{-8}) and was chosen to decrease the large number of SNPs to a reasonably manageable number (500–2000), but with as many potential biomarkers as possible. The machine learning phase starts with a step called pre-conditioning to account for the broad population structure. The result is an alteration of the observed outcomes to 'pre-conditioned' outcomes that are meant to incorporate more information about each patient. This is performed using supervised principal component analysis (SPCA): principal components (PCs) are computed using highly ranked SNPs (a few hundred) in association with the original binary outcomes on training data. The resultant few PCs are weighted within logistic regression, resulting in the adjusted 'pre-conditioned outcomes' that are used in random forest regression modeling. The idea is to make the outcomes more informative by changing the binary outcome to something more like an expected average outcome. The approach PRFR has demonstrated superior predictive performance over other alternative methods in several GWAS of cancer treatment-associated outcomes, including late rectal bleeding (Oh *et al.*, 2017), erectile dysfunction (Oh *et al.*, 2017), genitourinary toxicity (Lee *et al.*, 2018) in prostate cancer, breast cancer treatment-induced fatigue (Lee *et al.*, 2020), and RT-associated induction of contralateral breast cancer (Lee *et al.*, 2020).

Figure 1 illustrates the performance comparison of PRFR with alternative methods for rectal bleeding, erectile dysfunction, and genitourinary toxicity (weak stream) in prostate cancer. For all endpoints, PRFR achieved the highest performance and smallest standard deviation, suggesting its reliability. Note that all models were tested against set-aside validation data (not used in the modeling). Patients were sorted based on the predicted outcomes and binned into six groups with one being the lowest risk group and 6 being the highest risk group. As shown in Fig. 2, for all endpoints, the comparison between the predicted and observed incidences had a good level of agreement and showed promising odds ratios.

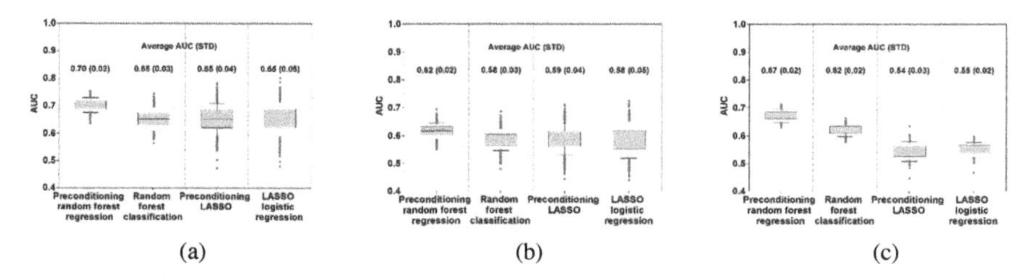

Fig. 1. Performance comparison of PRFR (pre-conditioned random forest regression) with alternative methods on the set-aside validation data for (a) rectal bleeding, (b) erectile dysfunction, and (c) genitourinary toxicity (weak stream) in prostate cancer patients. STD: standard deviation; AUC: area under the curve; LASSO: least absolute shrinkage and selection operator. Reprinted from Oh *et al.* (2017) with permission.

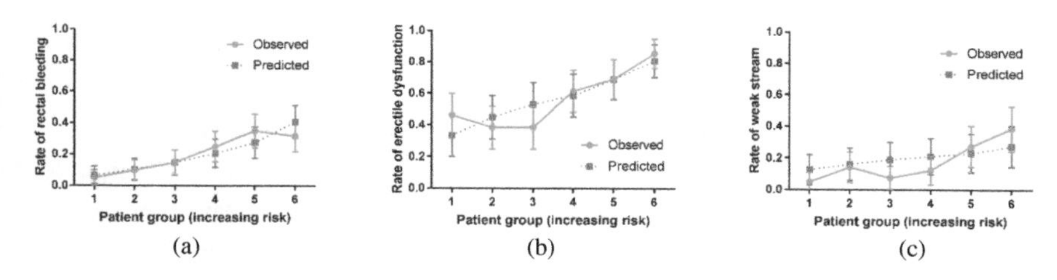

Fig. 2. Comparisons of the predicted and actual incidence rates for (a) rectal bleeding, (b) erectile dysfunction, and (c) genitourinary toxicity (weak stream) on the validation data set. The error bar indicates the standard error. Reprinted from Oh *et al.* (2017) with permission.

2.4. *Integration of dose-volume and genetic factors into NTCP models*

To better guide RT treatment planning, the development of accurate NTCP predictive models is vital, using complementary information from genetic risk factors in addition to RT dose. A few studies have proposed methods that incorporate the effect of SNPs as dose modifying factors (DMFs) in NTCP models (Coates *et al.*, 2015; Tucker *et al.*, 2013). Incorporating information about SNPs into a predictive model adjusts the effect of RT dose and the combined information is likely to yield better predictive power. Coates *et al.* (2015) proposed a method that integrates genetic variations into a Lyman–Kutcher–Burman (LKB) NTCP model as a DMF to build predictive models of RT-induced rectal bleeding and erectile dysfunction in prostate cancer, using copy number variation (CNV) and the SNP rs5489 in the *XRCC1* gene (Coates *et al.*, 2015). The integrated model led to increased cross-validated predictive power. Tucker *et al.* (2013) developed a predictive model for radiation pneumonitis in lung cancer, incorporating 16 SNPs from 10 genes (*XRCC1, XRCC3, APEX1, MDM2, TGFβ, TNFα, TNFR, MTHFR, MTRR,* and *VEGF*) in an LKB model as DMFs, demonstrating that SNPs significantly improved the LKB model (Tucker *et al.*, 2013). Note that these studies analyzed only a small number of selected SNPs, and in some cases it is not clear if they were selected from a larger number of SNPs. Clearly, the integration of many SNPs (hundreds or thousands) and RT dose in machine learning-based methods remains underexplored.

In multi-omic predictive modeling, it is important to consider the different nature of genomic data and conventional dosimetric or clinical data. Genomic data are much higher dimensional, which means that much more genomic features can be identified as significant by random chance. Moreover, clinical and dosimetric variables are often curated based on previous studies or mechanistic understanding of the endpoint. Therefore, rather than merely integrating RT dose into genetic modeling, a more sophisticated approach may be needed to assess the effect of genetics in combination with RT dose. For example, the predictive power represented by an odds ratio in a genetic machine learning model could be added into an existing RT dose-volume model, which would allow for assessing the effect size of integrated genetic factors. Figure 3 illustrates a general workflow in building a dose-volume-genetic predictive model.

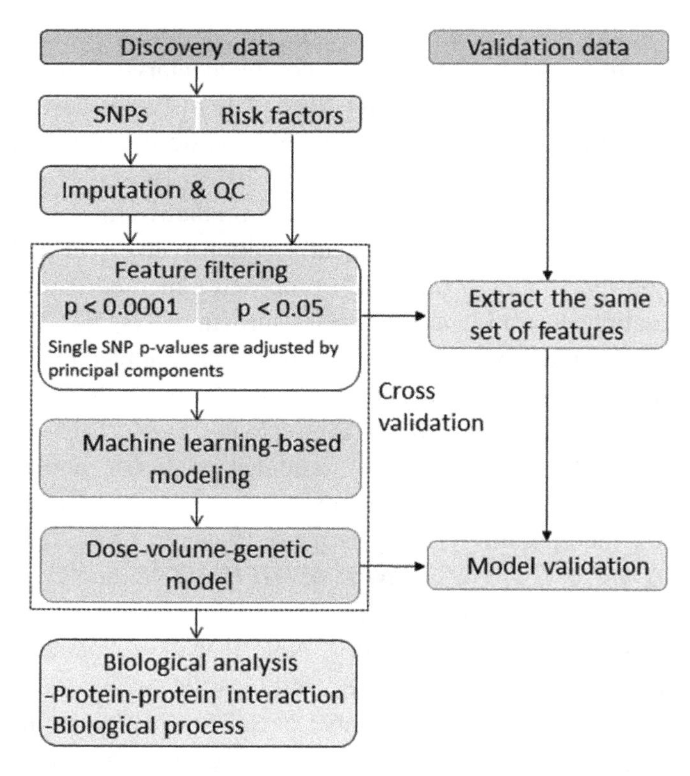

Fig. 3. A general workflow for building dose-volume-genetic predictive models.

3. The Identification of Biological Correlates Associated with Toxicity: A Key Advantage of Machine Learning Signatures in GWAS

After predictive modeling, the functional annotation of key SNPs exploiting bioinformatics techniques is essential to gain insights into biologic functions associated with RT-induced toxicities (Lee *et al.*, 2018, 2020; Oh *et al.*, 2017). For biological analysis at a gene level, SNPs should be mapped to the genes that are putatively causal to the phenotype of interest. There are two major methods for SNP-gene mapping. First, SNPs can be assigned to genes based on physical proximity within the genome. However, there is no clear threshold for the proximity, possibly introducing false-positive mapping. In another approach, SNPs are mapped to genes using tissue-specific eQTL effects. An eQTL is a region that has been identified as driving the genetic variation in gene expression patterns, and eQTL SNPs are often overrepresented in regulatory regions (Fagny *et al.*, 2017; Miller *et al.*, 2015). A disadvantage of this approach is that not all eQTL effects have been investigated. Once a list of genes for the key SNPs has been identified, gene ontology or protein–protein interaction analysis can be performed to recognize key biological processes in which the genes act together, which characterizes the functional effects of SNPs. To this end, enrichment analysis can be conducted to test the statistical significance of the enrichment of a group of genes or ontology. The resultant enrichment p-values indicate the significance of those biological processes identified in association with RT-induced toxicity. Several databases provide gene ontology analysis tools, including AmiGO 2 (http://amigo.geneontology.org/amigo), DAVID (https://david.ncifcrf.gov/), and the commercial database MetaCore (https://portal.genego.com/). Lamparter *et al.* (2016) presented a powerful tool, called Pathway scoring algorithm (Pascal), to compute gene and pathway scores from GWAS association summary statistics (Lamparter, Marbach, Rueedi, Kutalik, & Bergmann, 2016). This tool enables the identification of key pathways associated with phenotypes in the lack of genotype data.

In the following, we sketch the biological analysis after machine learning-based modeling on GWAS. In a bioinformatic analysis after PRFR modeling, Oh *et al.* (2017) identified ion transport activity as a key

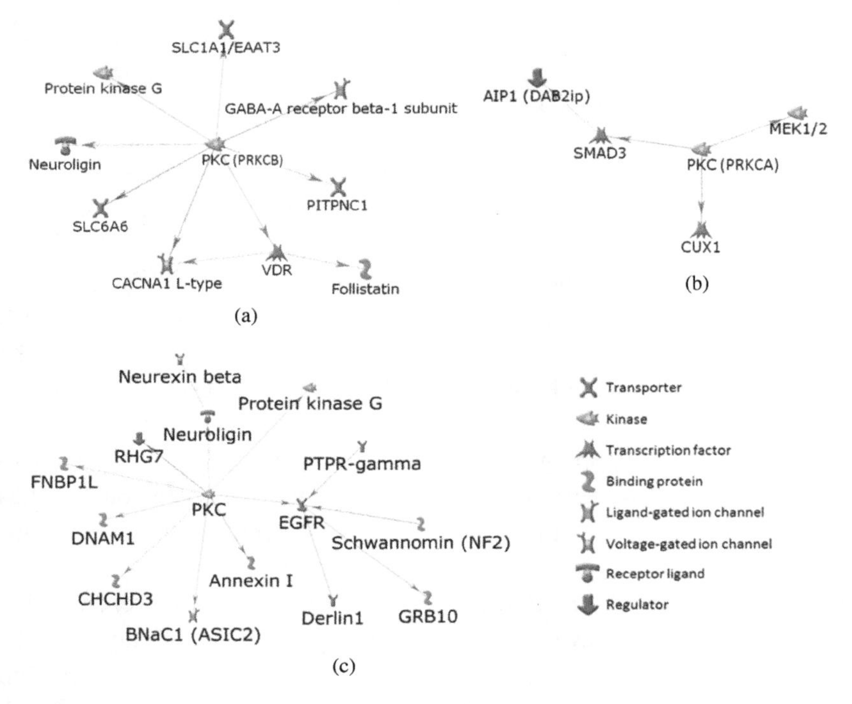

Fig. 4. Post-model bioinformatics analyses to identify key protein–protein interaction networks based on information derived from random forest modeling for (a) rectal bleeding, (b) erectile dysfunction, and (c) genitourinary toxicity (weak stream). Connections indicate known interactions. For all three endpoints, some of the interacting genes have previously been identified as relevant to the endpoint. Reprinted from (Oh *et al.* (2017) and (Lee *et al.* (2018) with permission.

biological process associated with RT-induced rectal bleeding in prostate cancer patients (Oh *et al.*, 2017); this process has been shown to be critical to the repair of rectal mucosa damage in several mouse model studies (McCole *et al.*, 2005). Figure 4 shows directly connected protein–protein interaction networks identified using the corresponding genes for important SNPs. In pre-clinical models, the results of several studies have shown that vitamin D receptor (VDR) deficiency is associated with rectal bleeding (Figure 4(a)) (Froicu *et al.*, 2003; Kong *et al.*, 2008). For erectile dysfunction, the top two biological processes identified were the negative regulation of heart contraction and the negative regulation of blood circulation. Figure 4(b) shows a protein–protein interaction network likely associated with erectile dysfunction. Several pre-clinical studies have previously found PKC (Wingard *et al.*, 2007) and SMAD3 (Zhang *et al.*, 2008) to be associated with erectile dysfunction. For genitourinary toxicity in the same cohort, Lee *et al.* (2018) identified a significantly enriched functional group, consisting of 9 gene ontology terms, strongly associated with neurogenesis. This is a plausible biological process since the lower urinary tract is innervated by various peripheral nerves (Lee *et al.*, 2018). Among the proteins identified through further network analysis, seven proteins, including protein-kinase C (PKC), annexin I, protein kinase G, epidermal growth factor receptor (EGFR), schwannomin, acid-sensing ion channel 2, and neurexin, have previously been associated with lower urinary tract syndrome (Fig. 4(c)). In another study, Lee *et al.* (2020) found the cyclic adenosine monophosphate (cAMP)-mediated signaling pathway to be associated with RT-associated contralateral breast cancer (Lee *et al.*, 2020), which has been previously shown to promote RT-induced apoptosis in human lung cancer cells via interaction with the *ATM* gene (Cho *et al.*, 2014). In further protein–protein interaction analysis, two distinct clusters were identified, consisting of eight proteins. The literature survey indicated that all eight proteins have been reported to be associated with breast cancer, radiation, or both. In particular, four (CD63, Ephrin A, ERBB4, and Neuregulin 1) out of the eight proteins were found to be relevant to both radiation and carcinogenesis (Kaenel *et al.*, 2012; Shi *et al.*, 2015; Sundvall *et al.*, 2008; Tsai *et al.*, 2003). Clearly, one of the underlying ideas is that variations in closely related genes are more likely to contribute to phenotype variability. This means that network analysis can be combined with unbiased machine learning methods in GWAS to better understand biological mechanisms.

4. Conclusion

In summary, it is clear from the results presented that germline genetic variation is a significant contributor to the variability in radiotherapy toxicity response among patients. Fortunately, AI/machine learning methods represent a practical approach to using this information, even when it spreads across hundreds of SNPs. The integration of germline genetic variants and RT dose into advanced interpretable machine learning modeling has the potential to provide NTCP models with increased accuracy, thereby enabling a reduction of RT-induced complications in cancer survivors. Importantly, the use of bioinformatics techniques in connection with AI/machine learning in GWAS provides an unbiased and powerful method to identify key biological mechanisms. Despite the promise of this area of research, progress is slow due to the need to accrue GWAS data sets for each relevant endpoint. Hopefully, recent results will help spur acceleration.

Acknowledgments

This research was funded in part through the National Institutes of Health/National Cancer Institute Cancer Center Support Grant P30 CA008748, R21 CA234752 (PI: J.H. Oh), and a grant from Breast Cancer Research Foundation, BCRF-17-193.

References

Arloth, J., Eraslan, G., Andlauer, T. F. M., Martins, J., Iurato, S., Kuhnel, B., ... Mueller, N. S. (2020). DeepWAS: Multivariate genotype-phenotype associations by directly integrating regulatory information using deep learning. *PLoS Computational Biology, 16*(2), e1007616. https://doi.org/10.1371/journal.pcbi.1007616.

Azencott, C. A., Grimm, D., Sugiyama, M., Kawahara, Y., & Borgwardt, K. M. (2013). Efficient network-guided multi-locus association mapping with graph cuts. *Bioinformatics, 29*(13), i171–179. https://doi.org/10.1093/bioinformatics/btt238.

Bach, S., Binder, A., Montavon, G., Klauschen, F., Muller, K. R., & Samek, W. (2015). On pixel-wise explanations for non-linear classifier decisions by layer-wise relevance propagation. *PLoS One, 10*(7), e0130140. https://doi.org/10.1371/journal.pone.0130140.

Barrett, J. C. (2009). Haploview: Visualization and analysis of SNP genotype data. *Cold Spring Harbor Protocol, 2009*(10), pdb ip71. https://doi.org/10.1101/pdb.ip71.

Bohmanova, J., Sargolzaei, M., & Schenkel, F. S. (2010). Characteristics of linkage disequilibrium in North American Holsteins. *BMC Genomics, 11*, 421. https://doi.org/10.1186/1471-2164-11-421.

Botta, V., Louppe, G., Geurts, P., & Wehenkel, L. (2014). Exploiting SNP correlations within random forest for genome-wide association studies. *PLoS One, 9*(4), e93379. https://doi.org/10.1371/journal.pone.0093379.

Cheng, H., Garrick, D. J., & Fernando, R. L. (2017). Efficient strategies for leave-one-out cross validation for genomic best linear unbiased prediction. *Journal of Animal Science and Biotechnology, 8*, 38. https://doi.org/10.1186/s40104-017-0164-6.

Cho, E. A., Kim, E. J., Kwak, S. J., & Juhnn, Y. S. (2014). cAMP signaling inhibits radiation-induced ATM phosphorylation leading to the augmentation of apoptosis in human lung cancer cells. *Molecular Cancer, 13*, 36. https://doi.org/10.1186/1476-4598-13-36.

Coates, J., Jeyaseelan, A. K., Ybarra, N., David, M., Faria, S., Souhami, L., ... El Naqa, I. (2015). Contrasting analytical and data-driven frameworks for radiogenomic modeling of normal tissue toxicities in prostate cancer. *Radiotherapy and Oncology, 115*(1), 107–113. https://doi.org/10.1016/j.radonc.2015.03.005.

Cosgun, E., Limdi, N. A., & Duarte, C. W. (2011). High-dimensional pharmacogenetic prediction of a continuous trait using machine learning techniques with application to warfarin dose prediction in African Americans. *Bioinformatics, 27*(10), 1384–1389. https://doi.org/10.1093/bioinformatics/btr159.

Das, S., Forer, L., Schonherr, S., Sidore, C., Locke, A. E., Kwong, A., ... Fuchsberger, C. (2016). Next-generation genotype imputation service and methods. *Nature Genetics, 48*(10), 1284–1287. https://doi.org/10.1038/ng.3656.

Denham, J. W. & Hauer-Jensen, M. (2002). The radiotherapeutic injury — a complex 'wound'. *Radiotherapy and Oncology, 63*(2), 129–145. https://doi.org/10.1016/s0167-8140(02)00060-9.

Denisko, D. & Hoffman, M. M. (2018). Classification and interaction in random forests. *Proceedings of the National Academy of Sciences of the United States of America, 115*(8), 1690–1692. https://doi.org/10.1073/pnas.1800256115.

Fagny, M., Paulson, J. N., Kuijjer, M. L., Sonawane, A. R., Chen, C. Y., Lopes-Ramos, C. M., ... Platig, J. (2017). Exploring regulation in tissues with eQTL networks. *Proceedings of the National Academy of Sciences of the United States of America, 114*(37), E7841–E7850. https://doi.org/10.1073/pnas.1707375114.

Froicu, M., Weaver, V., Wynn, T. A., McDowell, M. A., Welsh, J. E., & Cantorna, M. T. (2003). A crucial role for the vitamin D receptor in experimental inflammatory bowel diseases. *Molecular Endocrinology, 17*(12), 2386–2392. https://doi.org/10.1210/me.2003-0281.

Hellwege, J. N., Keaton, J. M., Giri, A., Gao, X., Velez Edwards, D. R., & Edwards, T. L. (2017). Population stratification in genetic association studies. *Current Protocols in Human Genetics, 95*, 1 22 21–21 22 23. https://doi.org/10.1002/cphg.48.

Hendricks, A. E., Dupuis, J., Logue, M. W., Myers, R. H., & Lunetta, K. L. (2014). Correction for multiple testing in a gene region. *European Journal of Human Genetics, 22*(3), 414–418. https://doi.org/10.1038/ejhg.2013.144.

Hindorff, L. A., Sethupathy, P., Junkins, H. A., Ramos, E. M., Mehta, J. P., Collins, F. S., & Manolio, T. A. (2009). Potential etiologic and functional implications of genome-wide association loci for human diseases and traits. *Proceedings of the National*

Academy of Sciences of the United States of America, 106(23), 9362–9367. https://doi.org/10.1073/pnas.0903103106.

Hong, E. P. & Park, J. W. (2012). Sample size and statistical power calculation in genetic association studies. *Genomics & Informatics, 10*(2), 117–122. https://doi.org/10.5808/GI.2012.10.2.117.

Hyten, D. L., Choi, I. Y., Song, Q., Shoemaker, R. C., Nelson, R. L., Costa, J. M., ... Cregan, P. B. (2007). Highly variable patterns of linkage disequilibrium in multiple soybean populations. *Genetics, 175*(4), 1937–1944. https://doi.org/10.1534/genetics.106.069740.

Ilhan, I. & Tezel, G. (2013). How to select tag SNPs in genetic association studies? The CLONTagger method with parameter optimization. *OMICS, 17*(7), 368–383. https://doi.org/10.1089/omi.2012.0100.

Kaenel, P., Mosimann, M., & Andres, A. C. (2012). The multifaceted roles of Eph/ephrin signaling in breast cancer. *Cell Adhesion & Migration, 6*(2), 138–147. https://doi.org/10.4161/cam.20154.

Kang, J., Rancati, T., Lee, S., Oh, J. H., Kerns, S. L., Scott, J. G., ... Rosenstein, B. S. (2018). Machine learning and radiogenomics: Lessons learned and future directions. *Frontiers in Oncology, 8*, 228. https://doi.org/10.3389/fonc.2018.00228.

Kerns, S. L., Fachal, L., Dorling, L., Barnett, G. C., Baran, A., Peterson, D. R., ... West, C. M. L. (2020). Radiogenomics consortium genome-wide association study meta-analysis of late toxicity after prostate cancer radiotherapy. *Journal of the National Cancer Institute, 112*(2), 179–190. https://doi.org/10.1093/jnci/djz075.

Kerns, S. L., Kundu, S., Oh, J. H., Singhal, S. K., Janelsins, M., Travis, L. B., ... Rosenstein, B. S. (2015). The prediction of radiotherapy toxicity using single nucleotide polymorphism-based models: A step toward prevention. *Seminars in Radiation Oncology, 25*(4), 281–291. https://doi.org/10.1016/j.semradonc.2015.05.006.

Kim, J., Sohn, I., Kim, D. D., & Jung, S. H. (2013). SNP selection in genome-wide association studies via penalized support vector machine with MAX test. *Computational and Mathematical Methods in Medicine, 2013*, 340678. https://doi.org/10.1155/2013/340678.

Kong, J., Zhang, Z., Musch, M. W., Ning, G., Sun, J., Hart, J., ... Li, Y. C. (2008). Novel role of the vitamin D receptor in maintaining the integrity of the intestinal mucosal barrier. *The American Journal of Physiology-Gastrointestinal and Liver Physiology, 294*(1), G208–216. https://doi.org/:10.1152/ajpgi.00398.2007.

Koul, A., Becchio, C., & Cavallo, A. (2018). Cross-validation approaches for replicability in psychology. *Frontiers in Psychology, 9*, 1117. https://doi.org/10.3389/fpsyg.2018.01117.

Lamparter, D., Marbach, D., Rueedi, R., Kutalik, Z., & Bergmann, S. (2016). Fast and rigorous computation of gene and pathway scores from SNP-based summary statistics. *PLoS Computational Biology, 12*(1), e1004714. https://doi.org/10.1371/journal.pcbi.1004714.

Lee, S., Deasy, J. O., Oh, J. H., Di Meglio, A., Dumas, A., Menvielle, G., ... Vaz-Luis, I. (2020). Prediction of breast cancer treatment-induced fatigue by machine learning using genome-wide association data. *JNCI Cancer Spectrum, 4*(5), pkaa039. https://doi.org/10.1093/jncics/pkaa039.

Lee, S., Kerns, S., Ostrer, H., Rosenstein, B., Deasy, J. O., & Oh, J. H. (2018). Machine learning on a genome-wide association study to predict late genitourinary toxicity after prostate radiation therapy. *International Journal of Radiation Oncology, Biology, Physics, 101*(1), 128–135. https://doi.org/10.1016/j.ijrobp.2018.01.054.

Lee, S., Liang, X., Woods, M., Reiner, A. S., Concannon, P., Bernstein, L., ... Oh, J. H. (2020). Machine learning on genome-wide association studies to predict the risk of radiation-associated contralateral breast cancer in the WECARE Study. *PLoS One, 15*(2), e0226157. https://doi.org/10.1371/journal.pone.0226157.

Malhotra, A., Kobes, S., Bogardus, C., Knowler, W. C., Baier, L. J., & Hanson, R. L. (2014). Assessing accuracy of genotype imputation in American Indians. *PLoS One, 9*(7), e102544. https://doi.org/10.1371/journal.pone.0102544.

Marchini, J. & Howie, B. (2010). Genotype imputation for genome-wide association studies. *Nature Reviews Genetics, 11*(7), 499–511. https://doi.org/10.1038/nrg2796.

Marks, L. B., Yorke, E. D., Jackson, A., Ten Haken, R. K., Constine, L. S., Eisbruch, A., Bentzen, S.M., Nam, J., & Deasy, J. O. (2010). Use of normal tissue complication probability models in the clinic. *International Journal of Radiation Oncology, Biology, Physics, 76*(3 Suppl), S10–19. https://doi.org/10.1016/j.ijrobp.2009.07.1754.

McCole, D. F., Rogler, G., Varki, N., & Barrett, K. E. (2005). Epidermal growth factor partially restores colonic ion transport responses in mouse models of chronic colitis. *Gastroenterology, 129*(2), 591–608. https://doi.org/10.1016/j.gastro.2005.06.004.

Mieth, B., Rozier, A., Rodriguez, J. A., Hohne, M. M. C., Gornitz, N., & Muller, K. R. (2021). DeepCOMBI: Explainable artificial intelligence for the analysis and discovery in genome-wide association studies. *NAR Genomics and Bioinformatics, 3*(3), lqab065. https://doi.org/10.1093/nargab/lqab065.

Miller, C. L., Pjanic, M., & Quertermous, T. (2015). From locus association to mechanism of gene causality: The devil is in the details. *Arteriosclerosis, Thrombosis, and Vascular Biology, 35*(10), 2079–2080. https://doi.org/10.1161/ATVBAHA.115.306366.

Mittag, F., Romer, M., & Zell, A. (2015). Influence of feature encoding and choice of classifier on disease risk prediction in genome-wide association studies. *PLoS One, 10*(8), e0135832. https://doi.org/10.1371/journal.pone.0135832.

Naret, O., Chaturvedi, N., Bartha, I., Hammer, C., Fellay, J., & Swiss, H. I. V. C. S. (2018). Correcting for population stratification reduces false positive and false negative results in joint analyses of host and pathogen genomes. *Frontiers in Genetics, 9*, 266. https://doi.org/10.3389/fgene.2018.00266.

Nguyen, T. T., Huang, J., Wu, Q., Nguyen, T., & Li, M. (2015). Genome-wide association data classification and SNPs selection using two-stage quality-based Random Forests. *BMC Genomics, 16* (suppl 2), S5. https://doi.org/10.1186/1471-2164-16-S2-S5.

Nouira, A. & Azencott, C.-A. (2022). Multitask group Lasso for Genome Wide association Studies in diverse populations. *Pacific Symposium on Biocomputing, 27*, 163–174.

Oh, J. H., Kerns, S., Ostrer, H., Powell, S. N., Rosenstein, B., & Deasy, J. O. (2017). Computational methods using genome-wide association studies to predict radiotherapy complications and to identify correlative molecular processes. *Scientific Reports, 7*, 43381. https://doi.org/10.1038/srep43381.

Oti, M. & Brunner, H. G. (2007). The modular nature of genetic diseases. *Clinical Genetics, 71*(1), 1–11. https://doi.org/10.1111/j.1399-0004.2006.00708.x.

Pei, Y. F., Zhang, L., Li, J., & Deng, H. W. (2010). Analyses and comparison of imputation-based association methods. *PLoS One, 5*(5), e10827. https://doi.org/10.1371/journal.pone.0010827.

Pitter, K. L., Casey, D. L., Lu, Y. C., Hannum, M., Zhang, Z., Song, X., ... Setton, J. (2021). Pathogenic ATM mutations in cancer and a genetic basis for radiotherapeutic efficacy. *Journal of the National Cancer Institute, 113*(3), 266–273. https://doi.org/10.1093/jnci/djaa095.

Price, A. L., Patterson, N. J., Plenge, R. M., Weinblatt, M. E., Shadick, N. A., & Reich, D. (2006). Principal components analysis corrects for stratification in genome-wide association studies. *Nature Genetics, 38*(8), 904–909. https://doi.org/10.1038/ng1847.

Purcell, S., Neale, B., Todd-Brown, K., Thomas, L., Ferreira, M. A., Bender, D., ... Sham, P. C. (2007). PLINK: A tool set for whole-genome association and population-based linkage analyses. *American Journal of Human Genetics, 81*(3), 559–575. https://doi.org/10.1086/519795.

Schaid, D. J., Chen, W., & Larson, N. B. (2018). From genome-wide associations to candidate causal variants by statistical fine-mapping. *Nature Reviews Genetics, 19*(8), 491–504. https://doi.org/10.1038/s41576-018-0016-z.

Schurz, H., Muller, S. J., van Helden, P. D., Tromp, G., Hoal, E. G., Kinnear, C. J., & Moller, M. (2019). Evaluating the accuracy of imputation methods in a five-way admixed population. *Frontiers in Genetics, 10*, 34. https://doi.org/10.3389/fgene.2019.00034.

Shi, J., Ren, Y., Zhen, L., & Qiu, X. (2015). Exosomes from breast cancer cells stimulate proliferation and inhibit apoptosis of CD133+ cancer cells in vitro. *Molecular Medicine Reports, 11*(1), 405–409. https://doi.org/10.3892/mmr.2014.2749.

Spain, S. L. & Barrett, J. C. (2015). Strategies for fine-mapping complex traits. *Human Molecular Genetics, 24*(R1), R111–119. https://doi.org/10.1093/hmg/ddv260.

Stram, D. O. (2004). Tag SNP selection for association studies. *Genetic Epidemiology, 27*(4), 365–374. https://doi.org/10.1002/gepi.20028.

Sun, S., Dong, B., & Zou, Q. (2021). Revisiting genome-wide association studies from statistical modelling to machine learning. *Briefings in Bioinformatics, 22*(4), bbaa263. https://doi.org/10.1093/bib/bbaa263.

Sun, T., Wei, Y., Chen, W., & Ding, Y. (2020). Genome-wide association study-based deep learning for survival prediction. *Statistics in Medicine, 39*(30), 4605–4620. https://doi.org/10.1002/sim.8743.

Sundvall, M., Iljin, K., Kilpinen, S., Sara, H., Kallioniemi, O. P., & Elenius, K. (2008). Role of ErbB4 in breast cancer. *Journal of Mammary Gland Biology and Neoplasia, 13*(2), 259–268. https://doi.org/10.1007/s10911-008-9079-3.

Tsai, M. S., Shamon-Taylor, L. A., Mehmi, I., Tang, C. K., & Lupu, R. (2003). Blockage of heregulin expression inhibits tumorigenicity and metastasis of breast cancer. *Oncogene, 22*(5), 761–768. https://doi.org/10.1038/sj.onc.1206130.

Tucker, S. L., Li, M., Xu, T., Gomez, D., Yuan, X., Yu, J., ... Liao, Z. (2013). Incorporating single-nucleotide polymorphisms into the Lyman model to improve prediction of radiation pneumonitis. *International Journal of Radiation Oncology, Biology, Physics, 85*(1), 251–257. https://doi.org/10.1016/j.ijrobp.2012.02.021.

Wei, Z., Wang, K., Qu, H. Q., Zhang, H., Bradfield, J., Kim, C., ... Hakonarson, H. (2009). From disease association to risk assessment: An optimistic view from genome-wide association studies on type 1 diabetes. *PLoS Genetics, 5*(10), e1000678. https://doi.org/10.1371/journal.pgen.1000678.

Wei, Z., Wang, W., Bradfield, J., Li, J., Cardinale, C., Frackelton, E., ... International, I. B. D. G. C. (2013). Large sample size, wide variant spectrum, and advanced machine-learning technique boost risk prediction for inflammatory bowel disease. *American Journal of Human Genetics, 92*(6), 1008–1012. https://doi.org/10.1016/j.ajhg.2013.05.002.

West, C., Azria, D., Chang-Claude, J., Davidson, S., Lambin, P., Rosenstein, B., ... Yuille, M. (2014). The REQUITE project: Validating predictive models and biomarkers of radiotherapy toxicity to reduce side-effects and improve quality of life in cancer survivors. *Clinical Oncology (R Coll Radiol), 26*(12), 739–742. https://doi.org/10.1016/j.clon.2014.09.008.

West, C. & Rosenstein, B. S. (2010). Establishment of a radiogenomics consortium. *Radiotherapy & Oncology, 94*(1), 117–118. https://doi.org/10.1016/j.radonc.2009.12.007.

West, C., Rosenstein, B. S., Alsner, J., Azria, D., Barnett, G., Begg, A., ... Yarnold, J. (2010). Establishment of a radiogenomics consortium. *International Journal of Radiation Oncology, Biology, Physics, 76*(5), 1295–1296. https://doi.org/10.1016/j.ijrobp.2009.12.017.

Wingard, C., Fulton, D., & Husain, S. (2007). Altered penile vascular reactivity and erection in the Zucker obese-diabetic rat. *Journal of Sexual Medicine, 4*(2), 348–362; discussion 362–363. https://doi.org/10.1111/j.1743-6109.2007.00439.x.

Yang, J., Benyamin, B., McEvoy, B. P., Gordon, S., Henders, A. K., Nyholt, D. R., ... Visscher, P. M. (2010). Common SNPs explain a large proportion of the heritability for human height. *Nature Genetics, 42*(7), 565–569. https://doi.org/10.1038/ng.608.

Yang, S., Wen, J., Eckert, S. T., Wang, Y., Liu, D. J., Wu, R., ... Zhan, X. (2020). Prioritizing genetic variants in GWAS with lasso using permutation-assisted tuning. *Bioinformatics, 36*(12), 3811–3817. https://doi.org/10.1093/bioinformatics/btaa229.

Zhang, L. W., Piao, S., Choi, M. J., Shin, H. Y., Jin, H. R., Kim, W. J., ... Suh, J. K. (2008). Role of increased penile expression of transforming growth factor-beta1 and activation of the Smad signaling pathway in erectile dysfunction in streptozotocin-induced diabetic rats. *Journal of Sexual Medicine, 5*(10), 2318–2329. https://doi.org/10.1111/j.1743-6109.2008.00977.x.

Chapter 13

Utilization of Radiomics in Prognostication and Treatment Response

Michael J. Baine

Department of Radiation Oncology, University of Nebraska Medical Center, Omaha NE, USA

Abstract

The relatively new field of radiomics seeks to leverage previously under/unutilized aspects of diagnostic imaging as a clinically meaningful tool with promise to change the face of how imaging may be used in future clinical practice. Through analysis of features in individual voxels and how those features interact with similar features of surrounding voxels as well as establishing patterns within individual features or classifications of features throughout an imaging set, a vast amount of data can be generated and mined. Further, through the current field of radiogenomics, researchers are seeking to gain a better understanding as to what these individual radiomic features and patterns truly represent at a cellular and subcellular level. Since its inception, the concept of radiomics has promised the potential to provide actionable information through multiple aspects of clinical care.

To date, a majority of radiomic-related publications have focused on two aspects of potential use: Providing information that can act as an adjunct to clinical and pathological prognostic criteria for patients with newly diagnosed malignancies and producing radiomic feature signatures that can predict likelihood and degree of response to specific treatments. With these, the potential clinical utility is apparent. Providing patients with the most accurate prognostic information possible allows for a more thorough and realistic discussion regarding treatment options and will help to better optimize healthcare resources. Predicting treatment response in an accurate real-time manner allows for better decision-making regarding the need or lack thereof for individual therapies, determination of total duration of treatment, and help to further clarify which treatment or combination thereof provides the best likelihood of treatment response in each individual patient.

Of increasing interest, however, are two additional potential avenues through which radiomics can provide aid to treating clinicians. Using radiographic signals beyond apparent tumor size reduction to track response to ongoing treatments can provide vital information to patients and providers regarding whether a current treatment should be continued or abandoned for other options, particularly in tumors that are difficult to objectively assess using standard imaging techniques or show a mixed response on follow-up imaging. Further, the potential utility of radiomic signatures to provide information regarding histology, mutational status, or targetable receptor status with a high degree of accuracy could open an avenue for patients and clinicians to gain information on primary tumors and metastatic disease without the need for biopsies, reducing the associated risk and morbidity to patients in the process.

Through this chapter, we seek to offer a glimpse into the general state of knowledge gained from and current failures of modern radiomics with a focus on each of the four directions of radiomic research delineated above. Our desire is to provide a high-level overview of radiomics literature with commentary throughout, highlighting areas of consistent promise while additionally underscoring areas of inconsistency or shortcomings in the data. With this, we hope to illustrate the continued and growing excitement in this field and provide areas in need of further development, helping to guide readers in the consideration and design of the future research directions that will shape this field in the coming years. In keeping with the theme of this work as a whole, we will also offer commentary on how artificial intelligence has been incorporated into the development of radiomics signatures and the general themes that emerge when assessing this field in its totality. The primary uses of radiomics in cancer is summarized at the end of this chapter, in Table 1.

1. Radiomics as an Adjunct to Prognosis

In patients with newly diagnosed malignancies, understanding their prognosis is of paramount importance. This knowledge can help patients determine how aggressive they may like to be with their treatment, the risk and nature of side effects they may be willing to tolerate, and what decisions should be made outside of the clinic regarding home life, finances, travel, and beyond. Classically, prognosis was based primarily on the nature of the malignancy the patient was diagnosed with, their clinical stage, and, to some degree, pathological grade. As we have increased our knowledge with regards to various malignancies, new aspects have arisen that are also considered such as hormone receptor status of breast cancer, growth factor receptor mutations or amplification, the presence or absence of specific mutations such as in primary CNS malignancies, and general mutational signatures in cancers such as breast and prostate. The vast amounts of data that are generated through radiomics analyses promise to potentially provide an additional tool by which to assess patient prognosis that goes beyond any of the current clinical, pathological, or histological tools currently available. Used either alone or in conjunction with other prognostic tools available, these radiomic signatures may provide the most robust individual assessment of prognosis currently possible.

Of all malignancies in which radiomics has been considered for bolstering prognostic differentiation of patients, the most robust data exists in primary CNS malignancies and, more specifically, glioblastoma. When all glioblastoma associated radiomics papers are amassed and considered in concert, several consistent findings emerge. Various radiomics signatures using multiple types of MRI sequences have demonstrated the ability to predict progression-free survival, the presence of disease recurrence, and patient overall survival (Oltra-Sastre *et al.*, 2019). Beyond providing improved prognostic distinction at the time of diagnosis, Ammari and colleagues demonstrated that a combination of clinical and radiomic information extracted from pretreatment contrasted T1 and T2 flair MRIs are able to stratify patients by overall survival at 9, 12, and 15 months after initiation of bevacizumab in the setting of recurrent glioblastoma. Interestingly, while their algorithms were able to differentiate patients who survived 12 months or longer with an AUC of up to 0.85 in their test set, they were unable to reliably construct an algorithm to predict progression-free survival, a fact that is perhaps attributable to the difficulty in reliably determining disease progression of glioblastoma in the setting of bevacizumab (Ammrai *et al.*, 2021).

Interestingly however, and perhaps with significant implications for all radiomics studies regardless of application, Beig *et al.* demonstrated differing prognostic and predictive abilities of radiomics signatures derived from contrasted T1 MRIs across genders and within tumor subcompartments. These findings suggest that radiomic signatures are unlikely to represent a one size fits all scenario and that both demographic factors and exact location of analysis within a tumor must be accounted for if the true clinical utility of radiomics for gliomas is ever to be realized (Beig *et al.*, 2021).

Radiomics signatures have also demonstrated potential prognostic capabilities within the CNS outside of the setting of primary CNS neoplasms. For example, Bhatia *et al.* found that MRI-based radiomics features were able to predict overall survival in patients with intracranial metastatic disease from melanoma receiving treatment with immune checkpoint inhibitors on univariate analysis though upon multivariate analysis their findings became statistically nonsignificant (Bhatia *et al.*, 2019). It remains unclear if this loss of significance is due to low patient numbers in their training and test sets, overly restrictive feature extraction techniques, or a general failing of radiomics in this setting. Langenhuizen *et al.* expanded the field of intracranial radiomic prognostication beyond malignant diseases, demonstrating that a predictive model using pretreatment MRI-derived texture features in patients with acoustic neuromas treated with SRS was able to predict likelihood of future tumor growth with an AUC of 0.93 (Langenhuizen *et al.*, 2020).

The ability of radiomics to improve prognostic abilities have been investigated across myriad extracranial malignancies as well. Liu *et al.* combined clinicopathologic features and deep learning radiomic signature analyses based on pretreatment MRIs from multiple centers to construct a nomogram that was able to predict likelihood of development of distant metastatic disease in patients with locally advanced rectal cancer receiving neoadjuvant chemoradiotherapy followed by TME with negative margins. The derived nomogram was found to be significantly superior to analysis of clinical features along with a *p*-value of less than 0.001 (Liu *et al.*, 2021). Similar results have been found across multiple additional studies, suggesting that radiomic signatures based on pretreatment MRIs promise to provide significantly improved prognostication of rectal cancer patients in the future (Wang *et al.*, 2021). FDG PET-based radiomics signatures have been demonstrated to improve prediction of disease-free survival in non-small-cell lung cancer patients undergoing surgical resection beyond that afforded by clinical and histological features alone (Kirienko *et al.*, 2018). Huang *et al.* additionally found that a five feature radiomic signature could predict survival in patients with ALK-mutated non-small-cell lung cancer based on data from The Cancer Imaging Archive, however, their signature performed better in patients not treated with targeted therapies and demonstrated general poor performance in those treated with ALK-directed agents; again suggesting that clinical and demographic information will weigh heavily on the predictive abilities of radiomic signatures (Huang *et al.*, 2019). Others have demonstrated the predictive abilities of radiomics in gynecologic malignancies, showing both CT- and MRI-based radiomic models to provide better predictions of both progression-free and overall survival than is possible using clinical or pathological features alone in patients with ovarian cancer (Nougaret *et al.*, 2021) and that post-treatment clinical outcomes including local control, regional control, distant metastasis-free survival, and overall survival could be reasonably predicted in node positive cervical cancer patients treated with definitive chemoradiation using pretreatment MRI-based radiomics features (Park *et al.*, 2020). Similarly, radiomics have shown predictive potential in malignancies of the GI tract though the results have been quite variable across subsites of disease. Pretreatment radiomic features based on PET scans have been shown to be able to predict both disease-free survival and overall survival in esophageal squamous cell carcinoma patients undergoing trimodality therapy consisting of neoadjuvant chemoradiation followed by surgical resection. Importantly, however, the predictive ability of these radiological features appeared to be no better than changes in delta SUV or degree of pathologic response when used alone though it was better when used in concert with clinical parameters (Chen *et al.*, 2019). Radiomic signatures from pretreatment CTs in esophageal cancer patients have also been found to be able to stratify patients based on overall survival, though they did not hold up when tested against a validation set of patients. Further, the AUCs derived from these investigations have remained relatively modest, generally below 0.7, and it remains unclear as to how much the addition of these features may add to the predictive abilities of currently used demographic and clinical information (Larue *et al.*, 2018). In contrast, in a very large retrospective study consisting of almost 1600 consecutive patients, Jiang *et al.* found that a 19-feature radiomics signature provided a robust ability to predict both disease-free and overall survival in patients undergoing treatment for gastric cancer and was significantly superior to that directed by clinicopathologic nomograms or TNM staging (Jiang *et al.*, 2008). Additionally, our group demonstrated that a six-feature radiologic signature derived from treatment planning CT scans obtained after initial chemotherapy but prior to radiation treatment was superior to clinical models in predicting overall survival of pancreas cancer patients undergoing treatment with Stereotactic Body Radiotherapy (SBRT) and the further addition of clinical features to the radiomic feature model only slightly improved its predictive abilities. Additionally, a separate seven-feature signature was significantly better than routinely used clinical predictors at predicting disease-free survival (AUC of 0.78 versus 0.66) (Parr *et al.*, 2020).

While radiomics signatures have demonstrated the consistent ability to improve prognostication of patients beyond current clinically utilized methods, the signatures found across each of the associated studies are heterogenous in nature, even within specific diseases. Currently, little work has been performed comparing signatures with regards to ease of implementation or overall clinical utility. Thus, each of the published works to date has been relegated to demonstrations of proof of concept as opposed to providing something actionable in the near future.

2. Prediction of Treatment Response

As knowledge continues to increase with regards to therapeutic options in patients diagnosed with cancer, patients are currently often faced with multiple treatment options that they could potentially pursue. Further, as the drive continues toward personalized medicine, there is a general desire among clinicians to be able to provide patients in such situations with information regarding which treatment options may provide their best individual outcomes. Currently, however, neither clinicians nor patients have significant information to go on in this regard, creating a situation where the patient and provider choose a specific treatment paradigm based on general practice patterns or, often, best clinical salesmanship. To date, however, multiple studies have suggested that leveraging data from radiomics may provide increasing knowledge with regards to likelihood of response to specific treatments, thus potentially providing patients with an ability to weigh treatment options in a way that is truly specific to themselves.

One such malignancy with multiple treatment options is non-small-cell lung cancer. In patients diagnosed with locally advanced disease, current treatment paradigms include definitive chemoradiation as well as neoadjuvant chemoradiation or chemotherapy alone followed by resection. To date, there is little to guide optimal treatment strategy on a patient-to-patient basis, leading current guidelines to represent the most recently published large-scale clinical trials as opposed to a more fluid and individualized approach. Radiomics, however, offers the potential to help guide treatment strategies by providing pre-treatment insight into likely response to these various treatment strategies, allowing for an optimized treatment regimen to be selected. For example, radiomics features from pretreatment CT scans have demonstrated a remarkable ability to predict clinical response to upfront chemotherapy in patients with non-small-cell lung cancer, achieving an accuracy of 85.7% and AUC of 0.941. Such a model promises the potential for better patient stratification with regards to upfront treatment options prior to curative intent resection (Chang *et al.*, 2021). Further, a 13-feature model of intratumoral and peritumoral texture features on pretreatment CT scans was also demonstrated to be able to predict the likelihood of significant pathologic response following neoadjuvant chemoradiation followed by surgical resection in patients with stage IIIA non-small-cell lung cancer, achieving an AUC of 0.86. Importantly, the same model was associated with an increase in both disease-free survival and overall survival as well, suggesting its clinical utility could be quite robust in designing optimal treatment strategy and prognostication of such patients (Khorrami *et al.*, 2019). Radiomic signatures derived from metabolic tumor volumes from pre-chemoradiation FDG PET scans in patients with locally advanced non-small-cell lung cancer were also found to be able to predict regional disease response as noted on a second FDG PET obtained mid chemoradiotherapy course. Importantly, radiomics features with predictive abilities were variable across tumor regions with high or low respective SUVs; again demonstrating the necessity of precision with regards to radiologic feature measurement to provide consistent or reproducible results (Duan *et al.*, 2020). The potential utility of radiomics in the setting of non-small-cell lung cancer is not limited only to the locally advanced setting but also has been demonstrated in patients with metastatic disease, for whom many treatment options exist including cytotoxic chemotherapy, immunotherapy, and targeted agents. In this patient population, pretreatment FDG PET derived radiomic signatures consisting of six individual features from the imaged primary tumor was able to better predict future response to the immune checkpoint inhibitor pembrolizumab than was afforded with the currently used PD-L1 tumor proportion score (AUC = 0.9 vs 0.6) (Valentinuzzi *et al.*, 2020). Additionally, radiomic modeling using a deep learning semantics signature method has been found to predict post EGFR TKI progression-free survival, with those patients noted to be in the low risk of progression cohort having a 2-month improvement in PFS over those in the high-risk cohort as predicted by modeling from their pretreatment CT scans. This is particularly important as patients with stage IV non-small-cell lung cancer found to have targetable variants of EGFR continue to have heterogenous responses to EGFR tyrosine kinase inhibitors (Song *et al.*, 2020). Of paramount importance however is that fact that radiomic features appear to be specific not just to intra-tumoral regions but also how and when the associated radiographs were obtained. Highlighting this, our group investigated a panel of 841 radiomic features from 4-dimensional CTs to determine stability across various phases of the breathing cycle. Our data suggests that, while some features remain relatively stable with a less than 10% coefficient of variance across breathing cycles, approximately a quarter of the features were found to have significant variation and thus would likely not be reliable in a clinical setting. Further, when only stable features were used for prediction of overall survival in early stage non-small cell lung cancer patients undergoing SBRT, predictability was significantly enhanced over models in which all radiomic features were considered regardless of stability (Du *et al.*, 2019).

Similar studies have also underlined the potential utility of radiomics in patients embarking on treatment for newly diagnosed rectal cancers. For example, pretreatment MRIs of patients with rectal cancer undergoing upfront chemoradiation have been found to provide radiomic signatures that could reliably predict subsequent response with an AUC of 0.904 predicting good versus poor response and an AUC of 0.93 for predicting pathologic downstaging (Shayesteh *et al.*, 2019). This has been similarly shown in a multi center international study by Shaish *et al.* (Shaish *et al.*, 2020). In contrast, radiomics signatures have also been shown to be able to predict lack of response to neoadjuvant chemoradiation in patients receiving concurrent FOLFOX chemotherapy, thus potentially defining a patient population who should proceed directly to surgery after their diagnosis (Zhou *et al.*, 2019). Notably, the difference in chemotherapy used in this reported neoadjuvant regimen compared to what is generally used in American and European countries (5-fluorouracil or capecitabine alone) makes the generalizability of these findings difficult to interpret. However, others have conversely suggested that the ability of radiomic signatures from pretreatment MRIs to predict likely response to neoadjuvant radiation is no better than that provided through conventional radiological assessment by expert radiologists (van Griethuysen *et al.*, 2020). The ability to predict pathologic response following neoadjuvant chemotherapy alone without the addition of neoadjuvant radiation has also been demonstrated, noting that radiomic signatures based on pretreatment MRI are able to achieve an AUC of approximately 0.93 in such a patient population (Li *et al.*, 2020). Similar to pretreatment MRIs, pretreatment non-contrast CT-based radiomics signatures have also been shown to be able to predict the likelihood that a rectal cancer patient undergoing neoadjuvant chemoradiation will achieve a pathological complete response, a surrogate for overall prognosis and potentially signaling that subsequent surgical resection is unnecessary, with an accuracy of approximately 84% (Yuan *et al.*, 2020). Pretreatment MRI-based radiomics signatures have further been demonstrated to predict patient prognosis and likely benefit of adjuvant chemotherapy, the addition of which remains clinically controversial due to conflicting clinical trial results (Cui *et al.*, 2020). As in non-small-cell lung cancer, the utility of radiomics is not limited to local disease. In patients who have developed metastatic disease to the liver from HER-2 amplified cancers of the colon and rectum, pretreatment abdominal CT-based radiologic signatures demonstrated a significant ability to predict response to HER-2 directed therapy with a sensitivity of 92% and specificity of 86% (Giannini *et al.*, 2020). Such information will provide invaluable abilities for future physicians to guide upfront systemic therapy options including the potential for multimodality treatments to provide optimal response. Similar results have also been found in the ability for pretreatment CT-based radiomics signatures to predict response to FOLFIRI with or without cetuximab in patients with liver metastases from rectal cancer (Dercle *et al.*, 2020). Importantly, as a response to the various potential downfalls of radiomic signature reproducibility as suggested above, Cusumano *et al.* derived a pretreatment MRI-based radiomics signature that was able to predict pathological complete response rates following neoadjuvant chemoradiation in patients with locally advanced rectal cancer with an AUC of 0.72 regardless of field strength of the MRI utilized. However, while it was found that this signature was able to predict response across both 1.5 and 3.0 T field strengths, the accuracy of the signature was numerically better with the higher strength field (AUC 0.83 versus 0.70), suggesting that even among this data significant heterogeneity regarding signature interpretability remains (Cusumano *et al.*, 2021).

Other GI malignancies have additionally shown potential use of radiomics signatures though with more heterogenous results. Pretreatment CT-based radiomics features have been found to be able to predict the likelihood of achieving a clinical complete response in patients with squamous cell carcinoma of the esophagus undergoing definitive chemoradiation with a reliability far greater than that achieved by clinical parameters alone. However, the combination of radiographic features and clinical parameters into a single all-encompassing nomogram provided the greatest accuracy of all, once again suggesting that radiomics features, while likely of significance and potentially clinically relevant, are unlikely to stand on their own (Luo *et al.*, 2020). In contrast, however, another study found that pretreatment CT-based radiomics signatures could predict pathological complete response following neoadjuvant chemoradiation followed by surgical resection in patients with squamous cell carcinoma of the esophagus while no initial clinical or pathological features were able to provide the same (Yang *et al.*, 2019). The differences in these results can potentially be attributed to a lack of reliability in clinical complete response assessment, as supported by the clinical observation that esophageal cancer patients found to have a clinical complete response following chemoradiation and who do not undergo surgical resection ultimately have a high rate of local recurrence, as well as the general heterogeneity of radiomics results across studies, again highlighting the continued difficulty in making these results into clinically reliable tools. Additionally, in hepatocellular carcinoma, data showing radiomics ability to predict treatment outcomes remains sparse, however they have indeed been demonstrated in specific clinical situations. For instance, response of hepatocellular carcinoma to transarterial chemoembolization (TACE) remains quite heterogeneous though noncontrast CT-based radiomics features, combined with patient level clinical features, have demonstrated the ability to predict TACE response and, subsequently, overall survival in this patient population (Guo *et al.*, 2021).

Other high prevalence cancers for which radiomics have demonstrated potential utility to predict treatment response with salient clinical implications include breast cancer. Across multiple studies, pretreatment MRI radiomics-based features have been found to be able to predict likelihood of response to neoadjuvant cytotoxic chemotherapy in breast cancer patients, specifically for the potential achievement of a pathologic complete response (Bian *et al.*, 2020; Sutton *et al.*, 2020; Zhou *et al.*, 2020; Chen *et al.*, 2020; Liu *et al.*, 2019). Of note, however, while the ability to achieve a pathologic complete response is of great prognostic significance, it itself is not the most relevant endpoint for clinical decision-making at the time of initial patient diagnosis, particularly if the decision on neoadjuvant chemotherapy is being made in an attempt to provide the patient with a less extensive surgical resection that could not otherwise be achieved without reasonable treatment response. In this vein, radiomic features that could predict significant response, any response, or the ability to de-escalate surgical resection would likely be of greater clinical benefit. Regardless, while these specific signatures may not be of great clinical benefit, it does represent a proof of concept that chemotherapy response can be predicted based on radiomic features at the outset. Of particular interest in recent years, it has additionally been shown that pretreatment MRI-based radiomic signatures are able to predict likelihood of tumor response to neoadjuvant endocrine therapy in patients with newly diagnosed breast cancer (Hilal *et al.*, 2018). Other studies have attempted similar associations however with pretreatment PET-based radiologic signatures (Li *et al.*, 2020–2). While the radiomic signatures derived in this study achieved a reasonable AUC, especially when patient demographic features were also included, it is noteworthy that there were also significant associations between the radiomic features and both hormone receptor expression and tumor stage, both of which are independently known to be associated with likelihood of significant treatment response. Interestingly, another group attempted to derive a radiomics signature from ultrasound that could predict neoadjuvant chemotherapy response (DiCenzo *et al.*, 2020). While this endpoint is likely more clinically valid than those used in other studies as noted above, the true benefit of such a signature lies in the fact that the majority of breast cancer patients undergo ultrasound as part of their normal staging work-up whereas the addition of MRI and PET scan are often not clinically indicated and, thus, any such use of associated radiomics features would necessarily increase associated healthcare costs.

The ability of radiomics to predict treatment response has been shown in rarer malignancies as well. Multiple studies have suggested that preoperative imaging-based radiomics have the ability to predict response to neoadjuvant chemotherapy in patients with osteosarcoma (Zhong *et al.*, 2020). Such capacity could have significant ability to guide upfront treatment for these patients, shuttling some directly to surgery if upfront chemotherapy is unlikely to be helpful. Response to induction chemotherapy has also been demonstrated through radiomics signatures derived from pretreatment MRI imaging in patients with newly diagnosed cancer of the nasopharynx (Zhao *et al.*, 2020). Notably, however, the patient cohorts used for this study were from regions with endemic EBV infections and thus any potential extrapolation to nonendemic regions such as the Americas or Europe remains unclear. Preoperative MRI-based radiomics signatures have also demonstrated the ability to predict postoperative normalization of hormone levels in patients diagnosed with functional pituitary adenomas more reliably than clinical features, a finding that may help to guide recommendations for post-operative radiotherapy in future patients (Fan *et al.*, 2019). Going beyond solid malignancies, heterogeneity and radiomics signatures within pretreatment FDG PET scans in patients with newly diagnosed Hodgkin's lymphoma have also shown the ability to predict response to initial chemotherapy and, associated with this, both progression-free and overall survivals (Lue *et al.*, 2020). These findings may help to optimize escalation in chemotherapy regimens or predict who will likely require a future stem cell transplant.

Interestingly, it appears that the abilities for radiomics signatures to predict treatment response are not necessarily specific to individual diseases but rather may be able to predict response to specific drug classes regardless of the malignancy in which they are used. Prediction of likelihood of response to immune checkpoint inhibitors across many cancers has been demonstrated using radiomics features derived from pretreatment imaging including CTs, MRIs, and PET scans (Wu *et al.*, 2019). Additionally, and as well summarized by Wang *et al.* in 2021, radiomics signatures derived from both CT and PET imaging have also been established to identify pathologic features associated with immunophenotype and response to immunotherapy across myriad malignancies (Wang *et al.*, 2021–2). Importantly, however, the reliability of the signatures remained somewhat questionable with reported AUCs rarely rising above 0.8. Additionally, while this work represents the breadth of data generated in this regard, it is noteworthy that the number and nature of features included in each of the respective signatures derived from the individual studies varied widely and thus reproducibility and extrapolation to true clinical relevance remains murky.

Once again, regardless of if radiomics signatures are used to predict treatment response within specific malignancies or within a specific drug class across malignancies, the data to date is quite promising. However, as previously noted, there remains a general lack of uniformity across the patient populations studied, the methods used in each investigation, and in the radiomics signatures derived. Further, evidence suggests that features may vary wildly depending on where within the tumor the features are extracted, the type and quality of scan used, and the normal physiological and anatomical variations within the patient at the time the scan is conducted. Accounting for this will be paramount in transitioning the field of radiomics from a scene of scientific interest to that of true clinical value.

3. Tracking Treatment Response

Similarly, individualized treatment decision-making with regards to duration of treatment or whether a currently utilized treatment should be revisited in consideration of switching to a new treatment/paradigm is also an area in which radiomics has demonstrated a potential ability that goes beyond currently available methods. Such a concept is of particular importance in malignancies that are difficult to assess through standard radiographic methods. Specifically, in cancers treated with neoadjuvant therapy prior to attempted resection such as pancreas, esophagus, and rectal cancers, there is a general lack of ability to assess real-time treatment efficacy, thus making the neoadjuvant treatments standardized and not adapted to individual patients. As such, there is a proportion of patients who necessarily receive more neoadjuvant therapy than required while others would likely benefit from further extension of the preoperative treatments. Further, in cancers that have multiple treatment options such as newly diagnosed prostate cancer, the ability to assess treatment response in real-time in patients undergoing definitive radiation may allow for more optimal conversion to a potential surgical intervention if poor response is seen midway through the treatment course. This concept could prevent patients from undergoing unnecessary treatments while helping them to pivot to more efficacious treatments based on their individual responses, all utilizing noninvasive imaging tests with low associated healthcare costs.

One malignancy in which the ability to better track response is of vital importance is adenocarcinoma of the pancreas. This cancer is well known to be associated with a significant desmoplastic reaction within the tumor itself, which often does not change with therapy regardless of actual response seen within the sparse malignant cells interspersed throughout. As such, tumor size and shape often do not change significantly with neoadjuvant treatments, making it clinically difficult to determine when a sufficient number of neoadjuvant chemotherapy cycles has been delivered, when the addition of neoadjuvant radiation therapy should be considered, and when the patient may indeed have resectable disease after upfront therapy despite lack of objective tumor regression in the unresectable and borderline resectable settings. To date, multiple authors have demonstrated that changes in CT-based radiomic signatures over the course of neoadjuvant chemotherapy more robustly predict treatment response and ultimate surgical resectability than clinical radiologic criteria in patients with newly diagnosed adenocarcinoma of the pancreas (Zhang *et al.*, 2021). While the majority of these studies continue to show relatively modest differentiation capabilities and suffer from inter-study heterogeneity, the ability to use radiomic profiling to go beyond overt radiographic changes and provide a more accurate assessment than is currently afforded has a potential to offer a seismic shift in how such patients are assessed and how clinical decision-making is undertaken.

It has also been seen across multiple malignancies that radiomics features from imaging obtained both during and after completion of an upfront therapy as well as changes in the signatures during such therapies may have significant predictive abilities with regards to overall treatment response and patient outcomes. For example, changes in radiomic signatures between pretreatment and mid treatment PET scans in patients with stage III non-small-cell lung cancer undergoing definitive chemoradiation have demonstrated the ability to predict overall treatment response and progression-free survival more reliably than standard conventional imaging metrics such as tumor volume and SUV max value (Zhang *et al.*, 2020). Further, longitudinal changes in radiomics signatures derived from cone beam CT scans from patients actively undergoing chemoradiation for locally advanced non-small-cell lung cancer have demonstrated the potential to stratify patients based on overall survival, suggesting that differences in treatment response as notable by radiomic features may be able to progressively predict overall response to treatment and patient prognosis (Shi *et al.*, 2020). Additionally, changes in radiomic features based on CT scans before and after two cycles of immune checkpoint inhibitor therapy in patients with non-small-cell lung cancer has also been demonstrated to help differentiate those who will versus will not respond to this therapy with associated differences in overall survival also demonstrated accordingly (Khorrami *et al.*, 2020). In rectal cancer, delta radiomics from serial MRIs used for MRI guided radiation therapy has also been demonstrated to be able to reliably predict both clinical and pathologic complete response in patients undergoing neoadjuvant chemoradiation for locally advanced disease (Cusumano *et al.*, 2021). Similar results have also been shown from delta radiomic features derived from diagnostic quality MRIs obtained both pre and post neoadjuvant chemoradiotherapy (Li *et al.*, 2019). Treatment response to neoadjuvant chemotherapy in patients with bladder cancer has also been demonstrated using pre and posttreatment CT-based radiomic signatures (Cha *et al.*, 2017). However, it is noteworthy that this model primarily focused on differentiating patients who achieved pathologic complete response from those who did not which, itself, is only partially clinically meaningful. Patients who derive any significant response to upfront chemotherapy have improved prognosis compared to those who do not regardless of if that response is pathologically complete and, thus, such a differentiation should be the focus of future studies. In patients with newly diagnosed breast cancer, serial ultrasound derived radiomic signatures, particularly derived at treatment weeks 1 and 4, have also been demonstrated to predict and track response to neoadjuvant chemotherapy, however it is notable that it remains unclear as to whether this predictive ability is superior to conventional radiologic features and/or physical exam (Quiaoit *et al.*, 2020). Multiple studies have also demonstrated the ability of posttreatment or serial imaging derived radiomic signatures to accurately represent treatment response in patients undergoing definitive treatment for cancers of the head and neck, however, as discussed by Guha *et al.* and is true across most disease sites, heterogeneity among the designs and statistical methods utilized in the studies prevents a clear picture of the true clinical relevance or promise of radiomics from being apparent (Guha *et al.*, 2019).

4. Radiomics as a Surrogate for Pathologic Information

The potential utility of radiomic signatures to provide information currently reserved for histological or molecular testing would be of significant benefit, both in clinical decision-making and with regards to general healthcare costs. Identification of new or targetable mutations, understanding the amount by which a patient's tumor is evading the immune system through expression of PD-L1 and thus how likely they are to derive benefit from immune checkpoint inhibition, as well as the determination of if a new lesion represents the development metastatic disease/ metastatic progression versus being a benign entity or a second primary malignancy altogether are of paramount and ever-increasing importance. In the current clinical setting, however, answering these questions often requires obtaining new tissue from the lesion/lesions of interest, thus creating increased costs from the procedure as well as the increased cost and morbidity of any associated complications. As we improve our understanding as to the histological and molecular underpinnings of the radiomic signatures derived from various imaging exams, the potential for these signatures to reduce the requirement for, or replace entirely, such procedures becomes increasingly promising. To date, multiple studies have suggested that radiomics have the ability to provide histology level information with the potential to significantly impact clinical decision-making.

In some malignancies, improving the ability to noninvasively differentiate tumor subtypes or characteristics which impact treatment options available to patients is of paramount importance. For example, in non-small-cell lung cancer, a patient's candidacy for targeted therapies has great impact on both prognosis and treatment associated morbidity. Zhu *et al.* found that radiomic signatures derived from pretreatment CT imaging in patients with newly diagnosed locally advanced or metastatic adenocarcinomas of the lung could reliably differentiate tumors that were EGFR negative, EGFR positive but without mutation of p53, or had commutations in EGFR and p53 (Zhu *et al.*, 2021). This latter differentiation is of significant importance as the presence of commutations in EGFR and p53 is associated with reduced efficacy of EGFR TKIs as well as overall worsened patient prognosis. Thus, collectively, these results suggest that radiomics may be able to help guide use of targeted therapies in non-small-cell lung cancer without the time and expense of the added pathological evaluations. Further, Wang *et al.* demonstrated that radiomics features from CTs of patients ultimately diagnosed with adenocarcinoma of the lung were able to predict both tumor mutation burden status as well as the presence of EGFR and p53 mutations though with relatively modest AUCs which were collectively less than 0.7 (Wang *et al.*, 2019). While obviously not yet ready for prime time, this work acts as a further proof of concept that radiomics features can predict molecular/mutational characteristics with significant clinical impact. Jian *et al.* additionally reviewed many articles investigating the ability of radiomics signatures to determine the likelihood of IDH mutation, MGMT methylation, and 1p/19q codeletion in preoperative MRIs of patients with newly diagnosed gliomas (Jian *et al.*, 2021). This information is significant for patient prognosis, treatment response, and optimal systemic therapy utilized during primary and subsequent treatments. Li *et al.* demonstrated the ability of PET-based radiomics signatures to predict likelihood of LVSI in patients with early-stage squamous cell carcinoma of the cervix, a pathological feature with clinical importance in choosing optimal treatment paradigms (Li *et al.*, 2021). Importantly, however, while these radiomic features were found to have good reliability in the training set of patients, the reliability was significantly reduced in the validation set but subsequently improved with the addition of information regarding the presence of tenascin-C (TNC) and cyclooxygenase-2 (COX-2) in the pathologic specimen, thus reducing the true clinical utility of this finding. Further, Bos *et al.* found that radiomics features extracted from primary tumor volumes derived from pretreatment MRIs in patients with oropharyngeal cancer were able to predict the likelihood of HPV positivity on eventual pathologic assessment though, notably, were by themselves no better than clinical models including smoking status, T stage, and tumor morphology. However, when both clinical and radiomics models were combined, the predictive ability increased significantly, again suggesting that radiomics when combined with validated clinical features will likely provide the greatest predictive ability for most/all salient endpoints (Bos *et al.*, 2021).

Other cancer diagnoses are notable for having significant difficulty in differentiating benign entities from clinically significant malignancy, a distinction that radiomics has demonstrated the potential to overcome. For instance, Conti *et al.* provided an in-depth synopsis of current literature with regards to pathologic predictive abilities of radiomics derived from both mammography and MRI in the differentiation of benign versus malignant breast lesions as well as the abilities of these imaging techniques in addition to ultrasound to determine histologic tumor type and grade in those found to be malignant (Conti *et al.*, 2021). Collectively, through their thorough review of the literature the authors suggest that they believe it highly likely that radiomics signatures will be able to further classify patients based on likelihood of being diagnosed with a malignant tumor, thus potentially saving many women from unnecessary biopsies. Further, Abdollah *et al.* noted that radiomic features derived from T2 weighted MRI imaging were able to predict the Gleason score of patients with prostate cancer with a reasonable reliability (AUC 0.74) (Abdollahi *et al.*, 2019). While this, itself, does not provide evidence that ultimately would lead biopsies to be unnecessary, it again acts as a proof of concept with potential clinical relevance in the setting of prebiopsy MRIs in which such an ability could help to risk stratify patients regarding urgency or necessity of obtaining a subsequent tissue diagnosis.

As with the other aspects of radiomics previously described in this chapter, the concept of utilizing radiomics signatures in lieu of tissue level evaluation remains a hope of eventual clinical utility but is not yet ready for clinical application. However, as the landscape of oncology diagnosis and treatment continues to evolve, becoming ever more complex as we gain further understanding regarding histologic and molecular heterogeneity of each disease, the importance of radiomics' potential in this regard is becoming ever more apparent. While, to date, this portion of radiomics research remains less robust than the use of radiomics for predicting patient prognosis or predicting/tracking treatment response, this ability to noninvasively differentiate clinically meaningful differences within specific diagnoses likely represents the greatest promise of radiomics of all.

5. Artificial Intelligence in the Development of Clinically Focused Radiomics Signatures

Similar to the discussion regarding the field of radiomics as a whole across each of the four potential avenues of clinical utility, concise assessment of the role that artificial intelligence has played in the development of radiologic signatures to date is hobbled by an extreme lack of uniformity in methods used as well as the clarity of the written manuscripts. In total, of the 64 manuscripts referenced in this book chapter, a total of 20 clearly state that analytical methods using artificial intelligence were utilized in their productions with the remainder either using more conventional techniques or being unclear in the exact techniques used.

Of the studies that clearly discussed artificial intelligence methods utilized, exact methods used were again quite heterogeneous. In general, fewer studies utilized deep learning methods (examples: Liu *et al.*, 2021; Song *et al.*, 2021) than did various methods of supervised or unsupervised machine learning. Notably, when deep learning through a convolutional neural network was compared to machine learning using random forest, the latter emerged victorious in the assessment of treatment response in bladder tumors (Cha *et al.*, 2017). Of the studies that undertook various methods of machine learning for production of their radiomics signatures, several reported on a single method being used with the majority using random forest (Sutton *et al.*, 2020; Zhou *et al.*, 2020; Li *et al.*, 2020). Others, however, utilized multiple methods of machine learning in parallel and then chose whichever method provided the best performance for their final signature optimization (Ammari *et al.*, 2021; Chang *et al.*, 2021; Quiaoit *et al.*, 2020; Zhu *et al.*, 2021). In these settings, either random forest or support vector machine consistently beat out the other methods such as k-nearest neighbor and logistic regression, suggesting that these may be the most robust methods for development of further radiomics signatures going forward.

6. Conclusions and Future Directions

As discussed above, research into the clinical utility of radiomics, particularly with regards to patient prognostication, choice of treatment, and tracking treatment response, is simultaneously relatively robust and yet still in its infancy. Currently, the literature to date should be considered a general proof of concept that, with each subsequent publication, it is becoming increasingly proven. At this point, there is little doubt that the vast amounts of information derived through routine clinical imaging that is, otherwise, not clinically apparent hides within it many secrets that will improve our abilities to treat and observe our future patients. In this regard, the field of radiomics is both exciting and deserving of significant future investigations.

However, upon looking at the current literature collectively and with a critical eye, it is equally apparent that no current study has provided a clinically actionable tool that is useful outside of very specific contexts. While each study has sought to provide the most optimized radiomics signature within its specific data sets, the generalizability of these signatures, or even individual features within them, across different patient populations remains a mystery. Even in studies looking to answer highly similar questions, the consistency of the predictive abilities of specific radiomic signatures and the robustness of specific radiomics features across different images and physiologic contexts is unknown. As such, two separate research pathways must be followed going forward to bring the clinical promise of radiomics to fruition. (1) the most promising radiomic signatures with regards to predictive accuracy and clinical impact must be validated across multiple unrelated data sets to prove their abilities to be extrapolated to the studied populations as a whole and (2) the understanding of radiogenomics must be further improved to provide a better comprehension of what specific radiomics features represent at a histological, cellular, and subcellular level. With this, individual radiomics features with the greatest likely clinical impact and consistency across individual patients can be thoughtfully selected for future investigations. Of additional and near equal importance, establishment of the most consistently reliable methods for development of radiomics models, particularly those using artificial intelligence via either machine learning or deep learning, is required to improve efficiency and provide a framework for best practices in future projects.

Table 1. There are four primary areas of clinical promise for radiomics in cancer, including acting as an adjunct for patient prognosis, predicting treatment response, tracking treatment response, and providing further histological or pathological information.

Individual Avenues of Clinical Promise for the Field of Radiomics		
Promise	***Explanation and Importance***	***Examples***
Adjunct to prognosis	Radiomics promises to provide more robust information regarding patient prognosis than is currently afforded by standard clinicopathologic features. This will ultimately help to inform decisions regarding treatment aggressiveness as well as nonmedical decision-making such as those regarding finances, home life, travel, etc.	– Predicting PFS and OS in glioblastoma (Oltra-Sastre *et al.*, 2019; Ammari *et al.*, 2021) – Predicting local recurrence of acoustic neuromas after SRS (Langenhuizen *et al.*, 2020) – Predicting development of metastases in locally advanced rectal cancer (Liu *et al.*, 2021) – Predicting DFS in NSCLC (Wang *et al.*, 2021) – Predicting DFS and OS in stomach cancer (Jiang *et al.*, 2018)
Predicting response to treatment	By providing better prediction with regards to response to various aspects of individual treatment regimens as well as the relative efficacies for specific treatment options when multiple options exist, radiomics promises to allow for greater personalization of treatments for individuals diagnosed with cancer based on an optimized balance between effectiveness and toxicity reduction.	– Predict pathologic response rate following neoadjuvant CRT in NSCLC (Khorami *et al.*, 2019) – Predicting pathologic response rate following neoadjuvant CRT in rectal cancer (Shayesteh *et al.*, 2019; Shaish *et al.*, 2020) – Predicting response to TACE in HCC (Zhao *et al.*, 2019) – Predicting response of breast cancer to neoadjuvant chemotherapy (DiCenzo *et al.*, 2020) – Predicting response to chemotherapy in Hodgkin lymphoma (Fan *et al.*, 2019)
Tracking treatment response	Enhanced assessment of treatment response, as potentially afforded by radiomics, may allow for more optimized decision-making regarding	– Predicting pathologic response and resectability after neoadjuvant chemotherapy in pancreas adenocarcinoma (Zhang *et al.*, 2021)

	overall treatment duration as well as both the need and candidacy for further treatments in patients with diseases that are difficult to assess using standard clinical and radiographic means.	– Predicting pCR after neoadjuvant CRT in rectal adenocarcinoma based on changes during the treatment (Cusumano 2021) – Predicting response to neoadjuvant chemotherapy in newly diagnosed breast cancer (Quiaoit *et al.*, 2020)
Providing histopathological information	As treatment decision-making becomes increasingly complex based on the presence/absence of specific individual mutations or epigenetic alterations within a tumor as well as the overall mutational burden of a malignancy, the cost with regards to both patient-associated morbidity due to increasing need for further biopsies for tissue analysis and financial cost to healthcare system increases. Radiomics may provide the ability to forego a portion of this histopathologic testing with the ability to predict mutational status/burden using imaging features alone.	– Predicting mutational status of EGFR and p53 in newly diagnosed NSCLC (Zhu *et al.*, 2021) – Predicting IDH mutation, MGMT methylation, and 1p19q codeletion status in newly diagnosed gliomas Jian *et al.*, 2021) – Predicting the presence of LVSI in newly diagnosed early-stage cervical cancer (Li *et al.*, 2021) – Predicting if a new breast lesion is malignant vs benign in nature as well as histopathologic features of malignant lesions (Conti *et al.*, 2021)

Note: PFS; progression-free survival, OS; overall survival, SRS; stereotactic radiosurgery, DFS; disease-free survival, NSCLC; non-small-cell lung cancer, CRT; chemoradiotherapy, TACE; trans-arterial chemoembolization, HCC; hepatocellular carcinoma, pCR; pathological complete response, LVSI; lympho-vascular space invasion.

References

Abdollahi, H., Mofid, B., Shiri, I., Razzaghdoust, A., Saadipoor, A., Mahdavi, A., Galandooz, H. M., & Mahdavi, S. R. (2019). Machine learning-based radiomic models to predict intensity-modulated radiation therapy response, Gleason score and stage in prostate cancer. *Radiology Medicine*, *124*(6), 555–567. https://doi.org/10.1007/s11547-018-0966-4. Epub 2019 Jan 3. PMID: 30607868.

Ammari, S., Sallé de Chou, R., Assi, T., Touat, M., Chouzenoux, E., Quillent, A., Limkin, E., Dercle, L., Hadchiti, J., Elhaik, M., Moalla, S., Khettab, M., Balleyguier, C., Lassau, N., Dumont, S., & Smolenschi, C. (2021). Machine-learning-based radiomics MRI model for survival prediction of recurrent glioblastomas treated with bevacizumab. *Diagnostics (Basel)*, *11*(7), 1263. https://doi.org/10.3390/diagnostics 11071263. PMID: 34359346; PMCID: PMC8305059.

Beig, N., Singh, S., Bera, K., Prasanna, P., Singh, G., Chen, J., Saeed Bamashmos, A., Barnett, A., Hunter, K., Statsevych, V., Hill, V. B., Varadan, V., Madabhushi, A., Ahluwalia, M. S., & Tiwari, P. Sexually dimorphic radiogenomic models identify distinct imaging and biological pathways that are prognostic of overall survival in glioblastoma. *Neuro Oncology*, *23*(2), 251–263. https://doi.org/10.1093/neuonc/noaa231. PMID: 33068415; PMCID: PMC7906064.

Bhatia, A., Birger, M., Veeraraghavan, H., Um, H., Tixier, F., McKenney, A. S., Cugliari, M., Caviasco, A., Bialczak, A., Malani, R., Flynn, J., Zhang, Z., Yang, T. J., Santomasso, B. D., Shoushtari, A. N., & Young, R. J. MRI radiomic features are associated with survival in melanoma brain metastases treated with immune checkpoint inhibitors. *Neuro Oncology*, *21*(12), 1578–1586. https://doi.org/10.1093/neuonc/noz141. PMID: 31621883; PMCID: PMC7145582.

Bian, T., Wu, Z., Lin, Q., Wang, H., Ge, Y., Duan, S., Fu, G., Cui, C., & Su, X. (2021). Radiomic signatures derived from multiparametric MRI for the pretreatment prediction of response to neoadjuvant chemotherapy in breast cancer. *British Journal of Radiology*, *93*(1115), 20200287. https://doi.org/10.1259/bjr.20200287. Epub 2020 Sep 2. Erratum in: Br J Radiol. 2021 Nov 19; bjr20200287c. PMID: 32822542; PMCID: PMC8519645.

Bos, P., van den Brekel, M. W. M., Gouw, Z. A. R., Al-Mamgani, A., Waktola, S., Aerts, H. J. W. L., Beets-Tan, R. G. H., Castelijns, J. A., & Jasperse, B. (2021). Clinical variables and magnetic resonance imaging-based radiomics predict human papillomavirus status of oropharyngeal cancer. *Head Neck*, *43*(2), 485–495. https://doi.org/10.1002/hed.26505. Epub 2020 Oct 7. PMID: 33029923; PMCID: PMC7821378.

Cha, K. H., Hadjiiski, L., Chan, H. P., Weizer, A. Z., Alva, A., Cohan, R. H., Caoili, E. M., Paramagul, C., & Samala, R. K. (2017). Bladder cancer treatment response assessment in CT using radiomics with deep-learning. *Scientific Report*, *7*(1), 8738. https://doi.org/10.1038/s41598-017-09315-w. PMID: 28821822; PMCID: PMC5562694.

Chang, R., Qi, S., Yue, Y., Zhang, X., Song, J., & Qian, W. (2021). Predictive radiomic models for the chemotherapy response in non-small-cell lung cancer based on computerized-tomography images. *Frontiers in Oncology*, *11*, 646190. https://doi.org/10.3389/fonc.2021.646190. PMID: 34307127; PMCID: PMC8293296.

Chen, Y. H., Lue, K. H., Chu, S. C., Chang, B. S., Wang, L. Y., Liu, D. W., Liu, S. H., Chao, Y. K., & Chan, S. C. (2019). Combining the radiomic features and traditional parameters of ^{18}F-FDG PET with clinical profiles to improve prognostic stratification in patients with esophageal squamous cell carcinoma treated with neoadjuvant chemoradiotherapy and surgery. *Annals of Nuclear Medicine*, *33*(9), 657–670. https://doi.org/10.1007/s12149-019-01380-7. Epub 2019 Jun 19. PMID: 31218571.

Chen, X., Chen, X., Yang, J., Li, Y., Fan, W., & Yang, Z. (2020). Combining dynamic contrast-enhanced magnetic resonance imaging and apparent diffusion coefficient maps for a radiomics nomogram to predict pathological complete response to neoadjuvant chemotherapy in breast cancer patients. *Journal of Computer Assisted Tomography*, *44*(2), 275–283. https://doi.org/10.1097/RCT.0000000000000978. PMID: 32004189.

Conti, A., Duggento, A., Indovina, I., Guerrisi, M., & Toschi, N. (2021). Radiomics in breast cancer classification and prediction. *Seminars in Cancer Biology*, *72*, 238–250. https://doi.org/10.1016/j.semcancer.2020.04.002. Epub 2020 May 1. PMID: 32371013.

Cui, Y., Yang, W., Ren, J., Li, D., Du, X., Zhang, J., & Yang, X. (2021). Prognostic value of multiparametric MRI-based radiomics model: Potential role for chemotherapeutic benefits in locally advanced rectal cancer. *Radiotherapy & Oncology*, *154*, 161–169. https://doi.org/10.1016/j.radonc.2020.09.039. Epub 2020 Sep 22. PMID: 32976874.

Cusumano, D., Meijer, G., Lenkowicz, J., Chiloiro, G., Boldrini, L., Masciocchi, C., Dinapoli, N., Gatta, R., Casà, C., Damiani, A., Barbaro, B., Gambacorta, M. A., Azario, L., De Spirito, M., Intven, M., & Valentini, V. (2021). A field strength independent MR radiomics model to predict pathological complete response in locally advanced rectal cancer. *Radiology Medicine*, *126*(3), 421–429. https://doi.org/10.1007/s11547-020-01266-z. Epub 2020 Aug 24. PMID: 32833198; PMCID: PMC7937600.

Cusumano, D., Boldrini, L., Yadav, P., Yu, G., Musurunu, B., Chiloiro, G., Piras, A., Lenkowicz, J., Placidi, L., Romano, A., De Luca, V., Votta, C., Barbaro, B., Gambacorta, M. A., Bassetti, M. F., Yang, Y., Indovina, L., & Valentini, V. (2021). Delta radiomics for rectal cancer response prediction using low field magnetic resonance guided radiotherapy: An external validation. *Physical Medicine*, *84*, 186–191. https://doi.org/10.1016/j.ejmp.2021.03.038. Epub 2021 Apr 23. PMID: 33901863.

Dercle, L., Lu, L., Schwartz, L. H., Qian, M., Tejpar, S., Eggleton, P., Zhao, B., & Piessevaux, H. (2020). Radiomics response signature for identification of metastatic colorectal cancer sensitive to therapies targeting EGFR pathway. *Journal of the National Cancer Institute*, *112*(9), 902–912. https://doi.org/10.1093/jnci/djaa017. PMID: 32016387; PMCID: PMC7492770.

DiCenzo, D., Quiaoit, K., Fatima, K., Bhardwaj, D., Sannachi, L., Gangeh, M., Sadeghi-Naini, A., Dasgupta, A., Kolios, M. C., Trudeau, M., Gandhi, S., Eisen, A., Wright, F., Look Hong, N., Sahgal, A., Stanisz, G., Brezden, C., Dinniwell, R., Tran, W. T., Yang, W., Curpen, B., & Czarnota, G. J. (2020). Quantitative ultrasound radiomics in predicting response to neoadjuvant chemotherapy in patients with locally advanced breast cancer: Results from multi-institutional study. *Cancer Medicine*, *9*(16), 5798–5806. https://doi.org/10.1002/cam4.3255. Epub 2020 Jun 29. PMID: 32602222; PMCID: PMC7433820.

Du, Q., Baine, M., Bavitz, K., McAllister, J., Liang, X., Yu, H., Ryckman, J., Yu, L., Jiang, H., Zhou, S., Zhang, C., & Zheng, D. (2019). Radiomic feature stability across 4D respiratory phases and its impact on lung tumor prognosis prediction. *PLoS One*, *14*(5), e0216480. https://doi.org/10.1371/journal.pone.0216480. PMID: 31063500; PMCID: PMC6504105.

Duan, C., Chaovalitwongse, W. A., Bai, F., Hippe, D. S., Wang, S., Thammasorn, P., Pierce, L. A., Liu, X., You, J., Miyaoka, R. S., Vesselle, H. J., Kinahan, P. E., Rengan, R., Zeng, J., & Bowen, S. R. (2020). Sensitivity analysis of FDG PET tumor voxel cluster radiomics and dosimetry for predicting mid-chemoradiation regional response of locally advanced lung cancer. *Physics in Medicine and Biology*, *65*(20), 205007. https://doi.org/10.1088/1361-6560/abb0c7. PMID: 33027064; PMCID: PMC7593986.

Fan, Y., Liu, Z., Hou, B., Li, L., Liu, X., Liu, Z., Wang, R., Lin, Y., Feng, F., Tian, J., & Feng, M. (2019). Development and validation of an MRI-based radiomic signature for the preoperative prediction of treatment response in patients with invasive functional pituitary adenoma. *European Journal of Radiology*, *121*, 108647. https://doi.org/10.1016/j.ejrad.2019.108647. Epub 2019 Sep 7. PMID: 31561943.

Giannini, V., Rosati, S., Defeudis, A., Balestra, G., Vassallo, L., Cappello, G., Mazzetti, S., De Mattia, C., Rizzetto, F., Torresin, A., Sartore-Bianchi, A., Siena, S., Vanzulli, A., Leone, F., Zagonel, V., Marsoni, S., & Regge, D. (2020). Radiomics predicts response of individual HER2-amplified colorectal cancer liver metastases in patients treated with HER2-targeted therapy. *International Journal of Cancer*, *147*(11), 3215–3223. https://doi.org/10.1002/ijc.33271. Epub 2020 Sep 14. PMID: 32875550.

Guha, A., Connor, S., Anjari, M., Naik, H., Siddiqui, M., Cook, G., & Goh, V. (2020). Radiomic analysis for response assessment in advanced head and neck cancers, a distant dream or an inevitable reality? A systematic review of the current level of evidence. *British Journal of Radiology*, *93*(1106), 20190496. https://doi.org/10.1259/bjr.20190496. Epub 2019 Nov 6. PMID: 31682155; PMCID: PMC7055439.

Guo, Z., Zhong, N., Xu, X., Zhang, Y., Luo, X., Zhu, H., Zhang, X., Wu, D., Qiu, Y., & Tu, F. (2021). Prediction of hepatocellular carcinoma response to transcatheter arterial chemoembolization: A real-world study based on non-contrast computed tomography radiomics and general image features. *Journal of Hepatocellular Carcinoma*, *8*, 773–782. https://doi.org/10.2147/JHC.S316117. PMID: 34277508; PMCID: PMC8277455.

Hilal, T., Covington, M., Kosiorek, H. E., Zwart, C., Ocal, I. T., Pockaj, B. A., Northfelt, D. W., & Patel, B. K. (2018). Breast MRI phenotype and background parenchymal enhancement may predict tumor response to neoadjuvant endocrine therapy. *Breast Journal*, *24*(6), 1010–1014. https://doi.org/10.1111/tbj.13101. Epub 2018 Jul 31. PMID: 30066421.

Huang, L., Chen, J., Hu, W., Xu, X., Liu, D., Wen, J., Lu, J., Cao, J., Zhang, J., Gu, Y., Wang, J., & Fan, M. (2019). Assessment of a radiomic signature developed in a general NSCLC cohort for predicting overall survival of ALK-positive patients with different treatment types. *Clinical Lung Cancer*, *20*(6), e638–e651. https://doi.org/10.1016/j.cllc.2019.05.005. Epub 2019 May 11. PMID: 31375452.

Jian, A., Jang, K., Manuguerra, M., Liu, S., Magnussen, J., & Di Ieva, A. (2021). Machine learning for the prediction of molecular markers in glioma on magnetic resonance imaging: A systematic review and meta-analysis. *Neurosurgery*, *89*(1), 31–44. https://doi.org/10.1093/neuros/nyab103. PMID: 33826716.

Jiang, Y., Chen, C., Xie, J., Wang, W., Zha, X., Lv, W., Chen, H., Hu, Y., Li, T., Yu, J., Zhou, Z., Xu, Y., & Li, G. (2018). Radiomics signature of computed tomography imaging for prediction of survival and chemotherapeutic benefits in gastric cancer. *EBioMedicine*, *36*, 171–182. https://doi.org/10.1016/j.ebiom.2018.09.007. Epub 2018 Sep 14. PMID: 30224313; PMCID: PMC6197796.

Khorrami, M., Jain, P., Bera, K., Alilou, M., Thawani, R., Patil, P., Ahmad, U., Murthy, S., Stephans, K., Fu, P., Velcheti, V., & Madabhushi, A. (2019). Predicting pathologic response to neoadjuvant chemoradiation in resectable stage III non-small cell lung cancer patients using computed tomography radiomic features. *Lung Cancer*, *135*, 1–9. https://doi.org/10.1016/j.lungcan.2019.06.020. Epub 2019 Jul 5. Erratum in: Lung Cancer. 2019 Oct; 136:156. PMID: 31446979; PMCID: PMC6711393.

Khorrami, M., Prasanna, P., Gupta, A., Patil, P., Velu, P. D., Thawani, R., Corredor, G., Alilou, M., Bera, K., Fu, P., Feldman, M., Velcheti, V., & Madabhushi, A. (2020). Changes in CT radiomic features associated with lymphocyte distribution predict overall survival and response to immunotherapy in non-small cell lung cancer. *Cancer Immunology Research*, *8*(1), 108–119. https://doi.org/10.1158/2326-6066.CIR-19-0476. Epub 2019 Nov 12. PMID: 31719058; PMCID: PMC7718609.

Kirienko, M., Cozzi, L., Antunovic, L., Lozza, L., Fogliata, A., Voulaz, E., Rossi, A., Chiti, A., & Sollini, M. (2018). Prediction of disease-free survival by the PET/CT radiomic signature in non-small cell lung cancer patients undergoing surgery. *European Journal of Nuclear Medicine and Molecular Imaging*, *45*(2), 207–217. https://doi.org/10.1007/s00259-017-3837-7. Epub 2017 Sep 24. PMID: 28944403.

Langenhuizen, P. P. J. H., Zinger, S., Leenstra, S., Kunst, H. P. M., Mulder, J. J. S., Hanssens, P. E. J., de With, P. H. N., & Verheul, J. B. (2020). Radiomics-based prediction of long-term treatment response of vestibular Schwannomas following stereotactic radiosurgery. *Otology & Neurotology*, *41*(10), e1321–e1327. https://doi.org/10.1097/MAO.0000000000002886. PMID: 33492808.

Larue, R. T. H. M., Klaassen, R., Jochems, A., Leijenaar, R. T. H., Hulshof, M. C. C. M., van Berge Henegouwen, M. I., Schreurs, W. M. J., Sosef, M. N., van Elmpt, W., van Laarhoven, H. W. M., & Lambin, P. (2018). Pre-treatment CT radiomics to predict three year overall survival following chemoradiotherapy of esophageal cancer. *Acta Oncology*, *57*(11), 1475–1481. https://doi.org/10.1080/0284186X.2018.1486039. Epub 2018 Aug 1. PMID: 30067421.

Li, Y., Liu, W., Pei, Q., Zhao, L., Güngör, C., Zhu, H., Song, X., Li, C., Zhou, Z., Xu, Y., Wang, D., Tan, F., Yang, P., & Pei, H. (2019). Predicting pathological complete response by comparing MRI-based radiomics pre- and postneoadjuvant radiotherapy for locally advanced rectal cancer. *Cancer Medicine*, *8*(17), 7244–7252. https://doi.org/10.1002/cam4.2636. Epub 2019 Oct 22. PMID: 31642204; PMCID: PMC6885895.

Li, Z. Y., Wang, X. D., Li, M., Liu, X. J., Ye, Z., Song, B., Yuan, F., Yuan, Y., Xia, C. C., Zhang, X., & Li, Q. (2020). Multi-modal radiomics model to predict treatment response to neoadjuvant chemotherapy for locally advanced rectal cancer. *World Journal of Gastroenterology*, *26*(19), 2388–2402. https://doi.org/10.3748/wjg.v26.i19.2388. PMID: 32476800; PMCID: PMC7243642.

Li, P., Wang, X., Xu, C., Liu, C., Zheng, C., Fulham, M. J., Feng, D., Wang, L., Song, S., & Huang, G. (2020). ^{18}F-FDG PET/CT radiomic predictors of pathologic Complete Response (pCR) to neoadjuvant chemotherapy in breast cancer patients. *European Journal of Nuclear Medicine and Molecular Imaging*, *47*(5), 1116–1126. https://doi.org/10.1007/s00259-020-04684-3. Epub 2020 Jan 25. PMID: 31982990.

Li, X., Xu, C., Yu, Y., Guo, Y., & Sun, H. (2021). Prediction of lymphovascular space invasion using a combination of tenascin-C, cox-2, and PET/CT radiomics in patients with early-stage cervical squamous cell carcinoma. *BMC Cancer*, *21*(1), 866. https://doi.org/10.1186/s12885-021-08596-9. PMID: 34320931; PMCID: PMC8317359.

Liu, Z., Li, Z., Qu, J., Zhang, R., Zhou, X., Li, L., Sun, K., Tang, Z., Jiang, H., Li, H., Xiong, Q., Ding, Y., Zhao, X., Wang, K., Liu, Z., & Tian, J. (2019). Radiomics of multiparametric MRI for pretreatment prediction of pathologic complete response to neoadjuvant chemotherapy in breast cancer: A multicenter study. *Clinical Cancer Research*, *25*(12), 3538–3547. https://doi.org/10.1158/1078-0432.CCR-18-3190. Epub 2019 Mar 6. PMID: 30842125.

Liu, X., Zhang, D., Liu, Z., Li, Z., Xie, P., Sun, K., Wei, W., Dai, W., Tang, Z., Ding, Y., Cai, G., Tong, T., Meng, X., & Tian, J. (2021). Deep learning radiomics-based prediction of distant metastasis in patients with locally advanced rectal cancer after neoadjuvant chemoradiotherapy: A multicentre study. *EBioMedicine*, *69*, 103442. https://doi.org/10.1016/j.ebiom.2021.103442. Epub 2021 Jun 20. PMID: 34157487; PMCID: PMC8237293.

Lue, K. H., Wu, Y. F., Liu, S. H., Hsieh, T. C., Chuang, K. S., Lin, H. H., & Chen, Y. H. (2020). Intratumor heterogeneity assessed by ^{18}F-FDG PET/CT predicts treatment response and survival outcomes in patients with Hodgkin Lymphoma. *Academic Radiology*, *27*(8), e183–e192. https://doi.org/10.1016/j.acra.2019.10.015. Epub 2019 Nov 21. PMID: 31761665.

Luo, H. S., Huang, S. F., Xu, H. Y., Li, X. Y., Wu, S. X., & Wu, D. H. (2020). A nomogram based on pretreatment CT radiomics features for predicting complete response to chemoradiotherapy in patients with esophageal squamous cell cancer. *Radiation Oncology*, *15*(1), 249. https://doi.org/10.1186/s13014-020-01692-3. PMID: 33121507; PMCID: PMC7597023.

Nougaret, S., McCague, C., Tibermacine, H., Vargas, H. A., Rizzo, S., & Sala, E. (2021). Radiomics and radiogenomics in ovarian cancer: A literature review. *Abdominal* Radiology *(NY)*, *46*(6), 2308–2322. https://doi.org/10.1007/s00261-020-02820-z. Epub 2020 Nov 11. PMID: 33174120.

Oltra-Sastre, M., Fuster-Garcia, E., Juan-Albarracin, J., Sáez, C., Perez-Girbes, A., Sanz-Requena, R., Revert-Ventura, A., Mocholi, A., Urchueguia, J., Hervas, A., Reynes, G., Font-de-Mora, J., Muñoz-Langa, J., Botella, C., Aparici, F., Marti-Bonmati, L., & Garcia-Gomez, J. M. (2019). Multi-parametric MR imaging biomarkers associated to clinical outcomes in gliomas: A systematic review. *Current Medical Imaging Reviews*, *15*(10), 933–947. https://doi.org/10.2174/1573405615666190109100503. PMID: 32008521.

Park, S. H., Hahm, M. H., Bae, B. K., Chong, G. O., Jeong, S. Y., Na, S., Jeong, S., & Kim, J. C. (2020). Magnetic resonance imaging features of tumor and lymph node to predict clinical outcome in node-positive cervical cancer: A retrospective analysis. *Radiation Oncology*, *15*(1), 86. https://doi.org/10.1186/s13014-020-01502-w. PMID: 32312283; PMCID: PMC7171757.

Parr, E., Du, Q., Zhang, C., Lin, C., Kamal, A., McAlister, J., Liang, X., Bavitz, K., Rux, G., Hollingsworth, M., Baine, M., & Zheng, D. (2020). Radiomics-based outcome prediction for pancreatic cancer following stereotactic body radiotherapy. *Cancers (Basel)*, *12*(4), 1051. https://doi.org/10.3390/cancers12041051. PMID: 32344538; PMCID: PMC7226523.

Quiaoit, K., DiCenzo, D., Fatima, K., Bhardwaj, D., Sannachi, L., Gangeh, M., Sadeghi-Naini, A., Dasgupta, A., Kolios, M. C., Trudeau, M., Gandhi, S., Eisen, A., Wright, F., Look-Hong, N., Sahgal, A., Stanisz, G., Brezden, C., Dinniwell, R., Tran, W. T., Yang, W., Curpen, B., & Czarnota, G. J. (2020). Quantitative ultrasound radiomics for therapy response monitoring in patients with locally advanced breast cancer: Multi-institutional study results. *PLoS One*, *15*(7), e0236182. https://doi.org/10.1371/journal.pone.0236182. PMID: 32716959; PMCID: PMC7384762.

Shaish, H., Aukerman, A., Vanguri, R., Spinelli, A., Armenta, P., Jambawalikar, S., Makkar, J., Bentley-Hibbert, S., Del Portillo, A., Kiran, R., Monti, L., Bonifacio, C., Kirienko, M., Gardner, K. L., Schwartz, L., & Keller, D. (2020). Radiomics of MRI for pretreatment prediction of pathologic complete response, tumor regression grade, and neoadjuvant rectal score in patients with locally advanced rectal cancer undergoing neoadjuvant chemoradiation: An international multicenter study. *European Radiology*, *30*(11), 6263–6273. https://doi.org/10.1007/s00330-020-06968-6. Epub 2020 Jul 14. PMID: 32500192.

Shayesteh, S. P., Alikhassi, A., Fard Esfahani, A., Miraie, M., Geramifar, P., Bitarafan-Rajabi, A., & Haddad, P. (2019). Neo-adjuvant chemoradiotherapy response prediction using MRI based ensemble learning method in rectal cancer patients. *Physical Medicine*, *62*, 111–119. https://doi.org/10.1016/j.ejmp.2019.03.013. Epub 2019 May 15. PMID: 31153390.

Shi, L., Rong, Y., Daly, M., Dyer, B., Benedict, S., Qiu, J., & Yamamoto, T. (2020). Cone-beam computed tomography-based delta-radiomics for early response assessment in radiotherapy for locally advanced lung cancer. *Physics in Medicine and Biology*, *65*(1), 015009. https://doi.org/10.1088/1361-6560/ab3247. PMID: 31307024.

Song, J., Wang, L., Ng, N. N., Zhao, M., Shi, J., Wu, N., Li, W., Liu, Z., Yeom, K. W., & Tian, J. (2020). Development and validation of a machine learning model to explore tyrosine kinase inhibitor response in patients with stage IV EGFR variant-positive non-small cell lung cancer. *JAMA Network Open*, *3*(12), e2030442. https://doi.org/10.1001/jamanetworkopen.2020.30442. Erratum in: JAMA Netw Open. 2021 Feb 1;4(2):e211634. PMID: 33331920; PMCID: PMC7747022.

Sutton, E. J., Onishi, N., Fehr, D. A., Dashevsky, B. Z., Sadinski, M., Pinker, K., Martinez, D. F., Brogi, E., Braunstein, L., Razavi, P., El-Tamer, M., Sacchini, V., Deasy, J. O., Morris, E. A., & Veeraraghavan, H. (2020). A machine learning model that classifies breast cancer pathologic complete response on MRI post-neoadjuvant chemotherapy. *Breast Cancer Research*, *22*(1), 57. https://doi.org/10.1186/s13058-020-01291-w. PMID: 32466777; PMCID: PMC7254668.

Valentinuzzi, D., Vrankar, M., Boc, N., Ahac, V., Zupancic, Z., Unk, M., Skalic, K., Zagar, I., Studen, A., Simoncic, U., Eickhoff, J., & Jeraj, R. (2020). [18F]FDG PET immunotherapy radiomics signature (iRADIOMICS) predicts response of non-small-cell lung cancer patients treated with pembrolizumab. *Radiology & Oncology*, *54*(3), 285–294. https://doi.org/10.2478/raon-2020-0042. PMID: 32726293; PMCID: PMC7409607.

van Griethuysen, J. J. M., Lambregts, D. M. J., Trebeschi, S., Lahaye, M. J., Bakers, F. C. H., Vliegen, R. F. A., Beets, G. L., Aerts, H. J. W. L., & Beets-Tan, R. G. H. (2020). Radiomics performs comparable to morphologic assessment by expert radiologists for prediction of response to neoadjuvant chemoradiotherapy on baseline staging MRI in rectal cancer. *Abdominal Radiology (NY)*, *45*(3), 632–643. https://doi.org/10.1007/s00261-019-02321-8. PMID: 31734709.

Wang, X., Kong, C., Xu, W., Yang, S., Shi, D., Zhang, J., Du, M., Wang, S., Bai, Y., Zhang, T., Chen, Z., Ma, Z., Wang, J., Dong, G., Sun, M., Yin, R., & Chen F. (2019). Decoding tumor mutation burden and driver mutations in early stage lung adenocarcinoma using CT-based radiomics signature. *Thoracic Cancer*, *10*(10), 1904–1912. https://doi.org/10.1111/1759-7714.13163. Epub 2019 Aug 14. PMID: 31414580; PMCID: PMC6775017.

Wang, P. P., Deng, C. L., & Wu, B. (2021). Magnetic resonance imaging-based artificial intelligence model in rectal cancer. *World Journal of Gastroenterology*, *27*(18),

2122–2130. https://doi.org/10.3748/wjg.v27.i18.2122. PMID: 34025068; PMCID: PMC8117733.

Wang, J. H., Wahid, K. A., van Dijk, L. V., Farahani, K., Thompson, R. F., & Fuller, C. D. (2021). Radiomic biomarkers of tumor immune biology and immunotherapy response. *Clinical and Translational Radiation Oncology*, *28*, 97–115. https://doi.org/10.1016/j.ctro.2021.03.006. PMID: 33937530; PMCID: PMC8076712.

Wu, M., Zhang, Y., Zhang, Y., Liu, Y., Wu, M., & Ye, Z. (2019). Imaging-based biomarkers for predicting and evaluating cancer immunotherapy response. *Radiology Imaging Cancer*, *1*(2), e190031. https://doi.org/10.1148/rycan.2019190031. PMID: 33778682; PMCID: PMC7983749.

Yang, Z., He, B., Zhuang, X., Gao, X., Wang, D., Li, M., Lin, Z., & Luo, R. (2019). CT-based radiomic signatures for prediction of pathologic complete response in esophageal squamous cell carcinoma after neoadjuvant chemoradiotherapy. *Journal of Radiation Research*, *60*(4), 538–545. https://doi.org/10.1093/jrr/rrz027. PMID: 31111948; PMCID: PMC6640907.

Yuan, Z., Frazer, M., Zhang, G. G., Latifi, K., Moros, E. G., Feygelman, V., Felder, S., Sanchez, J., Dessureault, S., Imanirad, I., Kim, R. D., Harrison, L. B., Hoffe, S. E., & Frakes, J. M. (2020). CT-based radiomic features to predict pathological response in rectal cancer: A retrospective cohort study. *Journal of Medical Imaging and Radiation Oncology*, *64*(3), 444–449. https://doi.org/10.1111/1754-9485.13044. Epub 2020 May 9. PMID: 32386109.

Zhang, N., Liang, R., Gensheimer, M. F., Guo, M., Zhu, H., Yu, J., Diehn, M., Loo, B. W. Jr, Li, R., & Wu, J. (2020). Early response evaluation using primary tumor and nodal imaging features to predict progression-free survival of locally advanced non-small cell lung cancer. *Theranostics*, *10*(25), 11707–11718. https://doi.org/10.7150/thno.50565. PMID: 33052242; PMCID: PMC7546006.

Zhang, Y., Huang, Z. X., & Song, B. (2021). Role of imaging in evaluating the response after neoadjuvant treatment for pancreatic ductal adenocarcinoma. *World Journal of Gastroenterology*, *27*(22), 3037–3049. https://doi.org/10.3748/wjg.v27.i22.3037. PMID: 34168406; PMCID: PMC8192284.

Zhao, L., Gong, J., Xi, Y., Xu, M., Li, C., Kang, X., Yin, Y., Qin, W., Yin, H., & Shi, M. (2020). MRI-based radiomics nomogram may predict the response to induction chemotherapy and survival in locally advanced nasopharyngeal carcinoma. *European Radiology*, *30*(1), 537–546. https://doi.org/10.1007/s00330-019-06211-x. Epub 2019 Aug 1. PMID: 31372781.

Zhong, J., Hu, Y., Si, L., Jia, G., Xing, Y., Zhang, H., & Yao, W. (2021). A systematic review of radiomics in osteosarcoma: Utilizing radiomics quality score as a tool promoting clinical translation. *European Radiology*, *31*(3), 1526–1535. https://doi.org/10.1007/s00330-020-07221-w. Epub 2020 Sep 2. PMID: 32876837.

Zhou, X., Yi, Y., Liu, Z., Cao, W., Lai, B., Sun, K., Li, L., Zhou, Z., Feng, Y., & Tian, J. (2019). Radiomics-based pretherapeutic prediction of non-response to neoadjuvant therapy in locally advanced rectal cancer. *Annals of Surgical Oncology*, *26*(6), 1676–1684. https://doi.org/10.1245/s10434-019-07300-3. Epub 2019 Mar 18. PMID: 30887373; PMCID: PMC6510882.

Zhou, J., Lu, J., Gao, C., Zeng, J., Zhou, C., Lai, X., Cai, W., & Xu, M. (2020). Predicting the response to neoadjuvant chemotherapy for breast cancer: Wavelet transforming radiomics in MRI. *BMC Cancer*, *20*(1), 100. https://doi.org/10.1186/s12885-020-6523-2. PMID: 32024483; PMCID: PMC7003343.

Zhu, Y., Guo, Y. B., Xu, D., Zhang, J., Liu, Z. G., Wu, X., Yang, X. Y., Chang, D. D., Xu, M., Yan, J., Ke, Z. F., Feng, S. T., & Liu, Y. L. A Computed Tomography (CT)-derived radiomics approach for predicting primary co-mutations involving *TP53* and Epidermal Growth Factor Receptor (*EGFR*) in patients with advanced Lung Adenocarcinomas (LUAD). *Annals of Translational Medicine*, *9*(7), 545. https://doi.org/10.21037/atm-20-6473. PMID: 33987243; PMCID: PMC8105857.

Chapter 14

How AI can Help us Understand and Mitigate Error Propagation in Radiation Oncology

Ed Kline* and Srijan Sengupta†

*RadPhysics Services LLC, Albuquerque NM, USA
†North Carolina State University, Raleigh NC, USA

Abstract

The treatment workflow in radiation oncology involves a long chain of clinical and technical steps involving numerous subsystems, multiple vendors, and a variety of medical professionals. This complex workflow must be further customized for individual patients whose tumor size and locations can change during treatment. Therefore, medical errors can occur, and, crucially, such errors can propagate to future steps unless detected and addressed immediately. Understanding this error propagation is key to proactive error management. This chapter aims to discuss these issues and to provide guidelines toward an artificial intelligence (AI)-based analytical framework to analyze structured and unstructured incident reports. Such an analytical framework can be used to model error propagation and proactively identify points of weakness in radiation oncology pathways. Incorporating statistical learning and AI tools in this model may preemptively identify errors or trends in errors and suggest actions to prevent their recurrence.

1. Introduction

The Institute of Medicine (IOM), an authority at the intersection of medicine and society, released a report titled "To Err is Human: Building a Safer Health System" in November 1999. Its goal was to break the cycle of inaction regarding medical errors by advocating a comprehensive approach to improving patient safety. Based on two studies [conducted in 1984 and 1992], the IOM concluded that between 44,000 and 98,000 patients die every year in United States (U.S.) hospitals due to medical errors. Costs alone from medical errors were approximately $37.6 billion per year. About $17 billion were associated with preventable errors (Kohn *et al.*, 2000). Given the intense level of public and scientific reaction to the report, various stakeholders responded swiftly to take action. In February 2000, President Clinton announced a national action plan to reduce preventable medical errors by fifty percent within five years.[1] Congress mandated the monitoring of progress in preventing patient harm. In July 2004, a Healthgrades Quality Study asserted that IOM had in fact vastly underestimated the number of deaths due to medical errors, citing 195,000 deaths per year (Smith, 2005). In September 2013, a study covering the period 2008–2011 estimated preventable medical errors leading to patient deaths at 210,000 to 400,000 each year (James, 2013). Of $2.5 trillion spent on domestic healthcare costs in 2009, $765 billion (or 30%) was attributed to preventable errors (Olsen *et al.*, 2010). In May 2016, Johns Hopkins released a study suggesting more than 250,000 deaths per year were due to medical errors in the U.S. This figure made medical errors the third leading cause of death in the U.S. (Makary & Daniel, 2016). Today, preventable deaths due to medical errors are 10 times higher than the IOM estimate based on quality-adjusted life years. A 2012 study estimated that preventable medical errors may cost the U.S. economy up to $1 trillion in lost human potential and contributions (Andel *et al.*, 2012).

[1] https://clintonwhitehouse4.archives.gov/textonly/WH/New/html/20000222_1.html.

Government regulations have flourished in an attempt to reduce medical errors. Federal and state legislation was passed to establish safety standards and deter bad performance of healthcare providers. Medical providers and healthcare organizations spend significant resources and money to comply with federal quality and safety requirements to avoid civil penalties and reduced insurance reimbursement. A number of federal agencies and regulations[2] were created to promote quality of care and patient safety:

(1) The Healthcare Research and Quality Act required the Agency for Healthcare Research and Quality (AHRQ) to support research and build private–public partnerships,[3]
(2) The Patient Safety and Quality Improvement Act required patient safety organizations in each state to collect data and report on medical errors,[4]
(3) Patient safety advisory groups were created to promote patient safety,[5]
(4) The Joint Commission (JC) revised standards required all accredited hospitals to implement ongoing medical error reduction programs (Frankel *et al.*, 2013),
(5) A sentinel event policy was created requiring the identification of sentinel events, preventative actions, root cause analysis, and action plans (Levinson & General, 2010),
(6) The National Quality Foundation announced a list of serious ("never") reportable events where state federal insurance programs no longer reimburse providers for events (Editorial Board, 2009), and

[2] American Association of Physicists in Medicine. Government affairs: State Regulations and Licensure. http://aapm.org/government_affairs/licensure/default.asp. Accessed November 20, 2018.

American Society of Radiologic Technologists. Individual State Licensure Information. www.asrt.org/main/standards-regulations/state-legislative-affairs/individual-state-licensure-info. Accessed February 7, 2018.

[3] https://www.ahrq.gov/cpi/about/profile/index.html.

[4] https://www.hhs.gov/hipaa/for-professionals/patient-safety/statute-and-rule/index.html.

[5] https://www.nashp.org/state-patient-safety-centers-new-approach-promote-patient-safety/.

(7) AHRQ established safety indicators[6] while JC announced unannounced on-site evaluations.[7]

More recently, regulations were enacted that affect the finances of the hospital or healthcare provider. Under the Health Insurance Marketplace Quality Initiatives–Patient Protection and Affordable Care Act, health plan insurers are required to verify that hospitals use a Patient Safety Evaluation System (PSES) or else the Center for Medicare & Medicaid Services (CMS) will not reimburse the hospital for medical expenses.[8] The government also introduced incentives for providing better quality and patient safety. CMS announced quality incentives such as "Pay-for-Performance" and Physician Quality Reporting Initiative (PQRI) to reward good performance in the form of financial reward.[9] These incentives have further taken root in today's marketplace under the Medicare Access and CHIP Reauthorization Act of 2015 (MACRA) and Quality Payment Program (QPP) where CMS ties payments to quality and value. Financial penalties (–4 to –9%) and bonuses (+4 to +9%) apply in this program under the Merit-based Incentive Payment System (MIPS).[10] Further CMS proposed the Radiation Oncology (RO) Model to test whether prospective episode-based payments to designated providers reduce CMS expenditures while preserving or enhancing the quality of care for Medicare recipients. The RO Model would qualify as an Advanced Alternative Payment Model (Advanced APM) and a MIPS APM under the CMS QPP.[11]

Despite numerous regulations, resources, training courses, webinars, and standards, certain sentinel events continue to occur with alarming frequency. And although there has been an intense focus over two decades

---

[6] https://www.ahrq.gov/sites/default/files/publications/files/advancing-patient-safety.pdf.
[7] https://www.jointcommission.org/-/media/08c0024441f54848b8c212dd0b5dbeff.ashx.
[8] https://www.govinfo.gov/content/pkg/FR-2016-03-08/pdf/2016-04439.pdf.
[9] https://www.hhs.gov/guidance/document/provider-inquiry-assistance-program-overview-2010-physician-quality-reporting-initiative.
[10] https://go.cms.gov/QualityPaymentProgram.
[11] https://innovation.cms.gov/innovation-models/radiation-oncology-model.

to improve safety of medicine in the U.S., it appears little if any improvement has been made (Farokhzadian *et al.*, 2018).

2. Patient Safety in Radiation Oncology

The goal of radiation therapy is to deliver prescribed doses of lethal radiation as precisely as possible to the tumor while sparing the surrounding healthy tissue. Dosimetric benefits of precision radiotherapy allow for improved treatment quality in managing different cancer types such as breast, prostate, lung, head and neck, brain, and others. Focused radiotherapy is used for neuro-oncological applications such as radiation-based neuromodulation in treating cardiac tissue (ventricular tachycardia), trigeminal neuralgia (pain relief), and medically refractory Essential Tremor (movement disorder).

Radiotherapy treatment involves a long chain of specialized activities customized for individual patients whose tumor size and locations can change during treatment. This process can consist of as many as 300 or more steps involving numerous subsystems from multiple vendors and medical staff (e.g., radiation oncologist, nurses, dosimetrists, physicists, and administrative personnel). The specialized computer systems and devices used in this process often transfer data digitally between different subsystems. Automatic data transfer between subsystems may reduce manual data entry errors; however, it does not eliminate data use and transfer errors as a whole. Complexity of the entire system connected with inherent trust of digital transfers may result in data transfer errors not being identified (Siochi *et al.*, 2011). Procedural intricacies of accurate and timely radiation treatment add to further risk of making errors. Yet, various periodic checks are often performed manually using paper and spreadsheets. Ensuring the quality of checks to identify errors in the entire treatment process is difficult as treatment complexity continues to evolve in radiotherapy environments.

Human contributing factors resulting in preventable errors are on par with some of the most notable diseases in terms of their negative impact on human health (Weintraub *et al.*, 2021). Reducing avoidable medical errors involving human and machine interactions in the field of radiation oncology is a high priority for a growing audience of stakeholders. In 2020, an estimated 1.8 million new cancer cases were diagnosed in the U.S. which is the equivalent of approximately 4,950 new cases each day (Siegel *et al.*, 2020). Further, in the U.S., approximately 50% of cancer patients receive radiation therapy as part of their care at one of 2,322 radiation therapy centers (Bajaj, 2020). From a worldwide perspective, cancer diagnosis is projected to increase by 80% in low-income countries compared to 40% in high-income countries through 2030.[12] The global radiotherapy market is projected to reach $11.5 billion by the end of 2027, growing at a CAGR (compounded annual growth rate) of 7.3%.[13] The need for safe and reliable treatments in radiation oncology will continue to grow in the U.S. and worldwide.

In the U.S., most current data in radiation oncology suggests that approximately 0.04–4.7% of patients undergoing radiation therapy experience some operational and clinical shortcoming. Approximately 0.003–0.01% experience some level of harm per treatment. Approximately 100 and 500 patients experience some harm annually in the U.S. and worldwide, respectively. This figure corresponds to approximately 6–100 serious events per million treatments, of which some lead to death (Howell *et al.*, 2019; Ford *et al.*, 2012). Although the associated risk of mistreatment is estimated to be rare, the consequences of an error may be high (Ford & Terezakis, 2010). However, according to a *New York Times* article published in January 2010, radiation therapy accidents are chronically underreported, and some states do not require any error reporting.[14]

A patient safety reporting system (PSRS) is a risk management platform for collecting, investigating, examining, and learning from safety matters related to near misses and incidents (Ford *et al.*, 2012; Hutchinson *et al.*, 2009; Mazur *et al.*, 2015; Ford & Evans, 2018). Over the past 15 years, professional groups, accrediting organizations, governments, and others have responded with the development of PSESs or similar reporting systems using public databases such as Manufacturer and User Facility Device Experience (MAUDE), Vaccine Adverse Event Reporting

[12] https://www.grandviewresearch.com/industry-analysis/tumor-ablation-market.
[13] https://www.grandviewresearch.com/industry-analysis/radiation-oncology-market.
[14] https://www.nytimes.com/2010/01/24/health/24radiation.html.

System (VAERS), and FDA Adverse Event Reporting System (FAERS). More specific to the field of radiation oncology, voluntary incident reporting systems have been created in the U.S. and various countries. Many of these reporting systems in the U.S. are local, home-grown programs. The broader goal in radiation oncology is to improve the safe planning and delivery of radiotherapy by sharing safety-related events and safety analysis within respective countries and around the world. The most prominently known reporting systems worldwide in radiation oncology are as follows:

- ASTRO: Radiation Oncology–Incident Learning System (RO-ILS) (US)
- Radiation Oncology Safety Education and Information System (ROSEIS)(IRL)
- International Atomic Energy Agency (IAEA): Safety in Radiation Oncology (SAFRON)(AUT)
- Radiotherapy Incident Reporting & Analysis System (RIRAS)(US)
- Relir Othea (FR)
- National Reporting and Learning System (NRLS)(UK)
- National System for Incident Reporting in Radiation Therapy (NSIR-RT)(CAN).

Though progress has been made in identifying and correcting errors in radiation oncology pathways, significant weaknesses exist in PSRSs. Most if not all PSRSs are reactive reporting systems with limited flexibility and utilization. Errors are caught downstream, if at all (Mullins *et al.*, 2020; Mullins *et al.*, 2019; Ford *et al.*, 2009; Clark *et al.*, 2013). By the time users find the errors, they have already occurred and imparted their damaging effects. This strategy relies on hopes to stop the next types of similar errors from occurring by entering action plans typically using descriptors using free text. Further, there is no failure mode and effects analysis (FMEA) or comprehensive risk prioritization in these programs. Nor is there any automatic suggestion of corrective actions. Action plans do not drill down, nor do they offer a roadmap to correcting errors using credible root cause analysis (Rooney & Heuvel, 2004). If an adverse or medical event occurs that requires reporting to federal or state agencies in the U.S. or a country's regulatory authority, none of the PSRSs offer step-by-step guidance and reporting capabilities.[15] Barriers continue to exist in numerous PSRSs designed to promote a culture of safety and high reliability in radiation oncology. Open reporting culture is not acceptable. Fear of error is compounded by the manner in which error is investigated. The outcome inevitability results in an assessment of blame, blends liability with fault, and fails to promote a no-fault culture. In summary, local PSRSs are inadequate to investigate incidents, identify contributory factors, and implement and embed no-fault learning.[16] Large or enterprise reporting solutions benefit from collection of larger data pools and compilation of lessons learned; however, similar limitations plague their robust adoption and use.

The American Association of Physicists in Medicine (AAPM) looked at errors produced from failures in workflow and process in radiation oncology. AAPM Task Group 100 (TG-100) provided a systematic understanding of the likelihood and clinical impact of possible failures throughout a course of radiotherapy. TG-100 was designed to help effectively use limited quality management (QM) resources (Huq *et al.*, 2016). It established a framework for designing QM activities based on estimates of the probabilities of identified failures and their effect on the clinical process from radiotherapy planning to treatment delivery (Huq *et al.*, 2016). The strategies presented in TG-100 provide a mechanism to enhance quality and safety of patient care. Prospective QM techniques proposed by TG-100 include FMEA. FMEA provides a proactive approach to focus on identifying and addressing vulnerabilities before harm occurs. Simply stated, FMEA is a proactive, systematic method of identifying ways a process can go wrong and actions to address them (Spath, 2003).

A hazard analysis model known as System Theoretic Process Analysis (STPA) has been used to perform hazard analysis in radiation oncology (Pawlicki *et al.*, 2016). STPA uses a deductive hazard analysis method based on a Systems-Theoretic Accident Model and Process (STAMP). STAMP views safety as a system control problem rather than a component failure problem. STPA extends this model by detecting unsafe behaviors

[15] https://www.nrc.gov/reading-rm/doc-collections/cfr/part035/index.html.

[16] https://www.psqh.com/resource/the-cultural-cure-for-sentinel-events/

that can result in hazards and causal scenarios that identify the unsafe behavior.

TG-100, STPA, and other methodologies acknowledge the challenge in teaching a whole new way of thinking about quality and safety needs in relation to risk management. Buy-in and adoption of risk-based quality programs or hazard analysis techniques is difficult to establish and implement without proper tools. The historical, reactive approach to error mitigation and the challenging implementation of proactive methodologies makes it a key area for development of a predictive risk management tool. The complexity of the workflow makes this a difficult problem. Furthermore, errors can propagate from one step to the next in different care pathways. Hence, it is not only whether we can detect an error, but also, how quickly before they proceed downstream. A practical tool to foresee errors could improve patient safety, prevent errors, and drive efficiency in radiotherapy workflow.

3. The Radiation Oncology Workflow: Constructing a Reference Timeline

Predicting when and where errors occur in the entire treatment delivery process could provide an enhanced systematic understanding of risk management in patient safety and quality of care. Determining probability of failures in pathways could significantly help provide safe clinical workflows (Pillai *et al.*, 2019; Potters *et al.*, 2016; Weidlich & Weidlich, 2018; Chang *et al.*, 2017; Kalet *et al.*, 2015).

In our work, we chose to build upon an established, commercially available error reduction and regulatory compliance program called Medical Error Reduction Program (MERP©) (https://www.radphysics.com). MERP helps reduce preventable systems-related medical errors in radiation oncology. The MERP product is used in cancer center workflow to help minimize risk and improve patient safety by identifying errors, measuring improvement, and correcting causal factors with action plans. Errors are defined as failures in workflow or process to perform specific acts timely and/or correctly. Failures can include but are not limited to near misses, events, and violations. For our purposes, error data from multiple institutions were collected in MERP and fitted in various silos configured in the database. The silos comprise deep, multiple levels of categories. Each piece of data is characterized with specific identifiers and properties in the MERP database fields.

Figure 1 is a process tree that references a main timeline of steps in radiation oncology. The process tree works as an archetypical example for a typical patient undergoing external beam radiotherapy treatment. The temporal relationship between each step is shown from process start to end. Typical check points are shown on the main timeline. This main timeline represents a relative display of chronological events. It does not account for time from patient consultation to imaging (acquired before simulation) and diagnosis. The process tree shows the first part of this reference timeline for illustration. Here we do not show subsequent steps in the interest of space.

The bolded central arrow shows the entry of the patient into the process. The main steps are shown in bolded boxes along the central arrow.

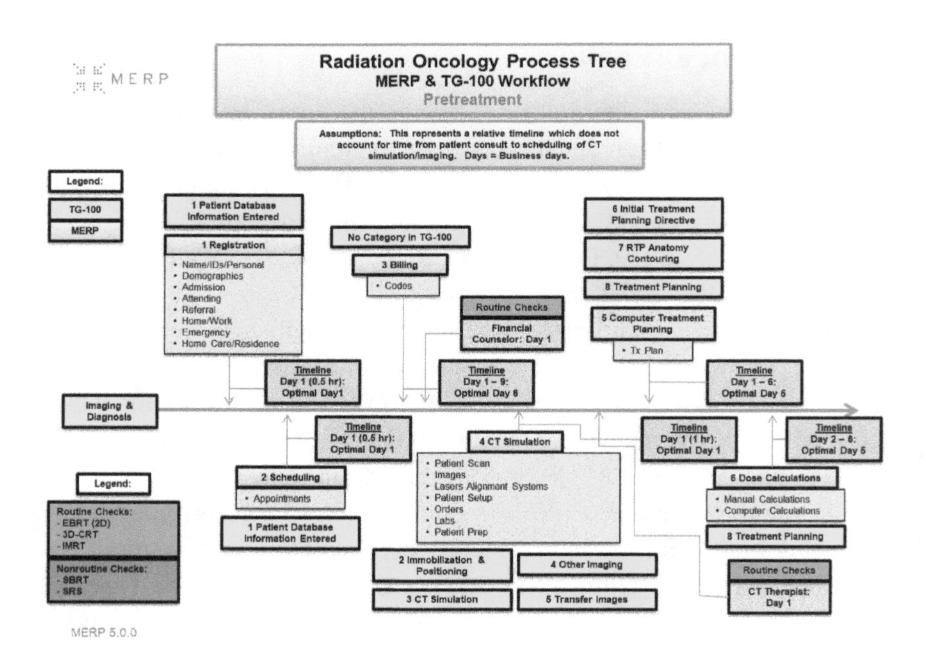

Fig. 1. A partial timeline of the different stages of the radiation oncology process.

Smaller vertical arrows point from each step to the central arrow. Each step is labeled with the step's name and a number representing the approximate chronological order of the step in the treatment process. Substeps show greater detail in regular boxes that appear below each step. Patient flow entering each step is shown with branches emerging horizontally from the smaller vertical arrows to boxes labeled "Step Time". Step Time boxes are bolded and show specific time intervals (a range of days with an optimal day) when the step should typically be performed in the treatment process. Typical checks (e.g., initial chart checks, dose calculation checks, etc.) for standard treatments (e.g., EBRT (2D), 3D-CRT, and IMRT) and non-routine checks for high-dose treatments (e.g., SBRT, SRS) along the main timeline are shown in bold boxes labeled "Routine Checks" and "Non-routine Checks", respectively. Each type of check shows the typical responsible individual who performs the check and when the check should generally be performed.

Key steps in our MERP process tree were compared to key steps in a process tree taken from TG-100 (Huq *et al.*, 2016) using color boxes. The orange shade boxes show steps and substeps in our MERP workflow. The yellow boxes show steps in the TG-100 workflow. The green shaded boxes in the MERP workflow show when steps should typically be performed. Routine and non-routine checks in MERP for standard treatments and high-dose treatments are shown in bright green and red shaded boxes, respectively. The lighter green shaded boxes under routine and non-routine checks in MERP show the responsible individual who performs the check and when the check should generally be performed in the process.

The process tree of steps in MERP compares favorably with similar steps in TG-100 and provides external validation of pathways used within our workflow. Steps in TG-100 (yellow boxes) matching similar steps in MERP (orange shaded boxes) are shown vertically in line with each other. For example, the step called "1 Patient Database Information Entered" in TG-100 matches similar steps called "1 Registration" and "2 Scheduling" in MERP. A comparison of remaining steps in TG-100 and MERP shows similar matches in both process trees.

The design and architecture of our MERP workflow expands the levels of "steps" and "substeps" found in the process tree into a deeper hierarchy of folders called "categories, subcategories, and attributes".

Pretreatment and posttreatment classifications were introduced, and new groupings called radiation safety, Quality Assurance (QA), and billing were added in MERP.

The MERP software design comprises a pre- and posttreatment timeline of 24 categories at level 1 hierarchy (first level of folders), 182 subcategories at level 2 hierarchy (second level of folders), and 1872 attributes at level 3 hierarchy. Each such category, subcategory, and attribute refers to the location where an error occurs in the radiotherapy process. When an error is identified (e.g., a particular task is not completed in a timely manner or correctly), the user (e.g., therapist, dosimetrist, physicist, physician, nurse, front desk, financial counselor, etc.) enters the error by selecting the error attribute from a hierarchy display of categories and subcategories that expand into various examples of error attributes. If the attribute is not shown on the list, a custom attribute may be created. When selecting or creating an error attribute, the MERP user selects the day of occurrence of the error (day when the error actually happened upstream) and the day when the error was identified (day when the error was found downstream). Note that at the time of this writing, MERP did not ask the user for the day of occurrence of the error. Natural language processing was subsequently used to derive this date from error data (discussed in what follows). Each attribute and location are mapped to the MERP database. Attributes are benchmarked against professional medical standards (e.g., American College of Radiology (ACR), American Society for Radiation Oncology (ASTRO), American College of Radiation Oncology (ACRO), etc.) and regulatory requirements (i.e., Conference of Radiation Control Directors, Inc. — Suggested State Regulations for the Control of Radiation, https://www.crcpd.org). MERP uses a scoring system (FMEA) and analyzes errors for which action plans (short- and long-term) are preconfigured and selected. New action plans can be created. Depending on the nature of the error, a Root Cause Analysis (RCA) can be performed to identify the causes of the event. MERP can launch dose analysis, sentinel event reports, and medical event reports for local and state reporting. Errors are routed through the network server to client workstations at the center level. Responsible parties are alerted to review and approve the proposed action plans. MERP allows for tracking, trending, and charting with dashboards and report writing capabilities. Procedures can be generated for action plans and retraining.

4. Creating a Prototype Statistical Model

To illustrate MERP, we created an error propagation model that models the likelihood that any single error is caught within a category and subcategory. The model would automatically flag potential high-risk failure points and errors in specific stages of the treatment, quality assurance, radiation safety, and billing processes before that specific process commences or proceeds downstream in the workflow. To illustrate our modeling strategy, we shall use an MERP data set from February 2006 to March 2008 with a total of 1121 error incidents. Each error incident has multiple fields, such as category level 1, category level 2, and attribute. The first two fields help us in determining the precise step in the radiation oncology process where the error was identified downstream. Furthermore, from each error incident we extracted two dates: (a) the date of error occurrence (the date when the error actually occurred upstream) from the free-text narrative (using natural language processing) and (b) the date of error detection downstream, which is assumed to be the same as the reporting date. Note the date when the error occurred upstream is the actual date when the incident took place in comparison to the date when the incident was subsequently discovered downstream. Any noted time difference between error detection and error reporting was kept at a minimum by daily oversight of error flow. The difference between the two dates described in (a) and (b) gives us the "detection lag" that passed between error occurrence and error detection.

Clearly, a large detection lag is problematic, as it implies that the error propagated for a long time before it was detected and a corrective action was taken. On the other hand, a small detection lag implies that the error was detected quickly. The most preferred outcome is that an error is detected on or during the first routine check. The next preferred outcome is that an error propagates undetected during the first routine check but gets detected on or during the second routine check. The worst possible outcome is that an error propagates undetected through both the first and second routine checks that were designed to catch it. To formalize this, we can flag each record with one of the following three labels:

1. Check 1: if detection lag is less than or equal to the gap between routine check 1 and day of occurrence
2. Check 2: if detection lag is greater than the gap between routine check 1 and day of occurrence, but less than or equal to gap between routine check 2 and day of occurrence
3. Neither: if detection lag is greater than the gap between routine check 2 and day of occurrence.

We now proceed to build a statistical model for error propagation with "flag" as the response variable and other fields as potential predictor/explanatory variables or features. Here, the "flag" variable is neither numeric nor categorical, but rather ordinal in nature. A "check 1" outcome is the best outcome, followed by "check 2", and "check 3" is the worst outcome. Therefore, we employ the ordered logit model, which is a well-known regression model for ordinal outcome variables. To analyze the full scope of the model, we consider a hierarchical framework that has three levels of aggregation:

(a) **Level-1 model** considers category-1 levels as the only explanatory variable,
(b) **Level-2 model** considers both category-1 and category-2 levels as the explanatory variables, and
(c) **Level-3 model** considers category-1 and category-2 levels as well as attributes and category-2 as the explanatory variables.

We fit these models using the Proportional Odds Logistic Regression (POLR) method in the statistical programming language, R. We briefly report the results from the level-1 and the level-2 models and skip further details in the interest of space.

Results for Level-1 model: We observed that the fitted probabilities show several interesting patterns. For example, errors related to patient docs/notes (e.g., documents or notes related to the patient's treatment) are very unlikely to be detected by either the first (2.4%) or the second check (9.6%). A similar observation holds for errors related to dose calculations (5.3% Check 1, 18.4% Check 2). On the other hand, errors related to registration (80.8% Check 1, 15.1% Check 2) and radiation safety (100% Check 1) are very likely to be detected within the first two checks. This helps us identify points of weakness and strength in the error detection process.

Results for Level-2 model: Now, we add level-2 categories in the mix. These results provide us with a deeper understanding of the error detection process. For example, from the level-1 model we saw that dose calculation errors are very likely to remain undetected, but the level-2 model tells us more — dose calculation errors related to computer calculations are quite likely to get detected, but others do not get detected in time. Thus, the level-2 model provides us with greater detail on the risk at various points of the radiation oncology treatment process. The following table shows a few selected results from this model.

Level-1 Category	**Level-2 Category**	**Check 1 (%)**	**Check 2 (%)**	**Neither (%)**
Scheduling (Appointments)	Appointments	89.0	7.5	3.5
Computer Treatment Planning	Treatment Plan	57.8	24.6	17.6
Dose Calculations	Computer Calculations	35.1	29.7	35.1
Treatment Delivery (Patient Setup)	Treatment Plan	12.2	19.9	67.9

This illustrative example shows the value of our modeling approach. The modeling framework is highly flexible and additional features (e.g., treatment stage, professional role, severity) can be easily integrated. By rigorously quantifying the risk patterns arising from various features we can objectively, efficiently, and effectively determine points of weakness in the care system.

5. Understanding Error Reporting Data in Our System: Past and Present

Figure 2 shows a simple example of a typical radiation oncology system with various subsystems and interfaces to external imaging, PACS, electronic medical record system, CT-simulation scanner, treatment planning system, record and verify system, linear accelerator, and other software services. Many of these systems may come from different vendors. These component subsystems from multiple manufacturers must communicate correctly for the safety and quality of treatment. Systematic errors could be a significant concern if communication flaws propagate undetected under a specific set of conditions. Data transfer is one of many error sources and can lead to poor productivity (Zietman *et al.*, 2012; Hendee & Herman, 2011; Siochi *et al.*, 2011). Efforts to improve data transfers are ongoing initiatives. Integrating Healthcare Enterprise – Radiation Oncology (IHE–RO)(https://aapm.org/IHERO/) is a non-profit organization and AAPM/ASTRO-sponsored initiative to develop a process of sharing data and a database standard for use cases to help eliminate issues with data transfers.

In our work, the error propagation model shows the likelihood that any single error is caught within a subsystem. For risk management, we are interested in analyzing the risk of failure to detect, which can be

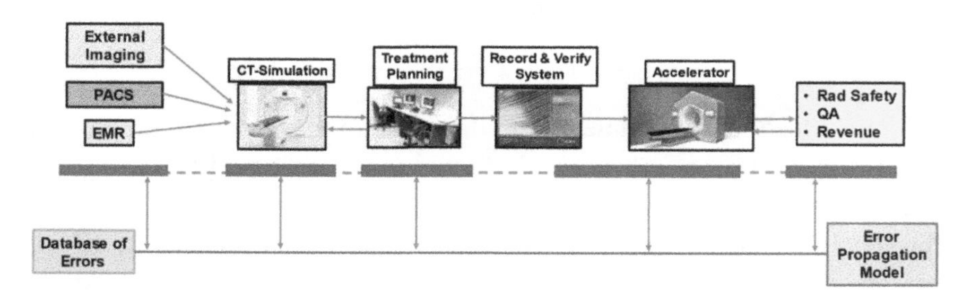

Fig. 2. Radiation oncology network system.

calculated as one minus the estimated probability from the statistical model that was previously discussed. Failures to detect errors at or before the first, second, and subsequent periodic checks are determined as a product of patient throughput. The primary subsystems of interest include external imaging, CT-simulation, treatment planning system, record and verify system, and linear accelerator. The secondary subsystems of interest include radiation safety (patient and worker regulatory compliance and safety), QA (quality requirements of machines, equipment, instruments, and clinical processes such as various physics and therapist checks, chart checks, chart rounds, etc.), and billing (charge capture for delivery of professional and technical services). As illustrated in the preceding section, by using MERP data collected from existing centers, our error propagation model recognizes which risk patterns exist for certain specific mixes of categories, subcategories, attributes, and subattributes at each stage.

6. Understanding Error Reporting Data: What's in the Future?

Upstream failure pathways influence workflow in all stages of the treatment delivery and task system (e.g., policies, procedures, schedules, checks). Corrective actions are often subjective to upstream latent failure pathways (contributory factors that may lie dormant for long periods of time) and active failure pathways (e.g., an error or oversight). Highly reliable organizations use this concept to identify latent and active failure pathways in their systems (Marks & Mazur, 2015). Identifying latent and active pathways of failure either in anticipation or before they occur can minimize and prevent errors and inefficiencies. Indications of a suspicious activity that falls outside the expected activity in one or more pathways can flag the action as a potential weakness or pending failure that will occur downstream at another point. Once a safety barrier (e.g., check point) is penetrated (error is detected), dependability in catching the error is compromised and risk of failure in the pathway increases. Measurable errors typically occur when one or more latent and active failure pathways intersect at some point downstream and proliferate through the treatment delivery process to cause a medical event or regulatory violation.

A tool that can provide a systematic understanding of the probability of an error occurring could measurably improve patient safety, compliance, and efficiency in the radiotherapy industry. Prospective identification of incidents in the treatment process could more effectively mitigate hazards and risks. Minimizing the probability of failure in quality assurance, radiation safety, and billing could expand the risk management model by tying verification of professional standards and regulatory compliance within the radiotherapy process.

An error propagation model can be very effective in radiation oncology if the model aims to integrate various subsystems from the perspective of error detection, error propagation, error reduction, and prevention. Ideally, the error propagation model would "sit" on top of various subsystems located in the clinical workflow process. The subsystem could interface with each machine or device by using an HL7 framework to exchange information. HL7 is a well-known standard for exchanging information between medical applications. The subsystem would let the error propagation model know the exact location where the patient or task resides in the overall clinical pathway.

The error propagation model can be designed to recognize which risk patterns exist for certain specific mixes of categories, subcategories, attributes, and subattributes at each stage. Because of this capability, the module could automatically flag potential high-risk failure points and true errors in specific stages of the treatment, radiation safety, QA, and billing processes before that specific process commences or proceeds downstream in the workflow. In the case of high-risk failure points, the alert can prompt the user if they want to evaluate the risk for potential corrective action or proceed to the next step. In the case of automatically flagging a predicted true error, risk could be automatically evaluated, assessed, and then scored for prioritization using FMEA. Scoring could be quantitatively expressed using a surrogate metric called the risk priority number. True errors of high severity could have a hard stop and warning deployed before allowing the user to proceed further in the process. The true error could next be routed for automatic processing of the corrective action plan. Escalation of any error to a status of high significance, such as sentinel event or medical event, could automatically launch a root cause analysis with reporting features.

In instances where the error propagation model does not catch the error but rather the user catches the error, the user could manually enter the error and action plan using a step-by-step roadmap provided in the error propagation model. In cases where a radiation oncology EMR system (i.e., record and verify) identifies an error as part of their verification checking process, the error propagation model could be alerted via an HL7 interface message and automatically capture the error. The same process could commence as described above. The error propagation model could ask if you want to correct the error before proceeding and allow for automatic processing of the corrective action plan.

The error propagation model could employ an automatic trigger tool developed that is powered by probability theory using sophisticated decision algorithms. Our approach to these algorithms is shown in what follows in the section "statistical modeling of error propagation". Dependability of the radiation therapy process could be the first function of the trigger tool. When a high-risk pattern presents, the trigger tool could automatically relay a notification to the user that a weak point or potential failure point has been identified. Error propagation model could have an automatic analytic and visualization system (dashboard) to display such results: (1) the estimated versus predicted "failure-to-detect" ratio for each checkpoint as a function of clinical stage within each subsystem for each patient in the treatment process, and (2) the estimated "failure-to-detect" ratios for each checkpoint displayed with a graduated color scale, ranging from a high to low, showing the chance of the error being detected. In our work, the estimated "failure-to-detect" ratio comes from existing MERP databases of errors. Predictability of dependability in process could be the second function of the trigger tool. In our work using MERP data and applying the predicted "failure-to-detect" ratio at each checkpoint based on patient volume at each clinical stage, one can predict near misses, probable hits, and direct hits. Thus, the estimated versus predicted "failure-to-detect" ratio can be determined for each stage. The automatic analytical and visualization system (dashboard) of the error propagation model could display the results: (1) pre and post-treatment errors produced, errors identified (caught), and errors missed by stages in the radiation therapy process; and (2) posttreatment errors that propagate through each stage and result in probable mistreatment of the patient.

With this knowledge, the error propagation model could perform two key roles in a real-time manner: (1) showing the effectiveness of checkpoints with both estimated and predicted "failure-to-detect" ratios for each stage within each subsystem, and (2) showing dependability of the radiation treatment process by targeting which errors propagate through stages of each subsystem and become near misses, probable hits, or direct hits. Confidence intervals for the "failure-to-detect" ratios can be adjusted on the fly for each clinical stage or combination of stages.

User validation for this process could be performed by comparing the estimated versus predicted "failure-to-detect" ratios at each checkpoint based on patient volume or tasks at each clinical stage. Prediction of process dependability is determined by using actual MERP data consisting of total error data and applying the predicted "failure-to-detect" ratio at each checkpoint. Based on patient volume at each clinical stage, one can make comparisons between predicting and recording near misses, probable hits, and direct hits. In addition, use cases with embedded errors could be sent through the pathways and error propagation model to measure the accuracy of the model in detecting errors.

Statistical regression modeling of past errors can help us identify the contributing factors and points of weakness in the treatment workflow. This is useful for understanding patterns and systematic issues at an operational level. In addition to this, it is also desirable to develop an automated tool to analyze individual incident reports, which are in the form of free-text narratives. In the next section, we cover this topic and outline current research as well as future directions.

7. Envisioning an AI-powered Error Mitigation System

Medical errors have traditionally been reported as free-text descriptions, which naturally results in a variety of responses as reporters use different levels of detail and types of vocabulary, and might have conflicting perspectives regarding the error itself. When the process was examined, one of the primary barriers to error reporting was the perspective on errors themselves (Soydemir *et al.*, 2017). Given these problems associated with the analysis of error reports and the process of error reporting itself, machine learning, specifically the branch of machine learning that deals with human language and speech — Natural Language Processing (NLP) — has become a key tool in the development of ways to improve error detection, reporting, and classification/analysis. Previous studies have demonstrated the ability of convolutional neural networks and multi-class classification models to accurately categorize errors and illuminate patterns in medical text (Young *et al.*, 2019; Yahia *et al.*, 2021).

One of the key benefits that NLP models have to offer for medical personnel and staff is the reduction in time required to report medical errors by streamlining the process and removing the need for reporters to essentially predict what caused the error despite their limited perspective. In these situations, reporters may end up using heuristics to save time and introduce experiential or contextual bias into the report. NLP offers a way to make the error reporting and analysis process more efficient by offering suggestions for reporters based upon what the natural language model has learned from previous reports, giving the reporters more time to focus on treatment and patient well-being. An added benefit of the model making suggestions is the removal of heuristic bias from error reports as these suggestions are being made. This is based on patterns observed across all reports and not just the experiences of one staff member.

The field of radiation oncology specifically is prone to errors due to the nature of the practice. Due to extensive planning and workflows that contain multiple steps involving multiple personnel at each step, highly accurate planning and treatment delivery inherently creates an error-prone environment. Errors due to miscommunication, inaccurate measures, and elongated timelines are frequent, and can have drastic effects on patient treatment outcomes. To date, the field of radiation oncology has received limited attention when it comes to the exploration of NLP as a tool to mitigate medical errors. Research shows promise in the ability of NLP to develop models that are effective in error labeling/classification (Mathew *et al.*, 2021; Syed *et al.*, 2020).

The general modeling framework is as follows. For each incident report, we are interested in predicting a certain variable, say y. The input data, x, consists of the free-text narrative of the incident report, which is converted into a numerical vector by leveraging NLP. The target variable y is "known" for the training data in the form of manual annotation by human experts. The goal is to construct a predictive model for y as a function of x by integrating NLP and statistical modeling. Two recent papers that have utilized this modeling framework are Mathew *et al.* (2021) and Syed *et al.* (2020). We now briefly describe their work and lay down future directions for this topic.

In Mathew *et al.* (2021), the authors collected a database of around 6000 incident reports from their own Safety and Incident Learning System (SaILS) as well as the National System for Incident Reporting — Radiation Treatment (NSIR-RT) managed by the Canadian Institute for Health Information (CIHI). There are three target (y) variables: (1) process step where the incident occurred, (2) problem type of the incident, and (3) the contributing factors of the incident. These three variables were chosen because human experts can typically derive these labels from the incident descriptions itself, without requiring additional information. To convert the free-text narrative to numerical vectors, they used the Term Frequency–Inverse Document Frequency (TF-IDF) vectorizer with unigrams (i.e., individual words) as well as selected bigrams (word pairs) and trigrams (groups of three words). A number of multilabel classification models were employed for the prediction task, of which the best three were selected. It was observed that this NLP-based strategy is much more accurate than the benchmark method based on label frequencies. Figure 3 provides a schematic representation of the modeling strategy.

In Syed *et al.* (2020), the authors collected a data set of around 1000 incident reports from Radiation Oncology facilities across the US Veterans Health Affairs (VHA) enterprise and Virginia Commonwealth University (VCU). In this work, the target variable of interest is incident severity, which has four possible values: A, B, C, and D, with A being the most severe to D being the least. Similar to [14C], the authors also used the Term Frequency–Inverse Document Frequency (TF–IDF) vectorizer to convert free text into numeric vectors. Next, they tested four classification

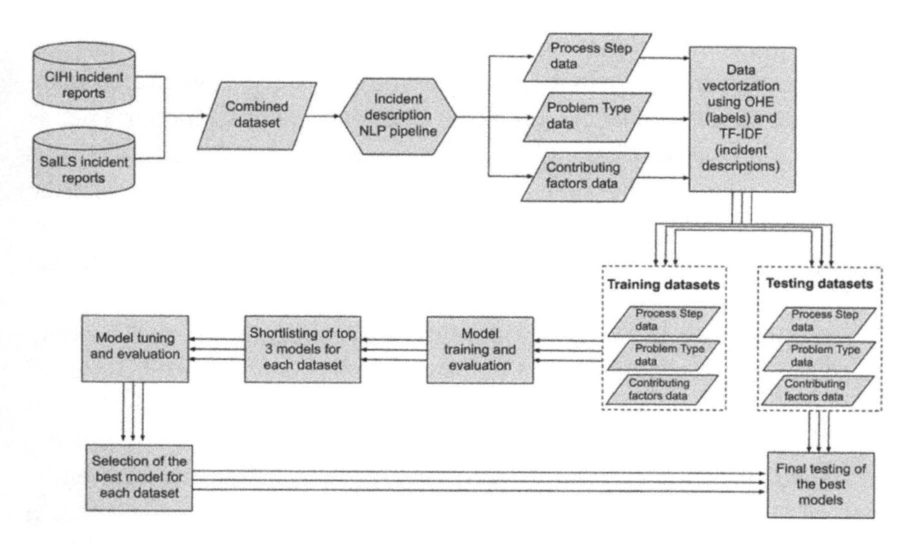

Fig. 3. Schematic representation of the method proposed in Mathew *et al.* (2021).

models: k-Nearest Neighbors (kNN), Logistic Regression (LR), Support Vector Machines (SVM), and Random Forests (RF). It was found that SVM with linear kernels performed the best.

Future research directions: The use of NLP to extract information from radiation oncology error incident reports is still in its infancy. The research so far is promising and there are several important paths to pursue. In what follows we outline some of the future research directions.

- In existing literature so far, the representation of free text as numerical vectors has been done through text-document matrices, which are known to be noisy, sparse, and high-dimensional. A better approach would be to use well-established vector embeddings such as word-2vec, GLOVE, or BERT (Mikolov *et al.*, 2013; Pennington *et al.*, 2014; Devlin *et al.*, 2018).
- So far, neural networks have not been used as classification models. Given the remarkable success of deep neural networks in other similar classification tasks (Ker *et al.*, 2017; Bakator and Radosav, 2018; Mohsen *et al.*, 2018), it is likely that deep neural networks will outperform the traditional models that have been used in the literature.

- The target variables for prediction so far considered in the literature are fairly simple, such as process step or severity. It would be more useful to set downstream corrective actions as the target variable, as this can lead to a truly automated system for handling errors. If this can be achieved, then the NLP-based system can directly predict the correct downstream action to address an error. Corrective actions can be categorized into two groups: (i) immediate or short-term and (ii) long-term or lasting corrective action. The first group of corrective actions arises in the scenario where a set process has a disruption, which needs to be undone. For example, this could happen because of an individual not performing their assigned task as an unintended oversight. The second group of corrective actions arises when the workflow itself needs to be improved for future patients. Currently, each incident report is manually analyzed to determine whether a short-term or a long-term corrective action is required. To be able to determine this automatically will be useful. A closely related task would be to automatically identify appropriate individuals to take a corrective action.
- There is a severe lack of high-quality, large, publicly available data sets that can be used as test beds for comparing different methods. So far, these methods have been applied on small and ad-hoc proprietary datasets. It is unclear whether the performance of a method on a particular data set can be generalized to other data sets. Most evident can be variations in model generalization caused by different data sets. The distribution of errors may be diverse for different institutions. For example, error data may vary due to different types of machines, scanners, EMR systems, and user types (e.g., physicians, physicists, dosimetrists, therapists, etc.). The model trained using the developer's data set may perform very differently on the workflow and process of a local user compared to an enterprise user. Developing a universal model could be a challenge. The curation of a national-level data set of radiation oncology error reports will be crucial for the training and development of AI systems.

8. The Challenges and Pitfalls of AI

The envisioned AI-powered system has several highly desirable benefits as it can be much more efficient and computationally scalable than current error mitigation systems based on human action. Furthermore, it has the potential to become a truly objective and quantifiable risk management system free from human subjectivity. This important benefit can help pivot the perspective on medical errors from a blame culture to a safety culture.

At the same time, we must be clear-eyed about the challenges and possible pitfalls of AI so that we can be proactive in avoiding them.

1. **Data quality:** Medical data in radiation oncology can be extraordinarily rich with information but also extremely complex. It is important to keep the garbage-in-garbage-out principle in mind when building an AI model. The quality of data inputted determines the reliability of outputted information. Building models to make predictions is significantly influenced by the structure of the data and data formatting. Sparse or incomplete data reduce the predictive power of AI algorithms. Missing data can introduce bias and false conclusions. Therefore, we must proactively build robust checks for data quality.
2. **Implicit bias:** It has been well documented that AI can suffer from bias (Panch *et al.*, 2019). In fact, it has been demonstrated that AI tools in healthcare not only reflect back social inequities but may ultimately make them worse (Panch *et al.*, 2019). AI tools must understand and account for potential sources of bias in the tools themselves, proactively looking for and evaluating for bias in models and monitoring results over time.
3. **Interpretability:** Convention and nomenclature usage can introduce problems in defining the terminology being used in the data pool. The use of terminology and their understanding changes between different institutions. This leads to variability in accuracy of terms used in training data sets. The end result is noise and lack of dependability of the AI-based algorithm.

Different technologies in radiation oncology can introduce different practices that change the patterns of the clinical process. This can exacerbate already existing interpretability challenges of AI outputs. Evaluating the quality of machine-learned models can be challenging. Thus, the frequency distributions of certain protocols evolve that effect the underlying assumptions of the AI algorithm. The AI model must evolve and relearn to reflect changes due to various technologies and clinical pathways.

4. **Statistical principles:** AI-powered systems are notorious for a "data first, theory later" approach, which flouts foundational statistical principles. For example, AI tools often ignore the statistical principles of multiple comparisons, colloquially known as the "Texas sharpshooter fallacy" (Smith, 2018). It is crucial to ensure that statistical principles are followed when building AI tools for healthcare. This includes all steps of algorithm development: from design to sampling to modeling and inference. Furthermore, we should carry out rigorous uncertainty quantification at all steps of statistical analysis.

AI should be able to help the medical professional make the best decision that ultimately benefits the treatment outcome and process. If the user does not know how the data predicts the outcome and how the information is combined, then the suggestion for an action to be taken can be unclear to the user, thus making the suggested decision difficult (accept or reject).

9. Conclusion

Preventable medical errors are one of the most critical problems of the U.S. healthcare system. While medical errors arise in all aspects of healthcare, they are particularly concerning in the case of radiation therapy due to complex treatment workflow involving several systems with fragile interconnectedness. As treatment complexity increases, the quality of data transfers becomes more problematic to produce errors. To address these problems, we first need to capture high quality incident report data in order to learn from past errors. Statistical modeling of such data can give us valuable operational insights into the entire treatment workflow and help identify points of weakness in a proactive manner.

The development of an error propagation model can be very effective in radiation oncology. Research on this issue is at a nascent stage, and there are several future directions to pursue. The error propagation model of the future should integrate various subsystems from the perspective of error detection, error propagation, error reduction, and prevention. The error propagation model can be designed to recognize which risk patterns exist for certain specific mixes of categories, subcategories, attributes, and subattributes at each stage. The error propagation model could employ an automatic trigger tool developed that is powered by probability theory using sophisticated decision algorithms.

Since medical errors are mostly reported in the form of free-text narratives, the use of NLP techniques can be transformational in our pursuit of an efficient, automated error mitigation toolbox. One of the key benefits that NLP models have to offer for medical personnel is the reduction in time required to report medical errors by streamlining the process and removing the need for reporters to essentially predict what caused the error despite their limited perspective. Research in this area has so far predicted simple target variables such as process step or severity. In the future, it would be more useful to set downstream corrective actions and designated roles as the target variables, as this can lead to a truly automated system for handling errors. Recent word embedding models (e.g., BERT) and deep learning-based classification methods can be valuable tools in this venture.

References

Andel, C., Davidow, S. L., Hollander, M., & Moreno, D. A. (2012). The economics of health care quality and medical errors. *Journal of Health Care Finance*, *39*(1), 39.

Bajaj, A. (2020). The impact of COVID-19 on radiation oncology department workflow in the United States. *Application Radiation Oncology*, *9*(2), 6–7.

Bakator, M. & Radosav, D. (2018). Deep learning and medical diagnosis: A review of literature. *Multimodal Technologies and Interaction*, *2*(3), 47.

Chang, X., Li, H., Kalet, A., & Yang, D. (2017). Detecting external beam radiation therapy physician order errors using machine learning. *International Journal of Radiation Oncology, Biology, Physics*, *99*(2), S71.

Clark, B. G., Brown, R. J., Ploquin, J., & Dunscombe, P. (2013). Patient safety improvements in radiation treatment through five years of incident learning. *Practical Radiation Oncology*, *3*(3), 157–163.

Consensus recommendations for incident learning database structures in radiation oncology. *Medical Physics*, *39*(12), 7272–7290.

Devlin, J., Chang, M. W., Lee, K., & Toutanova, K. (2018). Bert: Pre-training of deep bidirectional transformers for language understanding. arXiv preprint arXiv:1810.04805.

Editorial Board. (2009). A national survey of medical error reporting laws. *Yale Journal of Health Policy, Law, and Ethics*, *9*(1), 201–286.

Ekaette, E. U., Lee, R. C., Cooke, D. L., Kelly, K. L., & Dunscombe, P. B. (2006). Risk analysis in radiation treatment: Application of a new taxonomic structure. *Radiotherapy and Oncology*, *80*(3), 282–287.

Farokhzadian, J., Dehghan Nayeri, N., & Borhani, F. (2018). The long way ahead to achieve an effective patient safety culture: Challenges perceived by nurses. *BMC Health Services Research*, *18*(1), 1–13.

Ford, E. C. & Evans, S. B. (2018). Incident learning in radiation oncology: A review. *Medical Physics*, *45*(5), e100–e119.

Ford, E. C. & Terezakis, S. (2010). How safe is safe? Risk in radiotherapy. *International Journal of Radiation Oncology, Biology, Physics*, *78*(2), 321–322.

Ford, E. C., Fong de Los Santos, L., Pawlicki, T., Sutlief, S., & Dunscombe, P. (2012).

Ford, E. C., Gaudette, R., Myers, L., Vanderver, B., Engineer, L., Zellars, R., & DeWeese, T. L. (2009). Evaluation of safety in a radiation oncology setting using failure mode and effects analysis. *International Journal of Radiation Oncology* Biology* Physics* *74*(3), 852–858.

Frankel, A., Federico, F., Frush, K., Haraden, C., & Kaplan, G. S. (2013). *The Essential Guide for Patient Safety Officers*. M. Leonard (Ed.). Oakbrook Terrace, IL: Joint Commission Resources [and] Institute for Healthcare Improvement.

Hendee, W. R. & Herman, M. G. (2011). Improving patient safety in radiation oncology. *Medical Physics*, *38*(1), 78–82.

Howell, C., Tracton, G., Amos, A., Chera, B., Marks, L. B., & Mazur, L. M. (2019). Predicting radiation therapy process reliability using voluntary incident learning system data. *Practical Radiation Oncology*, *9*(2), e210–e217.

Huq, M. S., Fraass, B. A., Dunscombe, P. B., Gibbons Jr, J. P., Ibbott, G. S., Mundt, A. J., ... & Yorke, E. D. (2016). The report of Task Group 100 of the AAPM: Application of risk analysis methods to radiation therapy quality management. *Medical Physics*, *43*(7), 4209–4262.

Hutchinson, A., Young, T. A., Cooper, K. L., McIntosh, A., Karnon, J. D., Scobie, S., & Thomson, R. G. (2009). Trends in healthcare incident reporting and relationship to safety and quality data in acute hospitals: Results from the National Reporting and Learning System. *BMJ Quality & Safety*, *18*(1), 5–10.

James, J. T. (2013). A new, evidence-based estimate of patient harms associated with hospital care. *Journal of Patient Safety*, *9*(3), 122–128.

Kalet, A. M., Gennari, J. H., Ford, E. C., & Phillips, M. H. (2015). Bayesian network models for error detection in radiotherapy plans. *Physics in Medicine & Biology*, *60*(7), 2735.

Ker, J., Wang, L., Rao, J., & Lim, T. (2017). Deep learning applications in medical image analysis. *IEEE Access*, *6*, 9375–9389.

Kohn, L. T., Corrigan, J. M., & Donaldson, M. S. (Eds.). (2000). To Err is Human: Building a Safer Health System. Institute of Medicine (US) Committee on Quality of Health Care in America. National Academies Press (US).

Levinson, D. R. & General, I. (2010). Adverse events in hospitals: Methods for identifying events. Office of Inspector General, Department of Health and Human Services.

Makary, M. A. & Daniel, M. (2016). Medical error — the third leading cause of death in the US. *BMJ*, 353, i2139.

Marks, L. & Mazur, L. (2015). *Engineering Patient Safety in Radiation Oncology*. New York, NY: CRC Press, Taylor & Francis Group.

Mathew, F., Wang, H., Montgomery, L., & Kildea, J. (2021). Natural language processing and machine learning to assist radiation oncology incident learning. *Journal of Applied Clinical Medical Physics*.

Mazur, L., Chera, B., Mosaly, P., Taylor, K., Tracton, G., Johnson, K., ... & Marks, L. B. (2015). The association between event learning and continuous quality improvement programs and culture of patient safety. *Practical Radiation Oncology*, *5*(5), 286–294.

Mikolov, T., Chen, K., Corrado, G., & Dean, J. (2013). Efficient estimation of word representations in vector space. arXiv preprint arXiv:1301.3781.

Mohsen, H., El-Dahshan, E. S. A., El-Horbaty, E. S. M., & Salem, A. B. M. (2018). Classification using deep learning neural networks for brain tumors. *Future Computing and Informatics Journal*, *3*(1), 68–71.

Mullins, B. T., Mazur, L., Dance, M., McGurk, R., Schreiber, E., Marks, L. B., & Chera, B. S. (2020). Common error pathways in CyberKnife™ radiation therapy. *Frontiers in Oncology*, *10*, 1077.

Mullins, B. T., McGurk, R., McLeod, R. W., Lindsay, D., Amos, A., Gu, D., & Mazur, L. (2019). Human error bowtie analysis to enhance patient safety in radiation oncology. *Practical Radiation Oncology*, *9*(6), 465–478.

Olsen, L., Saunders, R. S., & Yong, P. L. (Eds.). (2010). The healthcare imperative: Lowering costs and improving outcomes: Workshop series summary. Roundtable on Evidence-Based Medicine — Institute of Medicine; National Academy of Sciences. pp. 2–3, 51.

Panch, T., Mattie, H., & Atun, R. (2019). Artificial intelligence and algorithmic bias: Implications for health systems. *Journal of Global Health*, *9*(2), 010318. https://doi.org/10.7189/jogh.09.020318.

Panch, T., Mattie, H., & Celi, L. A. (2019). The "inconvenient truth" about AI in healthcare. *NPJ Digital Medicine*, *2*(1), 1–3.

Pawlicki, T., Samost, A., Brown, D. W., Manger, R. P., Kim, G. Y., & Leveson, N. G. (2016). Application of systems and control theory-based hazard analysis to radiation oncology. *Medical Physics*, *43*(3), 1514–1530.

Pennington, J., Socher, R., & Manning, C. D. (2014, October). Glove: Global vectors for word representation. In *Proceedings of the 2014 Conference on Empirical Methods in Natural Language Processing (EMNLP)* (pp. 1532–1543).

Pillai, M., Adapa, K., Das, S. K., Mazur, L., Dooley, J., Marks, L. B., ... & Chera, B. S. (2019). Using artificial intelligence to improve the quality and safety of radiation therapy. *Journal of the American College of Radiology*, *16*(9), 1267–1272.

Potters, L., Ford, E., Evans, S., Pawlicki, T., & Mutic, S. (2016). A systems approach using big data to improve safety and quality in radiation oncology. *International Journal of Radiation Oncology, Biology, Physics*, *95*(3), 885–889.

Rooney, J. J. & Heuvel, L. N. V. (2004). Root cause analysis for beginners. *Quality Progress*, *37*(7), 45–56.

Siegel, R. L., Miller, K. D., & Jemal, A. (2020). Cancer statistics, 2020. *CA: A Cancer Journal for Clinicians*, *70*(1), 7–30.

Siochi, R. A., Balter, P., Bloch, C. D., Santanam, L., Blodgett, K., Curran, B. H., ... & Zhu, X. R. (2011). A rapid communication from the AAPM Task Group 201: Recommendations for the QA of external beam radiotherapy data transfer. AAPM TG 201: Quality assurance of external beam radiotherapy data transfer. *Journal of Applied Clinical Medical Physics*, *12*(1), 170–181.

Smith, D. S. (2005). Patient safety. *The Case Manager*, *16*(3), 74–79.

Smith, G. (2018). *The AI Delusion*. Oxford University Press.

Soydemir, D., Seren Intepeler, S., & Mert, H. (2017). Barriers to medical error reporting for physicians and nurses. *Western Journal of Nursing Research*, *39*(10), 1348–1363. Young, I. J. B., Luz, S., & Lone, N. (2019). A systematic review of natural language pro- cessing for classification tasks in the field of incident reporting and adverse event analysis. *International Journal of Medical Informatics*, *132*, 103971.

Spath, P. L. (2003). Using failure mode and effects analysis to improve patient safety. *AORN Journal*, *78*(1), 15–37.

Syed, K., Sleeman, W., Hagan, M., Palta, J., Kapoor, R., & Ghosh, P. (2020, September). Automatic incident triage in radiation oncology incident learning system. In *Healthcare* (Vol. 8, No. 3, p. 272). Multidisciplinary Digital Publishing Institute.

Weidlich, V. & Weidlich, G. A. (2018). Artificial intelligence in medicine and radiation oncology. *Cureus*, *10*(4), 1–5.

Weintraub, S. M., Salter, B. J., Chevalier, C. L., & Ransdell, S. (2021). Human factor associations with safety events in radiation therapy. *Journal of Applied Clinical Medical Physics*, *22*(10), 288–294.

Yahia, H. S. & Abdulazeez, A. M. (2021). Medical text classification based on convolutional neural network: A review. *International Journal of Science and Business*, *5*(3), 27–41.

Zietman, A. L., Palta, J. R., Steinberg, M. L., Blumberg, A., Burns, R., & Cagle, S., . . . Wazer, D. E. (2012). Safety is no accident: A framework for quality radiation oncology and care. *American Society for Radiation Oncology*.

Part 5

Assessment and Outcomes

Chapter 15

Ethics and Artificial Intelligence in Radiation Oncology

Megan Hyun* and Alexander Hyun†

**Department of Radiation Oncology, University of Nebraska Medical Center, Omaha NE, USA*
†Department of Arts and Humanities, Minerva University, San Francisco CA, USA

Abstract

In this chapter, we aim to overview the main ethical concerns that arise from the use of Artificial Intelligence (AI) in medicine, particularly those that apply to radiation oncology. We then examine some ethical concerns in greater detail, considering how the ethical principles of respect for autonomy, beneficence, nonmaleficence, and justice may apply when addressing these concerns at multiple stages of AI development and implementation. These considerations may provide some of the groundwork needed toward developing a more comprehensive, robust ethical framework for AI applications in radiation oncology as this technology becomes more prevalent in medicine.

1. Ethical Principles in Medicine

When considering ethical decision-making in artificial intelligence (AI) research, applications in medicine, or use in radiation oncology in particular, it is important to first understand the ethical principles that drive contemporary biomedical ethics. It would be difficult to present here a robust ethical framework to guide all of AI research and medical use in radiation oncology, partly because of the rapid advancements being made in the field and new dilemmas continually arising as a result. However, these basic ethical principles can and should guide ethical decision-making for scientists, medical practitioners, and other stakeholders in medical AI. In this section, we provide an overview of the four ethical principles that are widely accepted in contemporary biomedical ethics. In the remaining sections of this chapter, we will apply these principles to some pertinent dilemmas that impact the current or emerging use of AI in radiation oncology. We will then touch on some dilemmas that may arise from future use of AI as the technology advances and becomes more prevalent in this field. Our hope is that our treatment of these dilemmas may serve as an example for readers to further explore and understand how to apply these principles more broadly on this topic.

The four ethical principles that are widely accepted in contemporary biomedical ethics, as described by Beauchamp and Childress (2009), are as follows:

1. Respect for autonomy
2. Beneficence
3. Nonmaleficence
4. Justice.

While they may be presented in different terms elsewhere (e.g., in The Belmont Report, which combines beneficence and nonmaleficence together and places autonomy under "respect for persons"), the moral framework tends to be the same (*The Belmont report*, 1978). These basic principles lay the foundation on which Western medical ethics are built and are at the heart of the ethical codes held by many medical associations, organizations, and boards (Skourou *et al.*, 2019; Donaldson, 2017; Riddick, 2003). As we explore the ethics of AI in radiation oncology in this chapter, we will draw on these four principles, so we will first give a brief description of each.

1.1. *Respect for autonomy*

The principle of respect for autonomy holds that there is a moral obligation to "foster autonomous decision-making" (Beauchamp & Childress, 2009). For a patient's decision to be autonomous, it must be adequately free of coercive influence (e.g., from the attending physician) and be based on an adequate understanding of the facts pertinent to that decision. Since patients' level of understanding and freedom from coercive influence both come in degrees, the autonomy of patients' decisions also comes in degrees. As we understand it, the principle of respect for autonomy implies that healthcare providers have a moral duty to perform those actions that would increase the level of autonomy of patients' medical decisions. This would include actions that enhance the patient's understanding of relevant medical facts. The principle also implies that healthcare providers have a moral duty to refrain from those actions that would decrease the level of autonomy of a patient's medical decisions, such as actions that are aimed at coercing the patient to make a specific medical decision.

1.2. *Beneficence and nonmaleficence*

The principle of beneficence states that healthcare providers have a moral duty to act for the benefit of their patients. The principle of nonmaleficence, which stems from the Hippocratic Oath to "do no harm," states that healthcare providers have a moral duty to refrain from performing acts that harm their patients. These two principles are sometimes combined into a single ethical principle because the risk of harm must be considered alongside potential benefits of a treatment or research study. In general, providers and researchers should aim to maximize benefits and minimize harm to patients or research subjects.

1.3. *Justice*

The final principle, that of justice, is the most complex to apply in medicine. According to Beauchamp and Childress's influential account, justice is multifaceted: multiple principles of justice "arguably merit acceptance," and each of these principles identifies an approach to distributing benefits that there is at least some moral reason to follow (Beauchamp & Childress, 2009). An egalitarian principle of justice that Beauchamp and Childress (2009) call the "fair-opportunity rule" will be especially relevant in what follows. This principle states "that no persons should receive social benefits on the basis of undeserved advantageous properties (because no persons are responsible for having these properties) and that no persons should be denied social benefits on the basis of undeserved disadvantageous properties (because they also are not responsible for these properties)."

To illustrate, suppose that a society provides healthcare only to citizens with a high IQ. Having natural intelligence is an advantageous property that is undeserved, for those who have this property aren't responsible for having it. And healthcare is an example of a social benefit. So, the society that we are imagining has a policy that brings it about that some people receive a certain type of social benefit on the basis of their having a certain type of undeserved advantageous property. As we understand it, then, the fair-opportunity rule implies that there is a moral duty to change this policy.

It is important to note that the moral duties identified by these four principles are *prima facie* moral duties. A *prima facie* moral duty to perform an action is a moral consideration in favor of doing that action that has some weight, but that may be outweighed by competing moral considerations. To illustrate, suppose that a doctor knows that a patient is likely to make an imprudent medical decision if they are provided with some pertinent information about the possible treatments available to them. Out of concern for the patient's well-being, the doctor refrains from sharing this information with the patient. It may be that the principle of beneficence implies that the doctor had a *prima facie* duty to behave as they did, for their choice to conceal the information resulted in the patient having the benefit of making the prudent medical decision. This means that there is something to be said in favor of the doctor's act of concealment, from the moral point of view. But this *prima facie* moral duty conflicts with another *prima facie* moral duty to *refrain* from this act of concealment. This competing *prima facie* moral duty derives from the principle of respect for autonomy, for the patient's medical decision is less autonomous as a result of the doctor's act of concealment.

A *prima facie* moral duty should be distinguished from what we may call an *all-things-considered* moral duty. It is one's all-things-considered moral duty to perform a certain action when that action is favored by one's weightiest *prima facie* moral duties. In the example in the previous paragraph, it seems plausible upon reflection that the *prima facie* moral duty against concealing the pertinent information from the patient is stronger than the *prima facie* moral duty in favor of concealing it. So, it seems plausible that the doctor failed to do that which they had an all-things-considered moral duty to do despite the fact that they acted in accordance with one of their *prima facie* moral duties.

When we are trying to solve a difficult moral dilemma using Beauchamp and Childress's moral framework (2009), the first step is to identify all of the significant *prima facie* moral duties that are in play. The second step is to consider which of these *prima facie* moral duties is weightiest or ought to take priority in the context at hand.

2. Ethical Concerns for AI in Medicine and Radiation Oncology

In the bioethics literature, many authors have considered the implications of current and potential future use of AI in medicine, and we will overview these considerations before delving into some issues relevant to radiation oncology in particular. However, we must first draw an important distinction between ethical and legal considerations, which are often conflated. Ethical considerations relate to what is right and wrong in AI research or its applications in medicine, and the *prima facie* duties and responsibilities of researchers and providers according to the ethical framework we laid out in Section 1. These considerations may have legal ramifications when it comes to existing laws or future laws that ought to be put in place, but we will focus only on the application of the ethical framework. We will bracket legal considerations in this chapter, but we encourage readers to consider and read further on the legal ramifications of the ethics discussed here.

Two important studies provide a review of the ethics literature related to AI in medicine. Both studies analyzed more than 100 papers, summarizing and categorizing ethical considerations raised. While extraordinarily helpful, these reviews reveal the difficulty of developing ethical frameworks for new technologies. For example, Murphy *et al.* published their meta-analysis of 103 papers in 2021, but only looked at papers published before 2018 (Murphy *et al.*, 2021). In three years, additional important ethical dilemmas may have arisen that would be missed due to the rapidly advancing nature of the field.

Despite the difficulty of meta-analyses keeping up with advancements in AI, it is still worth examining their conclusions on the pertinent ethical considerations for the use of AI in medicine. The uses of AI considered by the majority of papers analyzed by Murphy *et al.* (2021) include "carer" robots, diagnostics, and precision medicine. For these uses, the main foci of AI bioethics literature have been concerns related to privacy, trust, accountability/responsibility, and bias. Importantly, an area they note is largely missing in the literature at the time of publication is considerations related to global health, particularly low- and middle-income countries (LMICs). We will consider some global health concerns related specifically to radiation oncology in Section 3.

Morley *et al.*, in a meta-analysis of 156 papers, divided AI-health-related ethical risks into six subcategories, including inconclusive evidence, inscrutable evidence, misguided evidence, unfair outcomes, transformative effects, and traceability concerns (Morley *et al.*, 2020). We will briefly overview each of these subcategories, connecting them to principles from the framework in Section 1.

2.1. *Inconclusive evidence*

In the era of big data, techniques such as machine learning are able to parse large amounts of patient information much more effectively than human practitioners, so it stands to reason that we should be able to rely on properly developed AI tools to make or support clinical decisions. However, the patterns detected by these algorithms do not necessarily indicate causality or draw meaningful conclusions. Morley *et al.* point to the prevalence of inconclusive results, lack of reproducibility, and lack of external validity in results in current AI health solutions (Morley *et al.*, 2020).

The principles of beneficence and nonmaleficence would apply to this category of ethical considerations. If an algorithm is poorly validated, does not translate to the setting of interest, or relies on a small sample size of training data, patients whose diagnosis or treatment is based on it could be harmed. Any potential benefit of the tool's use would need to be weighed against this risk of harm, which may be difficult to quantify.

2.2. *Inscrutable evidence*

Current AI technologies used in medicine tend to be "black box" solutions, especially to the patients whose care may be affected by the information or decisions generated from them, but perhaps also to many clinicians who may use or rely on them.

This concern relates to the principles of nonmaleficence and respect for autonomy. If the healthcare staff do not understand the algorithms or limitations of the AI tools they rely on, it will be difficult if not impossible to determine whether the tool produces an erroneous result, which could result in patient harm. Additionally, patient autonomy may be limited due to their lack of understanding. We will explore this potential lack of autonomy further in Section 4.

2.3. *Misguided evidence*

The quality of AI algorithms is heavily dependent on their underlying data. Morley *et al.* (2020) point out that current methods "suffer from overfitting due to small numbers of samples, meaning that the majority of results (e.g. patterns of disease risk factors, or presence of disease) are inconclusive." Additionally, many studies suffer from lack of reproducibility and translatability to other settings or populations (Morley *et al.*, 2020). For example, if patient data from the US is used to create a model that is then applied to patients in China, there may be unintended harm due to differences between these patient populations.

Because this ethical concern relates to potential harm, the principles of beneficence and nonmaleficence will certainly apply. Practitioners would need to evaluate whether the potential benefits of using these tools when caring for their patients would outweigh the potential harm.

2.4. *Unfair outcomes*

Even if efforts are made to broaden the data used to create new AI tools, there is a much larger volume of medical trial data for white males than other groups. This means that the translatability concerns we already discussed would generate *prima facie* duties related to justice considerations as well. If, out of consideration of potential harm, AI tools are limited to only the populations whose data informs the model (e.g., white males), other populations will be denied the potential benefits of these tools. We will explore this further in Section 3.

2.5. *Transformative effects*

AI has the potential to transform healthcare on multiple levels. It increases the importance of and reliance on large amounts of patient data, brings research and clinical practice into closer proximity, and may change the relationship between human healthcare providers and patients (Morley *et al.*, 2020). These transformative effects of AI in medicine may drive positive changes in the field, but they also generate ethical considerations that span all the ethical principles we have discussed. We will consider the role of the human practitioner further in Section 4.

2.6. *Traceability*

Finally, Morley *et al.* (2020) identify ethical concerns relating to traceability. As healthcare is transformed by the use of AI tools, it may become challenging to assign responsibility or liability when a patient or group is harmed. For instance, consider an AI tool intended to augment a radiologist's decision-making by detecting pancreatic cancer on magnetic resonance images. If this tool identifies pancreatic cancer in non-cancerous tissue, leading the radiologist to assign an erroneous cancer diagnosis to a patient, who is ultimately responsible for the misdiagnosis? Without a clear channel of responsibility for poor outcomes, such errors may continue to occur, causing harm and violating the principle of nonmaleficence.

Much less has been published regarding AI in radiation oncology compared to AI in the wider field of medicine. However, some specific considerations have been raised, including the "black box problem," the role of human practitioners, and bias and equity concerns (Smith & Bean, 2019; Bridge & Bridge, 2019).

Smith and Bean (2019) argue that because of the "black box" nature of deep learning tools like convolutional neural networks (CNNs), clinicians may be reluctant to adopt these technologies due to lack of trust in the accuracy of the CNN or concern for liability if the AI-recommended clinical decision resulted in harm. They also claim that, while a number of tasks in the radiation sciences can be automated through AI (such as nodule detection), human clinicians will continue to be needed for "clinical judgment," which they say cannot be performed by AI (Smith & Bean, 2019). Bridge and Bridge (2019) also emphasize the importance of human input in radiation oncology to provide creativity, innovation, and safe oversight. We will consider the impact of the black box problem and whether AI should replace human practitioners in Section 4 using the principles of respect for autonomy and beneficence.

Smith and Bean (2019) discuss the problem of bias and equity in the use of AI, noting the importance of mitigating bias in the design of machine learning tools in addition to carefully interpreting information relating to marginalized populations. We will discuss bias and distribution of outcomes in Section 3 using the principles of beneficence and justice.

Some suggestions have been proposed regarding how to approach ethical dilemmas in the use of AI in radiation oncology. Smith and Bean (2019) suggest both researchers and practitioners use a "life-cycle approach," which iteratively integrate ethical considerations into the development and implementation of new technologies. One life-cycle tool they suggest is the Transparency, Replicability, Ethics, and Effectiveness (TREE) approach, which asks 20 questions spanning every stage of AI development (Vollmer *et al.*, 2020). Similar to our approach using the principles laid out by Beauchamp and Childress (2009), Erkal *et al.* (2021) suggest evaluating AI applications in radiotherapy using a "four topics" approach. This approach, proposed by Jonsen *et al.* (2010), reorganizes the ethical principles in a way that, according to Erkal *et al.* (2021), is more understandable to radiation oncologists. The Royal Australian and New Zealand College of Radiologists (RANZCR) have proposed nine principles (*Ethical principles for AI*, 2019) to guide the development and use of AI in radiology and radiation oncology, including:

1. Safety
2. Privacy and protection of data
3. Avoidance of bias
4. Transparency and explainability
5. Application of human values
6. Decision-making on diagnosis and treatment
7. Teamwork
8. Responsibility for decisions
9. Governance.

Similarly, a joint multi-society statement published in *Radiology* (Geis *et al.*, 2019) emphasized the values of well-being, minimizing harm, just distribution of benefits, and transparency. While this statement focuses on the use of AI in radiology, the recommendations are also highly relevant to radiation oncology.

Many of these suggested approaches are rooted in the same fundamental ethical principles laid out by Beauchamp and Childress (2009). In this chapter, we will model the use of these four simple principles and the *prima facie* moral duties they generate to make ethical decisions in the development and use of AI in radiation oncology.

3. Emerging AI Tools in Radiation Oncology

3.1. *Adoption of AI tools with potential biases*

AI tools depend on the data used to generate the model that is then applied for the potential benefit of patients (e.g., image segmentation). In many cases, these data sets may include limited demographics, especially if the patient information comes from a single institution or region of the world. For example, Obermeyer *et al.* (2019) showed that a widely used algorithm — used by insurers to identify how "healthy" a patient is — would often erroneously identify Black patients as healthier than White patients who were just as sick. This type of limitation raises an ethical trilemma for healthcare institutions or practitioners considering using these tools. There are three main options:

A. Use these tools by offering them to patients of all demographic make-ups,
B. Use these tools by offering them only to patients matching the demographics of the data sets, or
C. Refrain from using these tools altogether.

Each option seems morally problematic in some respect. If option A is chosen, then patients with demographic make-ups not represented in the data sets may be harmed. If option B is chosen, then the use of the tool seems unfair since part of the population receives a privilege despite being no more deserving of it than the rest of the population. And if option C is chosen, then there are some patients (specifically, patients matching the demographics of the datasets) who are deprived of a significant medical benefit. Since there is a downside to all three options, it can be challenging to know what ought to be done with AI tools that are based on data sets that include limited demographics.

In the absence of a relevant example from the use of AI in radiation oncology, let us examine an example from the field of genetics that exemplifies the trilemma raised above. Ambry Genetics Corporation offered AmbryScore, a genetic screening test that offered some patients a metric to assess their genetic risks related to breast or prostate cancer. The patient populations used to develop AmbryScore were not ethnically diverse, and as a result, this test is known to be reliable only for a subset of Caucasian patients. This example is analogous to the use of AI in radiation oncology; just as the development of this genetic test depends on patient data that may be limited (e.g., in demographic diversity), many AI tools may likewise draw from limited patient data sets. The decision faced by Ambry Genetics is similar to that which will likely be faced by radiation oncology

AI developers and practitioners in the near future. Considering the ethical implications of this genetics case will allow us to better understand issues of bias affecting the use of AI tools in radiation oncology.

Ambry Genetics faced a decision between the three options listed above. (A) First, it could offer the use of AmbryScore to patients of all demographic make-ups. (B) Second, it could offer the use of AmbryScore only to patients with the kind of Caucasian background for which it is known to be reliable. (C) Third, it could refrain from offering AmbryScore altogether. Initially, Ambry Genetics favored the second option ("Ambry Genetics", 2018; "NorthShore University", 2018). Recently, it started favoring the third option, deciding to cease offering this screening to any patients outside clinical trials since it has "not been validated for use in patients of diverse backgrounds" ("AmbryScore discontinuation notice", 2021). The ethical issue of what ought to be done with AmbryScore is challenging because there are significant moral concerns about all options available to Ambry Genetics. Its initial policy faced the worry that it was unfair to non-Caucasian patients, while its current policy faces the worry that it deprives Caucasian patients of a significant medical benefit.

The moral framework presented in Section 1 helps to clarify the moral dimensions of the use of AmbryScore or relevantly similar AI tools. Each option available to Ambry Genetics is opposed by one of the four ethical principles. Option A is opposed by the principle of nonmaleficence, for choosing this option would risk causing harm to some non-Caucasian patients. Since the reliability of AmbryScore is uncertain for non-Caucasian patients, offering it to them poses two potential problems: it may lead some non-Caucasian patients to believe that they are not at increased risk of cancer when they actually are, and it may lead some non-Causcian patients to believe that they are at increased risk of cancer when they are not. The former possibility may harm patients by causing them to be less diligent than they ought to be at taking special steps to reduce their risk of breast or prostate cancer and to monitor themselves for symptoms of these types of cancer. And the latter possibility may harm patients by prompting them to pursue unnecessary prophylactic treatment that leaves them worse off. For example, a patient who is misled to believe that they are at a very high risk of developing breast cancer may end up having an unnecessary preventative double mastectomy. Another way that non-Caucasian patients may be harmed by being led to believe falsely that they are at increased risk of cancer is by experiencing unnecessary anxiety about their health.

Option B appears to be opposed by the principle of justice. Specifically, it seems to conflict with the fair-opportunity rule. As Beauchamp and Childress (2009) observe, "many studies in the United States indicate that blacks and women have poorer access to various forms of health care in comparison to white males." It is therefore plausible that being Caucasian is an advantageous property in the context of our society. And since one does not choose one's race, being Caucasian is an *undeserved* advantageous property. The fair-opportunity rule therefore implies that no one in our society should receive social benefits on the basis of being Caucasian. Access to information about one's risk of breast or prostate cancer is a type of social benefit. So, the fair-opportunity rule implies that no one in our society should receive access to information about their risk of breast or prostate cancer on the basis of being Caucasian. Implementing option B brings about that some patients receive access to this sort of information as a result of their being Caucasian. And so, the fair-opportunity rule seems to imply that there is a moral duty not to choose option B.

Finally, option C is opposed by the principle of beneficence, for choosing this option would involve a failure to provide some Caucasian patients with a significant medical benefit. Specifically, it would involve a failure to equip some Caucasian patients with the knowledge that they are at a higher risk of developing breast or prostate cancer. Having such knowledge would be beneficial because it would allow them to take special steps to reduce their risk of cancer and because it alerts them of the importance of being particularly alert for symptoms of these types of cancers.

Resolving this moral trilemma involves figuring out which of the *prima facie* moral duties identified above is the weightiest in this context. Let us consider an argument for the case that the weightiest *prima facie* moral duties favor option B, in which case Ambry Genetics has an all-things-considered moral duty to reverse course. This argument would go as follows.

Imagine a case in which a doctor has an interest in AmbryScore (or an analogous AI tool) and decides to test it out with the medical profile of a

Caucasian patient that the doctor is meeting with later that day. Because of the doctor's use of AmbryScore, they know that the patient is at increased risk of prostate cancer. It seems clear that it would be wrong for the doctor to refrain from sharing this information with the patient. And notice that the doctor's refraining from sharing this information would be very similar in morally relevant ways to Ambry Genetics's decision to discontinue AmbryScore. The main moral reason against the doctor's refraining from sharing the information (a moral reason deriving from the principle of beneficence) mirrors the main moral reason against Ambry Genetics's decision to discontinue Ambryscore. And the main moral reason in favor of the doctor's refraining from sharing the information (a moral reason deriving from the principle of justice) mirrors the main moral reason in favor of Ambry Genetics's decision to discontinue Ambryscore. In light of this moral parity, we have good reason to think that since the doctor's refraining from sharing the information would be wrong, Ambry Genetics's discontinuing AmbryScore is also wrong. In this sort of case, the weightest *prima facie* moral duties favor acting to benefit one's Caucasian patients.

There are ways to push back against this argument. Perhaps a defender of Ambry Genetics's actions could argue that an individual doctor is relevantly different from a company, such that their all-things-considered moral duties can diverge even when there is a lot of similarity between their *prima facie* moral duties. Or perhaps there are moral considerations against option B that we have not identified and factored into this deliberation. These suggestions are worthy of further investigation. Our main goal here is not to definitively resolve this moral trilemma and others like it, but rather to illustrate how to approach them using the moral framework laid out in Section 1.

A plausible balance between these conflicting *prima facie* moral duties may involve looking separately at the responsibilities of each party in the development chain. For instance, on the research end, decisions are made regarding how the data are collected and how the model is built. Perhaps at this stage, the principle of justice should win out: those who are developing AI tools ought to build them from data that include a broad range of demographics. For practitioners, however, the decisions center around whether to use a tool that may benefit some patients. Perhaps at this implementation stage, the principle of beneficence should win out: the practitioner should make use of the AI tool to benefit those patients who are members of the demographic group for which the AI tool is suited. This way of thinking underscores the need identified by Bridge and Bridge (2019) for an ethical framework that uses a "life-cycle approach."

3.2. *AI in radiation oncology and global health*

Global health considerations are largely missing from the bioethics literature on medical AI, so the radiation oncology community sorely needs to address the impact this technology has or may have on the world (Murphy *et al.*, 2021). While filling this gap is outside the scope of this chapter, we can raise one potential consideration related to the principle of justice.

Zubizarreta *et al.* (2015) showed that access to radiotherapy is incredibly limited in low-income countries, with more than 90% of their population lacking access to this critical component of cancer care as of 2015. Jaffray *et al.* (2015) note that, without intervention, this lack of access will only continue to worsen as the global cancer burden grows. It is clear that the global resource of radiation therapy is inequitably distributed.

Because new technological tools are often adopted by wealthy nations first, the potential benefits of AI will also likely be inequitably distributed as it achieves more widespread use in medicine. One of the interventions suggested by Jaffay *et al.* (2015) is simplified, "fault-proof" treatment delivery systems that can help ensure high-quality treatment access around the world. If this idea of simplicity limits newly developed, complex technologies such as AI tools from being implemented in low- and middle-income countries (LMICs), where radiation therapy is already a scarce resource, the use of AI in wealthy countries may widen the gap even further. This might suggest that there is a *prima facie* duty generated from the principle of justice for wealthier nations to refrain from adopting these tools until they can be more equitably distributed.

We argued in the section on bias that, even when AI tools and their benefits are only available for part of the population, practitioners have a *prima facie* duty to offer them to patients per the principle of beneficence. Similar argumentation could also be applied in this case, suggesting that wealthier nations (or at least practitioners within those nations) have stronger moral reasons to offer new and beneficial technology than they do to refrain on the basis of justice.

Additionally, it is possible that AI may actually help to close the gap in treatment access, which would shift the moral responsibilities generated by the principle of justice. Consider a tool like auto-segmentation, which can potentially improve contouring consistency between institutions. This type of tool would be particularly beneficial in LMICs, where resources are limited and staff may be under-trained. AI tools could potentially make years of accumulated experience from wealthier nations available in LMICs, facilitating the simplified, "fault-proof" systems envisioned by Jaffray *et al.* (2015). The main challenge is how to mitigate bias in data sets to allow tools to be generalizable where they are deployed. By our lights, it seems there are strong moral reasons, generated from the principles of justice and beneficence, for the global radiation oncology community to invest in AI tools and translate them to LMICs in a way that increases access to life-saving treatment and equitably distributes benefits around the world.

4. Ethics and the Future of AI in Radiation Oncology

In Section 3, we have considered two ethical concerns that impact the current or emerging use of AI in radiation oncology — namely, the issues of bias and global health. We will now consider the ethical implications of a potential future reality where AI tools may replace human practitioners for certain tasks in radiation oncology.

As AI technology improves, it may become possible to program an AI to produce reliable treatment recommendations to cancer patients. Those patients would then face the medical decision of whether to accept the AI's recommendation. It has been plausibly suggested that this type of use of AI in medicine is morally problematic for the following reason having to do with patient autonomy (Morley *et al.*, 2020). In order for a patient's medical decisions to be autonomous, they must be based on an understanding of the facts relevant to those medical decisions. The worse the patient's understanding of such facts is, the less autonomous their medical decisions are. Facts about how a treatment recommendation was determined seem relevant to the medical decision of whether to accept the recommendation. So, any policy that makes it harder for patients to understand how treatment recommendations are determined will also make it so that those patients' medical decisions are less autonomous than they otherwise would be. The policy of using AI-generated treatment recommendations makes it more difficult for patients to understand the reasoning behind these recommendations. This is because many patients lack the ability to understand "the underlying data, processes and technical possibilities" that would be involved in the generation of the AI-produced treatment recommendation (Morley *et al.*, 2020). So, such a policy makes it so that many patients' medical decisions are less autonomous than they otherwise would be. As we understand it, the principle of respect for autonomy implies that there is a *prima facie* moral duty for a healthcare provider to refrain from adopting policies that would decrease the level of autonomy of a patient's medical decisions. And so, the principle of respect for autonomy implies that there is a *prima facie* moral duty to refrain from relying on AI to produce treatment recommendations.

However, this moral objection to the use of AI to develop treatment recommendations is not decisive. First, it is worth considering whether the facts about "the underlying data, processes, and technical possibilities" that are involved in the generation of AI-produced treatment recommendations really do count as "pertinent" or "relevant" to the medical decision of whether to accept those recommendations. This is important because on Beauchamp and Childress's (2009) influential account of the principle of respect for autonomy, it is only understanding of facts relevant to a medical decision that are important for the autonomy of that medical decision. Central examples of facts that are relevant to the decision to accept a treatment recommendation are the patient's prognosis, expected side effects of the proposed treatment, and risks associated with forgoing treatment.

Technical facts about how an AI generates its treatment recommendation from the underlying data seem quite different from these paradigmatic examples of relevant facts. Notice that if a patient has a good understanding of the benefits and risks of an AI-generated treatment recommendation, of the alternatives to this recommendation, etc., then we would not be inclined to worry that the patient's decision to accept this treatment recommendation lacked autonomy by virtue of a deficiency of understanding. Since it is plausible that the facts about the technical details of how an AI generates its recommendations aren't relevant to the medical decision of whether to accept its recommendations, it is plausible that the principle of respect for autonomy doesn't entail that there is a *prima facie* duty to refrain from relying on AI to produce treatment recommendations.

Additionally, suppose these facts about the details of how an AI generates its recommendations actually *do* count as relevant to patients' medical decisions. This still would not mean that the principle of respect for autonomy implies that we ought to refrain from using AI to produce treatment recommendations in radiation oncology. Rather, this principle would imply only that if we do use AI in this way, then we also ought to take steps to ensure that patients have an opportunity to acquire an appropriate level of understanding of these technical facts. One way to accomplish this might be to offer patients consultations with medical physicists, as we have discussed in a previous paper (Hyun & Hyun, 2019). So, regardless of whether or not technical facts about the AI are relevant to patients' medical decisions, it seems that using AI-generated treatment recommendations should not violate the principle of respect for autonomy.

Patient autonomy is not the only relevant principle when considering a possible future where AI tools may replace human practitioners for some radiation oncology tasks. Imagine, for example, that the AI provides not only the treatment recommendation, but also the patient-facing roles traditionally held by human practitioners. This example could apply to both the initial consultation or on-treatment visits provided by the radiation oncologist, or dedicated consultation with the medical physicist.

In the book *Compassionomics*, Trzeciak *et al.* (2019) devote more than 100 pages to the evidence that compassion improves patient outcomes. They argue, with a staggering amount of supporting data, that incorporating compassion into medical care generates physiological and psychological benefits for patients, motivates patient self-care, and improves healthcare quality. The principle of beneficence would suggest, then, that hospitals have a *prima facie* duty to ensure their patients receive compassionate medical care.

Bridge and Bridge (2019) argue that, lacking a knowledge of the "self" and "the uniquely human viewpoint that enables us to understand how another person is feeling," an AI can "never understand what it means to act ethically," which "precludes the development of empathy." Since empathy and the expression of compassion are closely linked, it is quite possible that even the most advanced AI could never achieve the same level of compassion as a human practitioner. This suggests that hospitals have a *prima facie* duty to refrain from using AI to replace human practitioners in direct patient care.

Combining the considerations from autonomy and beneficence, it seems that hospitals may have strong moral reasons to adopt AI technology for assisting with treatment recommendations (perhaps providing additional education to patients if understanding the technology is relevant to decisions about their care). Yet, based on our current understanding of the limitations of AI, there are also strong moral reasons to refrain from using AI tools to completely replace human practitioners.

Acknowledgments

Many thanks to Dr. Dandan Zheng for providing helpful comments during the revision process.

References

Ambry Genetics. (2018, March 14). Ambry Genetics launches AmbryScore™ to assist health care providers in determining lifetime breast cancer risk. https://www.ambrygen.com/company/press-release/101/ambry-genetics-launches-ambryscoretm-to-assist-health-care-providers-in-determining-lifetime-breast-cancer-risk.

Ambry Genetics. (2021, May 20). AmbryScore discontinuation notice. https://info.ambrygenetics.com/take-a-brief-survey-for-entryinto-amazon-gift-card-drawing.

Beauchamp, T. & Childress, J. (2009). *Principles of Biomedical Ethics.* 6th ed. New York: Oxford University Press.

Bridge, P. & Bridge, R. (2019). Artificial intelligence in radiotherapy: A philosophical perspective. *Journal of Medical Imaging and Radiation Sciences, 50*(4), S27–S31. http://dx.doi.org/10.1016/j.jmir.2019.09.003.

Donaldson, S. S. (2017). Ethics in radiation oncology and the American Society for radiation oncology's role. *International Journal of radiation oncology Biology Physics, 99*(2), 247–249. https://doi.org/10.1016/j.ijrobp.2017.06.2446.

Erkal, E. Ẏ., Akpinar, A., & Erkal, H. Ş. (2021). Ethical evaluation of artificial intelligence applications in radiotherapy using the four topics approach. *Artificial Intelligence in Medicine, 115*(102055), 1–5. https://doi.org/10.1016/j.artmed.2021.102055.

Geis, J. R., Brady, A. P., Wu, C. C., Spencer, J., Ranschaert, E., Jaremko, J. L., Langer, S. G., Kitts, A. B., Birch, J., Shields, W. F., van den Hoven van Genderen, R., Kotter, E., Gichoya, J. W., Cook, T. S., Morgan, M. B., Tang, A., Safdar, N. M., & Kohli, M. (2019). Ethics of artificial intelligence in radiology: Summary of the joint European and North American multiscociety statement. *Radiology, 293*(2), 436–440. https://doi.org/10.1148/radiol.2019191586.

Hyun, M. A. & Hyun, A. B. (2019). Respecting patient autonomy in radiation oncology and beyond. In F. Allhoff & S. Borden (Ed.). *Ethics and Error in Medicine* (1st ed., pp. 103–117). New York, NY: Routledge.

Jaffray, D. A., Atun, R., Barton, M., Baumann, M., Gospodarowicz, M., Hoskin, P., Knaul, F. M., Lievens, Y., Rosenblatt, E., Torode, J., Van Dyk, J., & Vikram, B. (2015). Radiation therapy and the global health agenda. *Clinical Oncology, 27*(2), 67–69. http://dx.doi.org/10.1016/j.clon.2014.11.025.

Jonsen, A. R., Siegler, M., & Winsade, W. J. (2010). *Clinical Ethics: A Practical Approach to Ethical Decisions in Clinical Medicine.* 7th ed. New York, NY: McGraw-Hill.

Morley, J., Machado, C. C. V., Burr, C., Cowls, J., Joshi, I., Taddeo, M., & Floridi, L. (2020). The ethics of AI in health care: A mapping review. *Social Science & Medicine, 260*(113172), 1–14. https://doi.org/10.1016/j.socscimed.2020.113172.

Murphy, K., Ruggiero, E. D., Upshur, R., Willison, D. J., Malhotra, N., Cai, J. C., Malhotra, N., Lui, V., & Gibson, J. (2021). Artificial intelligence for good health: A scoping review of the ethics literature. *BMC Medical Ethics, 22*(14), 1–17. https://doi.org/10.1186/s12910-021-00577-8.

National Commission for the Protection of Human Subjects of Biomedical and Behavioral Research. (1978). *The Belmont Report: Ethical Principles and Guidelines for the Protection of Human Subjects of Research.* Bethesda, MD: The Commission.

Northshore University Healthsystem. (2018, September 25). NorthShore University HealthSystem, Ambry Genetics announce new prostate cancer risk test. https://www.eurekalert.org/news-releases/501950.

Obermeyer, Z., Powers, B., Vogell, C., & Mullainathan, S. (2019). Dissecting racial bias in an algorithm used to manage the health of populations. *Science, 366*(6464), 447–453.

Riddick, F. A., Jr (2003). The code of medical ethics of the American Medical Association. *The Ochsner Journal, 5*(2), 6–10.

Skourou, C., Sherouse, G. W., Bahar, N., Fairobent, L., Freedman, D. J., Genovese, L. M., Halvorsen, P. H., Kirby, N. A., Mahmood, U., Ozturk, N., Osterman, K. S., Serago, C. F., Svatos, M. M., & Wilson, M. L. (2019). Code of ethics for the American Association of Physicists in Medicine (Revised): Report of Task Group 109. *Medical Physics, 46*(4), e79–e93. https://doi.org/10.1002/mp.13351.

Smith, M. J. & Bean, S. (2019). AI and ethics in medical radiation sciences. *Journal of Medical Imaging and Radiation Sciences, 50*(4), S24–S26. https://doi.org/10.1016/j.jmir.2019.08.005.

The Royal Australian and New Zealand College of Radiologists. (2019). Ethical principles for Artificial Intelligence in medicine. Sydney, Australia: The Royal Australian and New Zealand College of Radiologists. https://www.ranzcr.com/documents/4952-ethical-principles-for-ai-in-medicine/file.

Trzeciak, S., Mazzarelli, A., & Booker, C. (2019). *Compassionomics: The Revolutionary Scientific Evidence that Caring Makes a Difference*. Pensacola, FL: Studer Group.

Vollmer, S., Mateen, B. A., Bohner, G., Kiraly, F. J., Ghani, R., Jonsson, P., Cumbers, S., Jonas, A., McAllister, K. S. L., Myles, P., Granger, D., Birse, M., Branson, R., Moons, K. G. M., Collins, G. S., Ioannidis, J. P. A., Holmes, C., & Hemingway, H. (2020). Machine learning and AI research for patient benefit: 20 critical questions on transparency, replicability, ethics and effectiveness. *British Medical Journal, 368*(I6927), 1–12. https://doi.org/10.1136/bmj.l6927.

Zubizaretta, E. H., Fidarova, E., Healy, B., & Rosenblatt, E. (2015). Need for radiotherapy in low and middle income countries — the silent crisis continues. *Clinical Oncology, 27*(2), 107–114. https://doi.org/10.1016/j.clon.2014.10.006.

Chapter 16

Evaluation of Artificial Intelligence in Radiation Oncology

Gretchen Purcell Jackson[*,†] and Roy Vergis[‡,§,¶]

**Intuitive Surgical, Sunnyvale CA, USA*
[†]Associate Professor of Surgery, Pediatrics, and Biomedical Informatics, Vanderbilt University Medical Center, Nashville TN, USA
[‡]Associate Partner and Clinical Leader, IBM Healthcare Consulting, London, UK
[§]Honorary Consultant in Clinical Oncology, Mount Vernon Cancer Centre, London, UK
[¶]Expert in Digital Health, World Health Organization, Geneva

Abstract

Artificial Intelligence (AI) has a wide variety of applications in radiation oncology, including patient assessment, treatment planning, and outcomes prediction. To ensure trust and foster adoption in clinical practice, both providers and patients want scientific evidence that demonstrates that AI tools are safe and effective. This chapter describes a framework for the evaluation of AI in healthcare, encompassing studies of technical performance, usability, and clinical impact. Similarities to and important differences from phases of clinical trials for drugs and medical devices are highlighted. Each phase of research is illustrated by examples of rigorous studies from the domain of radiation oncology.

1. Overview of AI in Radiation Oncology

AI could have particularly transformative applications in radiation oncology given the multifaceted and highly technical nature of this field, which relies heavily on digital data processing and computer software. AI platforms can recognize complex and unexpected patterns in medical data and provide both quantitative and qualitative insights. A wide range of AI tools have been developed to support therapy planning, treatment delivery, and quality assurance, and these applications have the potential to improve the accuracy, precision, efficiency, and overall quality of radiation therapy for patients with cancer.

2. A Framework for the Evaluation of AI in Healthcare

Whenever innovations are introduced into the healthcare environment, all stakeholders look for scientific evidence to show that those innovations offer clinical benefits and limit harm. To create such evidence, rigorous scientific studies that evaluate both performance and impact of AI solutions are needed.

The first step in evaluating an AI solution is the testing of the technical aspects. Developers should demonstrate that algorithms accurately perform their intended tasks, such prediction, or classification. Such evaluation is similar to performance testing for diagnostic tests and measures accuracy with metrics such as sensitivity, specificity, and area under the receiver operating characteristic curve. In this step, it is important to have clinicians involved in setting acceptable performance thresholds. Clinician expertise is needed to understand the consequences of false positive and false negative results and to determine acceptable tradeoffs.

The next step in AI tool evaluation involves ensuring the tool can be used and understood by its intended users in the appropriate clinical setting. This phase involves studies of usability, learnability, and satisfaction, and aspects of AI explainability or workflow transformation may be examined. Studies in this step often require qualitative research methodologies and team members with expertise in psychology, sociology, anthropology, and human factors engineering.

Finally, after ensuring adequate technical performance and usability, AI solutions should be evaluated for impact. Early evaluations may focus on intermediate or process outcomes, such as showing that tools influence clinical decisions or save time. Long-term studies are often needed to determine whether these systems affect clinical outcomes. Definitive studies to show clinical impact may use a randomized controlled trial design, and it is important to select an appropriate comparator. For AI tools that support clinicians, the study should compare clinicians with and without the assistance of the AI solution.

Evaluation of AI solutions shares some similarities with the phases of evaluation used for drugs and medical devices (Park *et al.*, 2020). Preclinical and phase I studies involve algorithm training, often with limited data sets, and testing of initial prototypes. Phase II studies should measure algorithm performance on enhanced data sets and study prototypes with relevant clinical users in real clinical environments to support safety and efficacy of the solutions. At this stage, it is particularly important to consider sources of bias in the underlying algorithm design, data used for training, or interface design, to ensure that AI solutions do not contribute to or worsen existing health disparities (Dankwa-Mullan I, 2021). It is important to note that AI solutions used by clinicians differ from drugs and devices, which tend to perform in a consistent manner. By contrast, the output of the AI algorithm must be understood, trusted, and applied to a specific context by a clinician. Phase III studies are larger, typically randomized trials or may use a pre–post implementation study design to provide evidence for effects. All AI tools warrant phase IV post-deployment surveillance to measure ongoing performance, especially when algorithms may learn with time (Petersen *et al.*, 2021).

3. AI Evaluations in Radiation Oncology

Some of the common practical applications of AI in radiation oncology and their performance evaluations are highlighted in what follows.

AI techniques have been applied to a wide variety of tasks in the Radiation Therapy (RT) planning process. Auto-contouring is an attractive concept in radiation treatment planning. Three of the top ten high-risk and high-severity failures in treatment planning are from "wrong" or inaccurate contouring, improper margins for the planning target volume, and "wrong" or inaccurate dosimetrist contours (Ford *et al.*, 2020). According to the AAPM Task Group 275, while automation cannot entirely replace human decision-making, it can "improve efficiency and effectiveness and allow physicists to focus more attention on the review tasks that require human judgment" (Ford *et al.*, 2020). Furthermore, automated tools can introduce standardization, a key component of error prevention. Smart planning tools in current clinical use can be summarized in three main categories: automated rule implementation and reasoning, modeling of prior knowledge in clinical practice, and multicriteria optimization (Wang *et al.*, 2019). Recently, Convolutional Neural Network (CNN)-based auto-segmentation models have been shown to improve consistency and efficiency of this process (van der Veen *et al.*, 2019; Lustberg *et al.*, 2018). In technical performance studies, these deep learning models are now outperforming traditional auto-contouring methods and reaching the accuracy range of manual delineations (Savenije *et al.*, 2020). There are AI studies related to the planning steps of RT, such as dose calculation, dose distribution, Dose-Volume Histogram (DVH), patient-specific dose calculation, Intensity Modulated Radiotherapy (IMRT) area determination, beam angle determination, real-time tumor tracking, and replanning in adaptive RT (Zhu *et al.*, 2020).

Target volume contouring is a labor-intensive step in the treatment planning flow in RT. Differences in manual contouring result from variability between contours, differences in radiation oncology education, or quality differences in imaging studies. Current automatic contouring methods aim to reduce manual workload and increase contour consistency but still tend to require significant manual editing (La Macchia *et al.*, 2012). The first example of a commercial release of a deep learning-based contouring tool to gain US FDA (510k) clearance was Mirada's DLCExpert (Mirada, 2020).in 2018. Other currently available solutions include Deep-Learning Segmentation solution from RaySearch Laboratories, Ethos, Varian's radiotherapy treatment system (Archambault *et al.*, 2020), and

Radiation Planning Assistant (RPA), which is an AI-based treatment planning platform developed by academic researchers and clinicians at MD Anderson Cancer Center (Court *et al.*, 2018). As part of the medical device regulatory process, both technical performance as well as workflow (i.e., workload) user studies are conducted.

Computer-Aided Detection (CAD) is another technique that leverages AI in treatment planning. Low Dose Rate (LDR) brachytherapy is extensively used in prostate cancer. The implementation and precise location of the implanted radioactive seeds are critical to the success of treatment. CAD has proven to be able to make accurate treatment plans for LDR brachytherapy that are comparable to those prepared by experienced treatment planners and radiologists, thus assisting in treatment delivery (Nicolae *et al.*, 2017).

Treatment modalities such as photon-based Volumetric Modulated Arc Therapy (VMAT) require a lot of planning before dose delivery, especially given the complex dose deposition. Machine learning algorithms have been shown to help to predict dose distribution for organs-at-risk and to plan target volume, enabling radiation oncologists to make better and more informed treatment decisions and to save significant time. One algorithm's accuracy was validated on 69 plans for lung Stereotactic Body Radiation Therapy (SBRT) and 121 plans for head-and-neck treatment with a mean error below 2.5 Gy. This shows the potential to be used as automated treatment plan in SBRT for lung and head and neck radiotherapy (Valdes *et al.*, 2017). Detection of intestinal air is critical to image guided radiotherapy in prostate cancer. Deep convolutional neural networks have been applied to this problem (Miura *et al.*, 2019). Kajikawa *et al.* compared a 3D Convolutional Neural Network (CNN) with the conventional machine learning method for predicting Intensity-Modulated Radiation Therapy (IMRT) dose distribution using only contours in prostate cancer. The CNN model could predict dose distributions that were superior or comparable with that generated by RapidPlan™ (Kajikawa *et al.*, 2019).

Quality Assurance (QA) is a critical step in the evaluation of radiotherapy planning and in the detection and reporting of errors. Features of RT QA programs such as error detection, error prevention, and treatment device QA have been found to be very suitable for AI applications (Valde *et al.*, 2017). This helps facilitate development of automated pretreatment validation workflows and provide a virtual assessment of treatment quality. For example, AI could play a role in current non-AI based steps in the treatment workflow as well as perform plausibility or sanity checks on the model outcome. For example, an independent, secondary algorithm can be used to benchmark the performance of the clinical (AI) model and point divergent behavior. Automatic case-specific QA tools can be utilized to facilitate the detection of outliers (Vandewinckele *et al.,* 2020). Finally, uncertainty estimates of the AI output can be used as a valuable tool to flag outcomes that require additional verification. It is important to note that these methods are under investigation and that supervision is currently the main application (Bragman *et al.*, 2018).

Radiation therapy may need to be adjusted during the treatment pathway to ensure proper implementation of the treatment plan. This may be necessitated due to either online factors such as the patient's pretreatment position, or longer-term factors related to anatomical changes and response to treatment. Images taken before treatment should be aligned with the images in the planning CT and kept in alignment. Based on anatomical and dosimetric variations such as shrinkage of the tumor, weakening of the patient, or edema, classifiers and clustering algorithms have been developed to predict the patients who will benefit most from updated plans during fractionated RT (Guidi *et al.*, 2016). However, it should also be kept in mind that these algorithms will mimic past protocols rather than determine the ideal time for replanning because AI learns from data about previous patients, their plans, and adaptive RT.

AI also has the potential to change the way radiation oncologists follow patients who have chosen definitive treatment. AI algorithms can be used to correlate image-based features with biological observations or clinical outcomes. Tseng *et al.* investigated deep reinforcement learning trained on historical treatment plans for developing automated radiation adaptation protocols in Non-Small-Cell Lung Cancer (NSCLC) patients; the goal was to maximize tumor local control at reduced rates of radiation pneumonitis. While these and similar studies demonstrate this is a promising approach for achieving similar results to those chosen by clinicians, these processes require customization (Tseng *et al.*, 2017). Furthermore, development of this framework into a fully credible autonomous system for clinical decision support would require further validation on larger multi-institutional data sets. A study by Cha *et al.* demonstrated the feasibility of radiomics-based predictive models using pre and posttreatment Computed Tomography (CT) images to potentially assist in assessing treatment response (Ha *et al.*, 2017).

The use of AI techniques for response and survival prediction in RT patients presents a significant opportunity to further improve decision support systems and provide an objective assessment of the relative benefits of various treatment options for patients (Tseng *et al.*, 2017).

There are several other potential applications for the use of AI in radiation oncology, and several studies of workflow have demonstrated significant time savings. CNNs and deep learning methods utilize AI-based methods compared to the traditional methods of creating synthetic CTs for optimum patient immobilization during the simulation process (Yakar & Etiz, 2021). Deep learning and AI can be novel game changers in the image registration and segmentation part of the treatment planning workflow, by facilitating the implementation process as well as improving accuracy in image registration. Manual segmentation of the Organs at Risk (OARs) is time consuming with a high degree of variability (Roques, 2014). Automatic segmentation using AI can reduce the inter-clinician variability and shorten the duration of radiation oncology planning (Sharp *et al.*, 2014). AI, particularly using CNNs, is a potential tool to reduce physician workload and define a standard segmentation. In recent years, deep learning methods have been widely used in medical applications such as organ segmentation in head-neck, lung, brain, and prostate cancers (Liang *et al.*, 2019; Savenije *et al.*, 2020). However, these methodologies will require further robust studies in real clinical settings and further quality assurance as well as a rigorous process of validation before they can be introduced into actual radiation oncology workflows.

Further advances of AI and deep learning will be driven by the availability of high-quality data, since most models in development by industry and academia rely on supervised learning approaches for radiotherapy treatment planning tools. As more tools become commercially available, their integration into clinical practice may largely depend on accessibility to annotated data sets and computational power.

4. Conclusions

AI has the potential to automate and accelerate the process of RT planning, treatment, and follow up. To deploy AI solutions safely and effectively in radiation oncology settings, scientific evidence demonstrating solution performance and accuracy, usability in clinical workflows, and clinical impact are necessary. Although preliminary studies of technical performance and time savings show promise, few solutions have undergone rigorous testing in clinical settings, and impact studies on short- and long-term clinical outcomes are limited. In addition, many AI learning methods require large, annotated data sets, and these are often not available, very expensive, or protected by intellectual property rights or privacy regulations. Additional research is needed to build the evidence base for AI transformation of RT.

References

Archambault, Y., Boylan, C., Bullock, D., Morgas, T., Peltola, J., Ruokokoski, E., *et al.* (2020). Making on-line adaptive radiotherapy possible using artificial intelligence and machine learning for efficient daily re-planning. *Medical Physics International Journal, 8*(2), 77–82.

Bragman, F. J. S., Tanno, R., Wenqi, Z. E., David, L., Ourselin, S., Alexander, D. C., *et al.* (2018). Quality control in radiotherapy-treatment planning using multi-task learning and uncertainty estimation. Proceedings from 1st Conference on Medical Imaging with Deep Learning (MIDL 2018). Amsterdam, the Netherlands.

Court, L. E., Kisling, K., McCarroll, R., Zhang, L., Yang, J., Simonds, H., *et al.* (2018). Radiation planning assistant — a streamlined, fully automated radiotherapy treatment planning system. *Journal of Visualized Experiments, 134*, 57411.

Dankwa-Mullan I, S. E., Matheny, M. E., Quintana, Y., Chapman, W. W., Jackson, G., & South, B. R. (2021). A proposed framework on integrating health equity and racial justice into the artificial intelligence development lifecycle. *JHCPU, 32*(2), 300–317. https://doi.org/10.1353/hpu.2021.0065.

Ford, E., Conroy, L., Dong, L., Fong de Los Santos, L., Greener, A., Kim, G. G., *et al.* (2020). Strategies for effective physics plan and chart review in radiation therapy: Report of AAPM task group 275. *Medical Physics, 47*(6), e236–e272.

Guidi, G., Maffei, N., Meduri, B., D'Angelo, E., Mistretta, G. M., Ceroni, P., Ciarmatori, A., Bernabei, A., Maggi, S., Cardinali, M., Morabito, V. E., Rosica, F., Malara, S., Savini, A., Orlandi, G., D'Ugo, C., Bunkheila, F., Bono, M., Lappi, S., Blasi, C.,

Lohr, F., & Costi, T. (2016). A machine learning tool for re-planning and adaptive RT: A multicenter cohort investigation. *Physical Medicine*, *32*, 1659–1666.

Ha, K. H., Hadjiiski, L., Chan, H. P., Weizer, A. Z., Alva, A., Cohan, R. H., Caoili, E. M., Paramagul, C., & Samala, R. K. (2017). Bladder cancer treatment response assessment in CT using radiomics with deep-learning. *Scientific Report*, *7*, 8738.

Kajikawa, T., Kadoya, N., Ito, K., Takayama, Y., Chiba, T., Tomori, S., Nemoto, H., Dobashi, S., Takeda, K., & Jingu, K. (2019). A convolutional neural network approach for IMRT dose distribution prediction in prostate cancer patients. *Journal of Radiation Research, 60*(5), 685–693.

La Macchia, M., Fellin, F., Amichetti, M., Cianchetti, M., Gianolini, S., Paola, V., Lomax, A. J., & Widesott, L. (2012). Systematic evaluation of three different commercial software solutions for automatic segmentation for adaptive therapy in head-and-neck, prostate and pleural cancer. *Radiation Oncology*, *7*, 160.

Liang, S., Tang, F., Huang, X., Yang, K., Zhong, T., Hu, R., Liu, S., Yuan, X., & Zhang, Y. (2019). Deep-learning-based detection and segmentation of organs at risk in nasopharyngeal carcinoma computed tomographic images for radiotherapy planning. *European Radiology*, *29*, 1961–1967.

Lustberg, T., van Soest, J., Gooding, M., Peressutti, D., Aljabar, P., van der Stoep, J. *et al.* (2018). Clinical evaluation of atlas and deep learning based automatic contouring for lung cancer. *Radiotherapy & Oncology*, *126*(2), 312–317.

Mirada. Mirada announces FDA clearance for its AI-powered Cancer Treatment Planning product DLCExpertTM | Mirada [Internet]. (2020 April, 21). https://mirada-medical.com/mirada-announce-fda-clearance-for-their-ai-powered-cancer-treatment-planning-product-dlcexpertold/.

Miura, H., Ozawa, S., & Doi, Y. (2019). Automatic gas detection in prostate cancer patients during image-guided radiation therapy using a deep convolutional neural network. *Physical Medica*, *64*(1), 24–28. https://doi.org/10.1016/j.ejmp.2019.06.009.

Nicolae, A., Morton, G., & Chung, H. (2017). Evaluation of a machine-learning algorithm for treatment planning in prostate low-dose-rate brachytherapy. *International Journal of Radiation Oncology, Biology, Physics*, *97*(4), 822–829. https://doi.org/10.1016/j.ijrobp.2016.11.036.

Park, Y., Jackson, G. P., Foreman, M. A., Gruen, D., Hu, J., & Das, A. K. (2020). Evaluating artificial intelligence in medicine: Phases of clinical research. *JAMIA Open, 3*(3), 326–331. https://doi.org/10.1093/jamiaopen/ooaa033.

Petersen, C., Smith, J., Freimuth, R. R., Goodman, K. W., Jackson, G. P., Kannry, J., ... Wright, A. (2021). Recommendations for the safe, effective use of adaptive CDS in the US healthcare system: An AMIA position paper. *Journal of the American Medical Informatics Association, 28*(4), 677–684. https://doi.org/10.1093/jamia/ocaa319.

Roques, T. W. (2014). Patient selection and radiotherapy volume definition — can we improve the weakest links in the treatment chain? *Clinical Oncology (R Coll Radiol)*, *26*, 353–355.

Savenije, M. H. F., Maspero, M., Sikkes, G. G., Van Der Voort Van Zyp, J. R. N., Alexis, A. N., Bol, G. H., *et al.* (2020). Clinical implementation of MRI-based organs-at-risk auto-segmentation with convolutional networks for prostate radiotherapy. *Radiation Oncology, 15*, 104.

Sharp, G., Fritscher, K. D., Pekar, V., Peroni, M., Shusharina, N., Veeraraghavan, H., & Yang, J. (2014). Vision 20/20: Perspectives on automated image segmentation for radiotherapy. *Medical Physics, 41*, 050902.

Tseng, H. H., Luo, Y., Cui, S., Chien, J. T., Ten Haken, R. K., & Naqa, I. E. (2017). Deep reinforcement learning for automated radiation adaptation in lung cancer. *Medical Physics, 44*, 6690–6705.

Valdes, G., Chan, M. F., Lim, S. B., Scheuermann, R., Deasy, J. O., & Solberg, T. D. (2017). IMRT QA using machine learning: A multi-institutional validation. *Journal of Applied Clinical Medical Physics, 18*, 279–284.

Valdes, G., Wojtowicz, L., & Pattison, A. J. (2017). OC-0253: Machine learning-based enables data-driven radiotherapy treatment planning decision support. *Radiotherapy & Oncology, 123*, S127–S128. https://doi.org/10.1016/s0167-8140(17)30696-5.

van der Veen, J., Willems, S., Deschuymer, S., Robben, D., Crijns, W., Maes, F. *et al.* (2019). Benefits of deep learning for delineation of organs at risk in head and neck cancer. *Radiotherapy & Oncology, 138*, 68–74.

Vandewinckele, L., Claessens, M., Dinkla, A., Brouwer, C., Crijns, W., Verellen, D., & van Elmpt, W. (2020). Overview of artificial intelligence-based applications in radiotherapy: Recommendations for implementation and quality assurance. *Radiotherapy and Oncology, 153*, 55–66.

Wang, C., Zhu, X., Hong, J. C., & Zheng, D. (2019). Artificial Intelligence in radiotherapy treatment planning: Present and future. *Technology in Cancer Research & Treatment, 18*, 1–11.

Yakar, M. & Etiz, D. (2021). Artificial intelligence in radiation oncology. *Artificial Intelligence in Medical Imaging, 2*(2), 13–31.

Zhu, J., Liu, X., & Chen, L. (2020). A preliminary study of a photon dose calculation algorithm using a convolutional neural network. *Physics in Medicine and Biology, 65*, 20NT02.

Index

CPSIA information can be obtained
at www.ICGtesting.com
Printed in the USA
JSHW041437130123
36111JS00002B/5